The Impact of Communication Disability Across the Lifespan

Judy Clegg
Human Communication
Sciences
University of Sheffield
J.clegg@sheffield.
ac.uk

Library of Congress Cataloguing in Publication Data
British Library Cataloguing in Publication Data
A catalogue record for this book is available from the British Library
Cover design: Jim Wilkie
Project management, typesetting and design: J&R Publishing Services Ltd, Guildford, Surrey, UK; www.jr-publishingservices.co.uk

The Publisher acknowledges with grateful thanks the work put into this book at proof stage by Nikky Twyman

Printed and bound by CPI Group (UK) Ltd, Croydon, CR0 4YY

The Impact of Communication Disability Across the Lifespan

Katerina Hilari

and

Nicola Botting

(Editors)

J&R Press Ltd

Contents

4 Developmental Speech Disorders 41
Barbara Dodd

5 Children with Learning Disabilities 61
Celia Harding

About the Editors

Nicola Botting is a Reader in the Department of Language and Communication Science, City University London and is also the Joint Editor of the *International Journal of Language and Communication Disorders*. She trained as a psychologist, completing a BSc Hons in Psychology (Hertfordshire) and an MA in Clinical Child Psychology (Nottingham), before then completing a PhD in Child Health (Liverpool). She has been researching language and communication difficulties for around 15 years. Nicola's main research interests are specific language impairment, pragmatic language difficulties, autistic spectrum disorders, cognitive development, longitudinal study of psychological development, and also psychological outcomes of very low birthweight, which was the subject of her PhD.

Katerina Hilari is a Psychologist and a Speech and Language Therapist (SLT). She is a Reader in the Department of Language and Communication Science, City University London and is also the Editor in Chief of the *International Journal of Language and Communication Disorders*. As an SLT, Katerina has worked with people with aphasia and other acquired disorders in both the acute and rehabilitation settings. She is a world expert on quality of life research in people with communication disabilities, with numerous peer-reviewed publications and invited conference presentations.

About the Contributors

Kathryn Bayles, PhD, CCC-SLP, is Professor and Chair of the Department of Speech-Pathology at the University of Central Arkansas. She is an internationally known expert on dementia-related cognitive-communication disorders and her research has received support from the National Institutes on Aging, Mental Health, Deafness and Other Communication Disorders and numerous foundations. Dr Bayles is a Fellow and Honors recipient of the American Speech-Language-Hearing Association and a Past President and Honors recipient of the American Academy of Neurologic Communication Disorders and Sciences. She is widely published and the co-author of three textbooks and two standardized tests for cognitive-linguistic disorders.

Abigail Beverly is a graduate of Central Saint Martins, gaining a distinction for her thesis 'How we understand words', based on having grown up with a speech and language disorder. This gave rise to her first exhibition in 2006 – 'Making Sense of the Puzzle' – where she used her art to try to convey her personal journey with 'words'. She is a volunteer with Afasic Youth Project, specializing in art workshops designed to encourage members to develop their language skills via creative activities. Abby's enthusiasm for art and craft has led her to develop her interest in quilting and sewing projects.

Susan Buell is a Lecturer in Speech and Language Therapy at the University of East Anglia. She has collaborated on research in the area of profound and multiple intellectual disability with a focus on SLT practice within the United Kingdom. More recently she has looked at improving the concept and the practice of 'participation' with people with disabilities and their families in Latin America.

Karen Bunning is a Reader at the University of East Anglia, where she contributes to the BSc (Hons) Speech and Language Therapy degree course. Her research interests lie in the field of severe to profound and multiple intellectual disability and the construction of partnership interaction. Recent and ongoing research has involved investigating rehabilitation provision for young people growing up with disability in a rural part of Kenya and the nature of interaction in the special needs classroom. Karen has written and contributed to a number of texts on the subject of intellectual disability.

Naomi Cocks is a Senior Lecturer in the Department of Language and Communication Science at City University London. Her research has covered a range of topics, including the impact of stroke on gesture production and comprehension. Prior to working as a lecturer, Naomi worked as a speech and language therapist in a range of settings, including acute, rehabilitation and community facilities. Her main role in these settings was the assessment and management of communication and swallowing disorders as a result of stroke, dementia or head injury.

Madeline Cruice is a Senior Lecturer in the Department of Language and Communication Science at City University London. She lectures in aphasia, professional studies and disability studies, works as a clinical tutor in the postgraduate Speech and Language Therapy programme, and supervises students in campus- and community-based clinical placements. Her research is focused on understanding and improving quality of life for people who have aphasia. Prior to her appointment at City University, Madeline worked clinically at the Royal Brisbane Hospital and lectured at the University of Queensland, in her native Australia.

Barbara Dodd is Professor of Child Speech at City University London. Over the last 40 years Barbara has worked in departments of Psychology, Linguistics and Speech-Language Pathology at universities in Australia and the United Kingdom. She has been involved in the development of new ways of educating speech and language therapists to maximize the link between theory and practice. Collaborations with practising clinicians has led to evaluations of intervention programmes that have influenced clinical practice. Barbara is best known for her research into the nature of spoken and written developmental speech disorders and how best to intervene cost-effectively.

Celia Harding is a Senior Lecturer and Clinical Tutor at the Department of Language and Communication Science, City University London. She is also a Speech and Language Therapist and continues to practise at the Royal Free Hospital as part of the paediatric gastroenterology team. She teaches in the areas of learning disability (which includes augmentative and alternative communication) and also paediatric dysphagia, both at pre-and post-registration level.

Lena Hartelius is Professor of Speech and Language Pathology at the University of Gothenburg, Sweden. The position is associated with clinical work at Sahlgrenska University Hospital. Her research, as well as clinical and teaching interests, is within the area of neurogenic communication disorders, for example, the speech and language disorders in multiple sclerosis, Parkinson's disease, Huntington's disease and stroke.

Ros Herman is a Speech and Language Therapist specializing in communication and deafness. She teaches at City University London and has carried out research on language development and assessment, communication interventions and reading in deaf children. She has developed two unique assessments of sign language acquisition and contributed to the UK Monitoring Protocol for Deaf Babies & Children and the standardization of the MacArthur Communicative Development Inventory in BSL. She has also collaborated in a major investigation of atypical language development in BSL and is currently leading a national study of reading and dyslexia in deaf children.

Tammy Hopper is a Speech and Language Pathologist and Associate Professor in the Department of Speech Pathology and Audiology at the University of Alberta in Edmonton, Canada. Her research is focused on interventions for cognitive-communication disorders of dementia as well as access to healthcare and rehabilitation services for people with dementia and their families. She has received research funding from local and national agencies, including the Canadian Institutes for Health Research, the Alzheimer's Association (USA), the Canadian Foundation for Dietetic Research, the CapitalCare Foundation (Edmonton), the Alberta Heritage Foundation for Medical Research and the Canadian Health Services Research Foundation.

Victoria Joffe is a Specialist Speech and Language Therapist and Reader in Developmental Speech, Language and Communication Difficulties in the Department of Language and Communication Science at City University London. Victoria's expertise is in the area of assessment and intervention of children and young people with developmental speech, language and communication difficulties. She is an experienced teacher and trainer and works in close collaboration with a range of educational and clinical professionals, people with speech, language and communication needs and their families, on best practice in enhancing the language, communication and learning of vulnerable children and young people.

Tess Lancashire lives in London and is the proud mother of a teenage son. For the past five years she has been the North London Aphasic Coordinator at Different Strokes. Different Strokes is a UK charity that was set up in order to support younger stroke survivors. In recent years, along with other members of the North London Different Strokes Group, she has been successful in obtaining funding to pay for a speech and language therapist to provide group and individual therapy. Tess had a stroke 22 years ago.

Marilyn Langevin is the Director of Research and interim Executive Director at the Institute for Stuttering Treatment and Research (ISTAR) and an Assistant Professor in the Department of Speech Pathology and Audiology at the Faculty of Rehabilitation Medicine, University of Alberta. She has over 23 years' experience in integrating research into clinical practice. She has made major contributions to the development of the Comprehensive Stuttering Programs for teens, adults and school-age children and the associated clinical training programmes. She also authored *Teasing and Bullying: Unacceptable Behaviour*, a school programme designed to educate school-age students about stuttering and change attitudes towards teasing and bullying. Her research interests include the social impact of stuttering on preschool and school-age children, evidence-based treatment and evidence-based clinical training practices.

James Law originally qualified in linguistics before training and practising as a Speech and Language Therapist. After obtaining his PhD from City University London in 1993, he has led a number of significant research projects in the UK, recently completing an ESRC-funded analysis of the BCS70 cohort entitled *The Mediating Effect of Language and Literacy Skills on the Cycle of*

Disadvantage – Following Five Year Olds into Adulthood. Between 2004 and 2009, he was Director of the Centre for for Integrated Healthcare Research in Scotland before moving to Newcastle University, UK, where he is Professor of Speech and Language Sciences. He is currently one of the four principal investigators on the Better Communication Research Programme (http://www.warwick.ac.uk/go/bettercommunication).

Mary T. Lee is a Speech and Language Therapist who trained in Canada at the University of British Columbia. Her area of clinical interest and expertise is Ears Nose and Throat (ENT), with a subspeciality in head and neck cancer. Mary worked in this area in Canada, Australia and Italy before joining the Department of Language and Communication Science, City University London. Research interests include functional outcomes in speech and swallowing after treatment for head and neck cancer, quality of life after total laryngectomy and quantifying changes in swallow function after total laryngectomy. Currently, she is involved in research investigating how changes in swallowing function affect quality of life and adjustment following treatment for head and neck cancer, as well as the impact of early therapeutic intervention on subsequent long-term swallowing recovery.

Skye McDonald is a neuropsychologist with 30 years of experience working with people with brain injury. She has developed new assessment and remediation techniques based upon theoretical approaches to understanding communication and social perception disorders and how these relate to brain function. Skye has 92 peer-reviewed publications, and 13 book chapters and edited volumes that focus on this research. She has developed the Awareness of Social Inference Test, which is used internationally to measure social perception in clinical conditions. She is the Director of the Master's (Clinical) Psychology Programme at the University of New South Wales.

Nidhi Mahendra is a bilingual Speech Language Pathologist and Assistant Professor in the Department of Communicative Sciences and Disorders at California State University East Bay. She conducts research on assessing and treating cognitive-communication disorders associated with dementia. She also investigates barriers experienced by culturally and linguistically diverse individuals in accessing speech language pathology services. Her research has been funded by grants from the American Speech-Language-Hearing Association, the Alzheimer's Association and the California State University Chancellor's Office.

Stuart Midgley lives in London. He has performed, written and directed fringe plays and storytelling since 1984. He has appeared at theatres throughout London, notably the Hen & Chickens Theatre Bar and Etcetera Theatre, and performed at Camden and Edinburgh Fringe Festivals. His work in the early 2000s included *Shame, Listen, Seepage, Winterval* and *Spinback*. In earlier days he was involved in children's storytelling around schools. He had a stroke five years ago. Since the stroke, he has taken up ceramics.

Nick Miller qualified as a Speech Language Therapist and worked in various hospital and clinical settings for many years before taking up a post in Newcastle in 1994. His main areas of teaching cover research methods and statistics, neuropsychology, motor speech disorders and dysphagia, and the university aphasia clinic. He has written major books on apraxia and on bilingualism and language disability, and published research in many fields, including swallowing, aphasia, dysarthria, apraxia of speech, bilingualism, gesture, foreign accent syndrome, conversation analysis and cerebral palsy. A particular area of interest in all these fields concerns the impact of neurological disorders on individuals and their families. He is a leading researcher in communication and swallowing in Parkinson's disease. He is also an adviser on motor speech disorders to the Royal College of Speech & Language Therapists.

Gary Morgan is Professor of Psychology in the Department of Language and Communication Science and Deputy Director of the Deafness, Language and Cognition Research Centre, City University London. His work focuses on the language and cognitive development of deaf children. He is a member of the Executive Committee of the International Association for the Study of Child Language and is a Governor of the Frank Barnes School for Deaf Children in London.

Mary, David and Felicity Morgan: Mary (75) and David (78) live in South London. They have a daughter, Felicity, and a son, as well as grandchildren and great-grandchildren. Mary was a principal dancer with the Royal Ballet. She had a stroke three and a half years ago. David spent 10 years in the Fleet Air Arm of the Royal Navy, and then became a theatre technician, coordinating specialist teams to ensure the hygiene of operating theatres across the United Kingdom. David and Felicity attend a regular stroke forum at the local hospital, where a volunteer visiting programme (befriending scheme) has now been implemented as a result of their suggestion.

Jennifer Oates is a Speech Pathologist with 32 years' experience as an academic and clinician in the field of the human voice and its disorders. She is an Associate

Professor in the School of Human Communication Sciences at La Trobe University in Melbourne, where she has been responsible for the education of speech pathology students in the area of voice for 22 years. Jenni is a co-founder of the Melbourne Voice Analysis Centre, a private multidisciplinary diagnostic service. Jenni holds a master's degree and a PhD from La Trobe University in addition to bachelor's degree qualifications in speech pathology. She is a Fellow of Speech Pathology Australia and a registered psychologist. She has published 50 journal papers and book chapters and presented more than 100 conference papers in Australia, New Zealand, Europe, Singapore and North America.

Mark Onslow is the Foundation Director of the Australian Stuttering Research Centre at the Faculty of Health Sciences, the University of Sydney. He leads a team that has twice been awarded multimillion-dollar research grants from the Australian National Health and Medical Research Council to develop treatments for stuttering. Professor Onslow's research interests are the epidemiology of early stuttering during early life, mental health of those who stutter, measurement of stuttering, and the nature and treatment of stuttering. The Australian Stuttering Research Centre has published the majority of the world's speech pathology clinical trials for stuttering treatment. Recently, work has begun at the Centre to adapt successful stuttering treatments for the internet. Mark has taught university courses about stuttering internationally, and currently teaches research methods to doctoral students at the Australian Stuttering Research Centre. He is a member of the international Lidcombe Program Trainers' Consortium and is in constant demand as a speaker internationally. With his colleagues, he has authored more than 250 publications dealing with stuttering, including journal articles, books and chapters.

Greg Pasco qualified as a Speech and Language Therapist in 1994 and has since specialized in the field of autism. After six years at the National Autistic Society, he moved into research, first at the International Molecular Genetics Study of Autism and then on a large-scale evaluation of the Picture Exchange Communication System. Following a brief stint as an SLT in East London, he returned to research, working on the Q-CHAT screening study at the Autism Research Centre (University of Cambridge), and is currently at the Centre for Research into Autism & Education (Institute of Education), working on the British Autism Study of Infant Siblings. His main clinical and research interests relate to the early identification, diagnosis and treatment of children with autism.

Lavinia Scott is 19 years of age and lives in East London with her mother and sister. She is studying for a Foundation Degree in Creative Industries at Redbridge College and the University of East London. Lavinia loves drawing and design and is working towards becoming an art therapist. She is a member of the Afasic youth group and represents Afasic on the Council for Disabled Children. She has been a carer since she was 9 years of age and does volunteer work for Barnardo's.

Vicky Slonims is a Speech and Language Therapist at Guy's and St Thomas' Hospital and holds an honorary senior lectureship at King's College London. She works in the service for children with complex needs, including learning difficulties, communication disorders and autism spectrum disorders. She is a member of the Research Autism: Scientific and Advisory Board (NAS) and the Strategic Research Group for the British Academy of Childhood Disability (BACD). She is an Associate Editor of the *International Journal of Language and Communication Disorders*. Her current research themes include early intervention in social communication and education outcomes for children with ASDs.

Leanne Togher is a Speech Pathologist who has worked for over 25 years in the area of communication disorders following brain injury. Leanne is a Senior Research Fellow of the National Health and Medical Research Council and a Principal Research Fellow of the University of Sydney. Leanne's current work at the University of Sydney has led to a new focus on the importance of providing communicative opportunities for people with brain injury. Leanne has worked with the New South Wales Police Service to improve police officers' interactions with people with brain injury, developed a training programme for staff in collaboration with the Attorney General's Department of NSW to improve access to legal services for people who cannot speak, and she has empirically evaluated a communication training programme for families and carers of people with traumatic brain injury called TBI Express.

1 Communication Disability Across the Lifespan

The Importance of Documenting and Sharing Knowledge about Wider Impacts

Nicola Botting and Katerina Hilari

City University London, UK

Communication disorders are wide-ranging and extend across the entire lifespan. Yet research into speech and language impairment is relatively young, with the literature focusing primarily on the nature of the impairment and interventions to address it. As we discover more about speech-language disorder, the more important it becomes to investigate and report the impact of communication disorders on people's lives. Understanding this impact is the only way for clinicians to make their interventions relevant to their clients' lives and to incorporate their clients' perspective into clinical decision-making.

The World Health Organization (WHO) has developed the *International Classification of Functioning, Disability and Health* (*ICF*; WHO, 2001), which addresses the notion of impact in a number of different areas. A key area is that entitled 'activity and participation'. Within this category, among other possible impacts the ICF lists communication, and others that are affected by communication such as learning, interpersonal interactions and relationships, community, social, and civic life and domestic life.

This impact on life caused by communication impairment is the focus of the current text. We use 'impact' to encompass the ideas of quality of life (QoL) – a term which has gained ground in recent literature, particularly for adult populations, but without some of the conceptual difficulties associated with this specific phrase. In 1995, Cummins reported that there were over 500 different definitions of the term 'QoL'. Thus, we feel that 'impact' better describes the wide range of different underlying causes, associations and effects of communication disability. In adult populations alone, a variety of different challenges arise from differing sources. From the effects of laryngectomy (Lee, Chapter 15) and voice disorders (Oates, Chapter 14), through motor speech disorder (Miller & Hartelius, Chapter 11) and acquired language impairment from traumatic brain injury (McDonald & Togher, Chapter 13) and stroke (Hilari, Chapter 9), to learning disabilities (Bunning & Buell, Chapter 12) and dementia (Bayles, Mahendra and Hopper, Chapter 10), communication is often one of the most impacting skills affected. It results in difficulties with employment; changes in family dynamics and relations; loss of friends; and a decline in social activities, emotional wellbeing and QoL. For adults there is a sense of loss for the skills and lifestyle that the individuals once enjoyed. Clients often feel isolated and under-resourced, as these chapters superbly indicate.

In contrast, in the developmental communication literature, the term 'QoL' is seldom used (notable exceptions are Markham, van Laar, Gibbard & Dean, 2009), but there has been much interest in the emotional and social challenges that associate with language and communication problems. In these developing populations, the challenges may be both similar and different. For example, children growing up with communication needs have never experienced life any differently, which brings the advantage of not 'losing' something, but also the disadvantage of having had more limited opportunity to build up strong communication experience, knowledge and support systems. In actual fact, little or no research has been conducted exploring the overlap of impact between these two groups. Within childhood disorders, it is also less clear the extent to which wider effects of communication disability are part of the neurological aetiology, or a psychosocial outcome of living with poor communicative skills. Developmental communication difficulties can also take many forms, from speech (Dodd, Chapter 4) and stuttering (Onslow & Langevin, Chapter 6), through young people with primary and persistent language impairments (Law, Chapter 2), and autism (Pasco & Slonims, Chapter 3), to those children with concomitant deafness (Herman & Morgan, Chapter 7) or learning disability (Harding, Chapter 5). For young people with communication needs, the overlap between disorders is also much less distinct, with many children receiving several diagnoses or experiencing concurrent difficulties. Rather than representing a medical truth, we need to view developmental diagnostic categories (even the quite wide ones presented in this volume) as dynamic and fluid constructs which best serve to describe and support individuals at a particular point in time.

This book is aimed at professionals, students, parents and academics who wish to discover more about the wide impact on life that communication impairments have. It was put together to address the lack of current texts focusing on the *impact* of communication difficulties rather than the nature of the disorders themselves.

Structure of the book

The volume is split into two halves: chapters dedicated to developmental disorders, and those discussing adult issues. Of course, the children and young people discussed grow up, and adult outcomes for those impairments are included in the first half (with the exception of adults with learning disabilities). We have asked authors to give relatively brief outlines of the disorders and populations themselves – there are numerous books outlining the nature of these, and in this volume they only serve as a background to further reading or clinical experience. Furthermore, although many of the impact themes are common in different chapters, we did not impose a set format for each client group in order that experts in the field could present and discuss the areas of impact most relevant to that particular communication difficulty. We have also decided not to include an index, since many of the themes of impact appear repeatedly throughout and across each chapter, and many different terms may be used to discuss the same aspect of impact. Instead, the table of contents gives each chapter's themes in more detail than usual. We felt that this was the most effective route for readers to identify the information they required.

The voice of people with communication disabilities

One aspect of reporting which is conspicuous in its absence from the literature is text written from the client's perspective or by those experiencing communication difficulties. This is not wholly surprising in that the medium of most dissemination is verbal and this makes personal narratives from people with communication impairments difficult to present in a straightforward way. We believe that this volume is the first academic text to offer people with communication disabilities the opportunity to share their experiences. Two chapters offer unique personal insights into the lives of young people with communication difficulties (Joffe, Beverly & Scott, Chapter 8) and the impact of aphasia on adults (Cruice, Cocks, Lancashire, Midgley, Morgan, Morgan & Morgan, Chapter 16). The first of these chapters is accompanied by expressive artwork by two of the young people to help convey their experiences.

Clinical implications

It is vitally important that, as well as problem-solving around the communication impairment itself, researchers and clinicians identify key areas of impact and work to manage and alleviate the challenges that arise. Educational needs is a key theme arising in the chapters on young people. McLeod and McKinnon (2010) conducted a large-scale cohort study (n=4845) examining support for groups of young people with educational needs. Importantly, of the nine areas of educational need identified, communication impairment was the strongest predictor of the teacher requesting additional classroom support.

For adults with communication disabilities, often physical or medical needs are the focus of attention. In their review of controlled trials with this population, Xiong, Bunning, Horton and Hartley (in press) report that 53% of outcome measures relate to the ICF category of 'bodily functions', compared with 36% addressing 'activity and participation'. For the clients discussed throughout this book, the impact of communication disability may require resources not only for educational, medical and health-related issues, but also support for the more subtle social and emotional needs that they experience. This is essential, as such needs (e.g. low mood and depression) can affect the client response to rehabilitation and their long-term outcomes. Although a substantial body of evidence is emerging on the complex impact of communication impairment in people's lives, much less attention has been devoted in the literature on what interventions best address this impact. The chapters in this book all include sections on the clinical implications, which aim to bring together this evidence for practising clinicians. They also identify gaps in our knowledge which highlight what future research should focus on.

It is important to note, whilst reading this volume, that many people with communication disorders or language needs would not describe themselves as disabled and would also identify positive impacts of the communication disorders on their lives. For example, people with aphasia sometimes mention having more time to spend with family and having a better perspective of what really matters in life; many young people with language impairment experience little or no impact on their everyday lives. Nevertheless, we hope the chapters on all the populations featured here are balanced and insightful, and give a useful window into the types of impact that different or limited communication needs can create.

References

Cummins, R.A. (1995) Assessing quality of life. In R.I. Brown (Ed.) *Quality of Life for Handicapped People*. London: Chapman & Hall.

Markham, C., van Laar, D., Gibbard, D. and Dean, T. (2009) Children with speech, language and communication needs: Their perceptions of their quality of life. *International Journal of Language and Communication Disorders, 44*, 748–768.

McLeod, S. and McKinnon, D.H. (2010) Support required for primary and secondary students with communication disorders and/or other learning needs. *Child Language Teaching and Therapy, 26(2)*, 123–143.

World Health Organization (WHO) (2001) *International Classification of Functioning, Disability and Health (ICF)*. Geneva: World Health Organization.

Xiong, T., Bunning, K., Horton, S. and Hartley, S. (in press) Assessing and comparing the outcome measures for the rehabilitation of adults with communication disorders in randomised controlled trials: An International Classification of Functioning, Disability and Health approach. *Disability and Rehabilitation*, DOI:10.3109/09638288.2011.568666

Section I
The Impact of Communication Disorders in Childhood

2 Developmental Language Impairment

James Law
Newcastle University, UK

Introduction

The term 'developmental language impairment' (henceforth 'DLI') is used to describe a group of children who are identified as having difficulties learning language.

How important is DLI to society? This question can be answered in terms of both its immediate and long-term impact. On the one hand it is important for parents and practitioners (educational psychologists, speech and language therapists, public health nurses, teachers, etc.) to raise concerns about a child's communication skills at any given point in a child's development. Yet on the other hand it is critical to understand the long-term impact that DLI has on children's outcomes and what, if anything, can be done to affect that impact. This chapter concentrates on the latter, asking two questions:

- What are the long-term (adult) impacts of DLI identified in early childhood?
- What factors influence the course of development?

We will start with a discussion of the nature of outcomes that are commonly associated with the measurement of impact in this field. We will then provide an overview of the association between early difficulties and identifiable concerns in adulthood before going on to identify some specific predictors of those outcomes.

The assessment of 'outcome' at different time points

Our understanding of relevant outcomes would be limited if it were restricted to communication alone. One of the key features of DLI is the level of co-morbidity associated with it. By co-morbidity we mean significant factors which co-occur sufficiently frequently that they appear to be part of the phenomenon itself. The two key examples are literacy and behaviour. Although delays in the development of oral language commonly predate identifiable literacy difficulties, they continue to interact one with another across time, the child with DLI coping better in school if they are able to develop reading skills (Catts, Fey, Zhang & Tomblin, 2001). Similarly, a substantial proportion of children with DLI are likely to have associated behaviour and literacy difficulties (Im-Bolterm & Cohen, 2007), with poor attention and listening at one end of the spectrum through to substantive aggressive and antisocial behaviours at the other. This association is likely to be especially pronounced for the children with externalising difficulties (Nelson, Benner, Neil & Stage, 2006). Yet whether we are talking about literacy, behaviour or oral language skills, we are still talking about what might be termed 'within-child' variables. And this takes us to a conceptual framework which has the potential to have considerable bearing on our understanding of outcomes for this group, namely the *International Classification of Functioning, Disability and Health* (ICF –WHO 2001; Estella, Threats & Worrall, 2008). Of particular significance is that the ICF makes it possible to discriminate between the type of within-child characteristics described above and the implications that these may or may not have for the day-to-day activities of the child. Thus the child may not perform well on a particular standardized measure of language, but does this really interfere with their ability to express themselves or have their needs met? If it does not, can we really say that the child's level of activity is restricted? The ICF emphasizes the impact that these 'skill' assessments have on the child's capacity to participate in relevant social structures, the family, the classroom, the peer group and as an adult to live healthy, productive lives.

Adult outcomes

A number of early studies followed samples of children with DLI through various periods in their early development. Only relatively few have considered the adult implications and have tended to be rather partial in the sense that their sample size was small or ascertained in such a way as to suggest potential bias. In a telephone follow-up of young adults who had been through a special school for children with DLI in the UK, Haynes and Naidoo showed that those concerned often found it difficult to find employment and, when they did, almost invariably took jobs that were below the level anticipated given their family background (Haynes & Naidoo, 1991). But such approaches are largely anecdotal and often difficult to interpret. One of the most commonly cited studies concerns a group of 17 men identified in primary school as having severe receptive language difficulties and who were followed through to 35 years (Clegg, Hollis, Mawhood & Rutter, 2005). They were compared with their siblings and a comparison group of men matched for IQ and social background from the National Child Development Study, a birth cohort of children born in 1958. Relative to both comparison groups, those concerned had poorer language, phonological processing skills and weaker theory of mind skills at follow up. Importantly, the study measured participation in a variety of ways: employment, living at home, having a partner, etc. Again we see these early difficulties being associated with prolonged unemployment and fewer close friendships, and four had very serious mental health problems. By way of illustration, 65% had experienced more than one year's unemployment relative to 6% and 10% in the two comparison groups. Indeed, by their mid-30s only 41% lived away from the parental home. The highest language scores for the group reached an age equivalent of 13 and years 10 for language and literacy respectively. The authors accept that it may be difficult to generalize from such a relatively small group of the most extreme cases.

A second follow-up of a clinical sample of approximately half the children originally identified by Bishop and Edmundson (1987) has recently reported outcomes for a proportion of the original group (Whitehouse, Watt, Line & Bishop, 2010). Although many of the participants were still in education or training, the authors examined the employment profile of the remainder. The young people were compared to a small group (n=8) of typically-developing individuals also identified as children. Subdividing their group into those with specific language impairment (SLI), pragmatic language impairment (PLI) and autism, they reported that the children with SLI were most likely to pursue jobs that did not require high levels of language skills. By contrast, the PLI young people had higher levels of education and were employed in much more skilled professions. The autistic young people were less independent and, in this study, were less likely to be employed. Although the results from these studies are important, it may be difficult to generalize from a relatively small group of the most extreme cases. We see similar findings in the Manchester Language Study followed through to post compulsory schooling in the UK (Conti-Ramsden & Botting, 1999; Conti-Ramsden, Durkin, Simkin & Knox, 2009; Durkin, Simkin, Knox & Conti-Ramsden, 2009) and a third in the US derived from a population sample (Tomblin, Records, Buckwalter, Zhang, Smith & O'Brien, 1997).

Fortunately, two other large-scale studies of DLI have reported adult outcomes in substantive community ascertained populations.

The first of these is the Ottowa-Carleton study in Canada, which has been reported at 5, 12, 19 and most recently at 25 years (Johnson, Beitchman & Brownlie, 2010). In this case the children were identified as 'cases' if their language or speech scores fell more than one standard deviation below the norm for the test. In the most recent follow-up study, 112 young people with this history of speech and language difficulties were compared with a comparable group from the original sample who had no such history. The young people differed significantly on all objective measurements of communication behaviour. In each case, those with DLI were different from both of the typically developing comparison group and the early speech delayed group, suggesting that the outcomes from DLI are much more pronounced than for early speech difficulties. The types of occupations differed markedly across the groups, with the comparison group most commonly going into sales and retail, the speech and the DLI groups going into trades and construction and, curiously in the case of the DLI group, specifically food processing. The authors do not report the gender split on these data, which may also have a role to play. There is no indication that the outcomes are comparable as far as employability or home life (partners, children, etc.) with the data from the Clegg et al. (2005) study above, although there was a curious finding that members of the DLI group were much more likely to have started families by the age of 25 than either of the other groups. Significantly, there was no difference in the perceived wellbeing of the groups, which was more closely linked to the social networks of those concerned than the objective measurement of communication performance.

Finally, we turn to a UK national birth cohort, the 1970 British Cohort Study (BCS70), one of Britain's richest research resources for the study of human development and a specific set of analyses associated with long-term outcomes for DLI (Law, Rush, Schoon & Parsons, 2009). The British Cohort Study takes as its participants 17,196 persons living in Great Britain who were born in one week in 1970. Although data are available about the cohort members at birth, 5, 10, 16, 26, 30 and, most recently in 2004, when aged 34 years, the data are much less consistent than those in the Ottawa-Carleton study, in part because it was not set up to address issues associated with language. For the purposes of this analysis the study included those whose first language was English and whose ethnicity was white European. The study included two baseline measures at 5 years, namely the English Picture Vocabulary Test (EPVT) (Brimer & Dunn, 1962), and the Copying Design Test (CDT) (Osborn, Butler & Morris, 1984). We then identified two groups of children with difficulties. The first (n=195) had vocabulary scores that fell below two standard deviations from the mean and their non-verbal performance was below one standard deviation – i.e. below average. These children were then designated as having 'non-specific language impairment' or N-SLI. A second group (n=211) had comparable language but non-verbal performance within the normal range. This was designated the 'specific language impairment' group (SLI). These two groups were then compared with a much larger (n=8726) typically developing group of children. Three domains were assessed at 34 years, namely literacy, mental health and employment, and for each the outcomes were split according to whether they were above or below a predetermined level of difficulty. The literacy assessment was split at Level 2 literacy (with poor literacy being defined as being equivalent to a grade D or lower in the national GCSE exam in the UK). Adult mental health was assessed using four measures: a shortened version of the Rutter Malaise Inventory; a measure of general satisfaction with life; a measure of how much feeling of control over life the individual has; and a measure of self-efficacy. The individual was considered to have mental health difficulties if they had difficulties in three or more of these areas. Finally, unemployment was defined as being out of employment for more than a year before the age of 33 years.

In addition, a series of distal and proximal risk factors were tapped prior to 5 years (Schoon, 2006). Distal risks represent risks perceived to be likely influences on child development over which there is no direct control. Those adopted in this study were gender, whether the child's mother left school before the age of 16 and whether the mother was a single parent. Proximal risks are those factors which might be considered modifiable in the sense that a parent might be encouraged to take literacy classes, to read more to their child or to change a child's accommodation. Those adopted in this study were a measure of overcrowding in the home (the person-per-room ratio), whether the child had experienced preschool of any sort, whether either parent reported reading to the child and whether the parent reported themselves to be a poor reader. We also included a number of biological and developmental health risks. Those adopted in this study were whether the mother had smoked during pregnancy, whether the child was born small for gestational age (calculated as a function of birthweight and gestation, namely with weight below 2515 grams and gestational age over 259 days) and whether the child had neurotic or antisocial behavioural difficulties as measured on the Rutter Behaviour Scale.

The first question to be addressed using these data is whether performance at 5 years was associated with performance at 34 years once the proximal and distal factors were taken into consideration. The results are presented in detail in Law et al. (2009) but can be summarized as follows: Adult literacy difficulties were predicted by the 5-year-old child being in either the N-SLI group (Odds Ratio (OR) 4.35) or the SLI group (OR 1.59) after controlling for demographic and other variables. Adult mental health difficulties were associated with the child being in the SLI group in all but the final model, whereas being in the N-SLI group continued to be strongly associated with adult mental health irrespective of what else was included in the analysis (OR 2.9). Being in either group was significantly associated with low employment. Interestingly, and counter to the pattern for the other two outcomes, the association was higher for the SLI group (OR 2.24) than for the N-SLI group (OR 1.88).

Of course, it is one thing to identify associations, another to look at these associations at an individual level. The figures for individuals scoring at different levels of the EPVT are provided for the three adult outcomes together with the productivity figures (Sensitivity and Specificity) for the principal threshold (+/- 1 SD) in Tables 2.1–2.3 below. It is important to acknowledge that the denominator in each table changes across tables, reflecting the response rate for the test items concerned.

Table 2.1 The relationship at an individual level between receptive vocabulary at 5 years and literacy at 34 years.

	Vocabulary performance at 5 years				
		−2 SD and below	−1.9–1.5 SD	−1.49–1.0 SD	WNL*	Total
Literacy at 34 years	Level 2	25	43	54	443	565
	+ Level 2	91	146	212	4116	4565
	Total	116	189	266	4559	5130
	Sensitivity=.21; Specificity=.9 *Within normal limits					

Table 2.2 The relationship at an individual level between receptive vocabulary at 5 years and mental health at 34 years.

	Vocabulary performance at 5 years				
Mental health at 34 years		−2 SD and below	−1.9–1.5 SD	−1.49–1.0 SD	WNL	Total
	3–4 signs	75	83	100	433	691
	No signs	204	334	434	7102	8074
	Total	279	417	534	7535	8765
	Sensitivity=.29; Specificity=.94					

Table 2.3 The relationship at an individual level between receptive vocabulary at 5 years and employment at 34 years.

	Vocabulary performance at 5 years				
		−2 SD and below	−1.9–1.5 SD	−1.49–1.0 SD	WNL	Total
Employment 34 years	+ 1 year	29	36	43	485	593
	−1 year	151	260	358	5633	6402
	Total	180	296	401	6118	6995
	Sensitivity=.12; Specificity=.92					

These data indicate fairly conclusively that a relatively straightforward measure of receptive language at 5 years has the potential to identify those who are likely to have normal literacy and mental health in adulthood together with relatively low levels of unemployment. By contrast, the sensitivity figures suggest that such scales do not work very effectively at an individual level at identifying those children who will go on to have difficulties later on. Indeed, we find that 61% of children with low language scores have developed into competent readers by 10 years and that those who are competent by this stage remain so through into adulthood (Parsons, Schoon, Rush & Law, 2009). This is supported by a range of analyses that have tested children's language and literacy performance in much greater detail. This is probably not surprising given the relatively long intervening period. Indeed, it might be more reasonable to express concern that these figures are as high as they are given this 29-year gap.

To check whether these findings were a function of the results of the thresholds adopted, we looked at literacy and mental health outcomes of the group of children whose scores fell above and below one standard deviation (i.e. those falling below the 16th centile), the threshold used in the Ottawa-Carleton study. The results are strikingly similar, with 5-year performance remaining in the model once all the other social and demographic variables have been controlled for (Schoon, Parsons, Rush & Law, 2010a, 2010b). While it would be reasonable to predict that the child with a language score below the second centile was a 'case' irrespective of whether they were referred or not, the same is probably not true for the more liberal cut point.

Potential mechanisms across childhood

Having established that there is a demonstrable risk from DLI across childhood and into adulthood, the key questions then become:

(a) Is it possible to consistently identify additional factors which are associated with elevated risk? and

(b) Can we identify different mechanisms at different time developmental points?

It is clear from cohort studies such as the BCS70 that environmental factors are fundamentally associated with both early language skills and language as it emerges over time. For example, we see consistent associations with a composite measure of social disadvantage which includes variables such as housing type and tenure and maternal educational level. Similarly, we see associations with parental engagement with the child – book reading, for example, or engagement with schooling. There are also likely to be factors such as maternal tobacco use during pregnancy, which can be shown to be associated with early language difficulties but that are no longer associated once socio-demographic factors are taken into consideration (Tomblin, Hammer & Zhang, 1998). Interestingly, a tension appears to be emerging in the literature between those who make the case that the environmental differences are determining the child's earliest performance (Hart & Risley, 1995) and that genetic/intrinsic factors start to take effect in middle childhood and those who assert that environment factors start to take effect once highly determined developmental effects have played their part (Reilly et al., 2007, 2010; Zubrick, Taylor, Rice & Slegers, 2007) – biology giving way to environmental factors or vice versa. For many years familial studies have reiterated the assumption that DLI is genetically determined to a considerable degree although generally less than reading skills. Heritability has also attracted considerable interest. DLI clearly runs in families (Bishop, North & Donlan, 1995; Tallal, Hirsch, Realpe-Bonilla, Miller, Brzustowicz et al., 2001), the more severe the difficulty, the more pronounced the genetic contribution. Results from the Twins Early Development Study (TEDS) have refined our understanding of this process, suggesting that DLI associated with low IQ or speech difficulties has a much higher genetic loading than slow language acquisition alone. Furthermore, the heritability is relatively constant over time and its impact is much higher for speech/phonological tasks than it is for non-phonological tasks such as vocabulary and syntax. A recent analysis of the relative contribution of environmental and genetics factors to the route from phonological development on the one hand and non-phonological development on the other from preschool through to 10 years of age (Hayiou-Thomas, Harlaar, Dale & Plomin, 2010) suggests that there is a moderate and stable genetic association between both speech and language and reading at 7 years and that this declines slightly up to 10 years. Interestingly, the relative role of genetic and environmental influence changes with severity, the genetic influences becoming more marked at the lower end of language ability. However, it is important to stress, as these authors do, that the ability to detect heritability from twin studies is not the same as demonstrating the mechanism by which oral language skills influences reading. It is likely that we will be discussing for some time to come whether the genetic association with early speech and language skills feeds into literacy directly or whether literacy, speech and language have a fourth common antecedent – perhaps it is determined by a generalist gene for which the impact is systemic (Plomin & Kovas, 2005).

But it is invidious to see this discussion as simply a distinction between nature and nurture, because what would appear, at face value, to be an environmental influence, for example parental book reading, may really be a proxy for parental capacity for reading. Thus the parent with better reading skills may be more inclined to this type of activity, suggesting a genetic as much as an environmental transmission. An interesting example of this interaction between constitutional and environmental factors is gender. For a long time it has been assumed that gender is a factor causing language learning difficulties but again it depends on how populations are ascertained and how language is measured. Thus, while there are consistent gender effects, invariably with a preponderance of boys over girls if we look at clinical samples and if we include measures of vocabulary in young children or phonological/reading activities in older children, community samples and especially those which use measures of receptive vocabulary consistently fail to find this association (Law, Rush, Schoon & Parsons, submitted).

Another issue, which is of primary importance as a potential mediator of outcomes, is intervention. While parental concerns about child difficulties are often an element of a child's history, detailed information about receipt of intervention rarely is – and even if it is included, this type of information is more related to parental concern and level of difficulty than intervention. Indeed, in our analysis of the BCS70, referral to speech and language therapy services was significantly associated with whether the children had a language difficulty (Law et al., 2009). Superficially rather alarming, such a finding points to the severity of the identified condition rather than the response to those services. Alternatively, it may be more associated with the more obvious aspects of communication difficulties, namely speech difficulties, which tend to be the main reason that many children receive services (Zhang & Tomblin, 2000). The only way of establishing whether intervention has the potential to contribute to the long-term outcomes of children with DLI is to follow up groups of children once they have received specific interventions, comparing them with control groups who did not receive that intervention. While there are a number of reasonably well-controlled studies and these have been reviewed and, in some cases, been meta-analyzed (Law, Garrett & Nye, 2004), the review conclusions suggest that, for speech and for expressive language, the results are relatively positive, but there is much less that can be said about children with receptive language difficulties – i.e. those often presenting as being most at risk in follow-up studies. Similarly, we know less about children with pragmatic difficulties. These studies have mostly been carried out within a relatively narrow developmental window – between 3 and 6 years – and they tend to be relatively short (6–10 weeks) with limited follow-up periods of six months or less. There are no studies which have completed lifespan or at least childhood follow-ups in the way that we have seen for children going through Head Start in the US or similar programmes for children who are from socially disadvantaged backgrounds. Such programmes tend to be relatively intensive and sustained and clearly show important long-term societal impacts (Campbell, Pungello, Miller-Johnson, Burchinal & Ramey, 2001). So we can say that such interventions may have the potential to reduce the long-term impact of DLI, but there are no specific data to support such a proposition at this stage. While we know that environmental factors are highly associated with adult outcomes, we are less clear that environmental modifications can be shown to influence clearly the course of DLI.

The service implications of changes across time

It is important to return to the practical implications of these continuities and discontinuities over time. Long-term follow-up studies are powerful for the data they provide but we need to exercise care in their interpretation in terms of service delivery – what was routine 30 years ago may not be routine today. That said, we can draw some conclusions about the process of identification. While there is a consensus that early identification is important, care has to be taken that we do not assume that early detection and management will be sufficient. Put simply, as the data above indicate, the methods of detection which we currently have at our disposal work in terms of population risk but are relatively imprecise at an individual level. Unfortunately, this is as true when the gold standard measures are administered immediately after the screening procedure as it is when the intervening period is much wider. Routine developmental screening is not currently recommended because of the difficulties associated with underidentification illustrated above but demonstrated in a much more comprehensive fashion elsewhere (Law, Boyle, Harris, Harkness & Nye, 1998; Nelson, Nygren, Walker & Panoscha, 2006). What would be helpful would be early identification procedures which account for development and are able to detect difficulties across time, but such procedures have been elusive to date.

The alternative is for services to be especially vigilant across critical transitions: when the child goes to school, transferring between nursery and primary school (age 5), primary and secondary school (age 11) and, of course, secondary education to employment (age 16–18). Children are always vulnerable at these points and it would be reasonable to assume that this is especially true for the child that does not speak as well as their peers. The challenge at a population level is: how do we know which children to monitor? If the child has already been identified this should be feasible, but it is not practical to do this for all children (except by introducing specific monitoring procedures). It might be argued that children's needs change across time and that their speech and language may not be the main priorities as the child gets older. Indeed, we see a steep decline in children being described as having 'speech, language and communication needs' (SLCN) in the UK between primary and secondary school. Thus in England the proportion of children with special needs who have speech and language difficulties as their primary need drops from around 25% in primary school to 7% in secondary school (Department for Education, 2010), a pattern which has been consistent for a number of years. Although it might be argued that children who have a difficulty in primary school have grown out of it by the time they reach the end of primary school – i.e. the data are real – it is probably more likely that oral language simply becomes less of a priority in many secondary school environments despite the fact that these are the very skills which facilitate adult outcomes. Although the early literature has tended to report within-child skills across time, there is an increasing interest in longer-term, more social outcomes such as employment and mental health. While such studies rarely characterize those difficulties in terms of the WHO criteria discussed above, it is clear that measures like mental health and employment are much closer to concepts such as 'participation' in terms of what they measure. It is not sufficient to see oral language as the primary outcome of interest because, by its very nature, oral language is the means by which we engage with others around us, negotiate with our boss, ask for help, form relationships, etc.

Summary and conclusions

DLI clearly interacts with other risk factors and can be associated with a variety of poor long-term outcomes. We need to know more about the impact of DLI both on economic outcomes such as income and employment and on outcomes that might be more closely associated with the ICF concept of 'participation' such as social inclusion and social mobility. Similarly, we need to know the extent to which such outcomes persist across the whole lifespan, not just into an individual's thirties. But it is important to stress both that these models are associative not causative and that many children who are slow to start do manage well in school and beyond, especially if they are able to compensate with their literacy skills. Children constantly demonstrate a startling capacity for resilience and there are those, who seem to be especially vulnerable, who do cope well across time. Similarly, there are those who seem to be relatively advantaged who do not have good outcomes. But as data from the BCS70 cohort demonstrate well we are looking at a risk factor which is clearly there at a group level but which is not deterministic in the sense that the outcome is inevitable. This would appear to be true across childhood but seems to be especially pronounced in the preschool period, declining over primary school.

Although this chapter has focused primarily on the long-term outcomes for the child with DLI, of course the pattern of vulnerability is common to groups of children with other developmental difficulties. For many of such groups we know that early identification and relevant evidence-based interventions are the key to better outcomes for children's development and emotional wellbeing, although the link between such knowledge and policy is not always as strong as it should be (Shonkoff, 2004). While it is tempting to think that what these children need is access to specific interventions at specific points in their development, the reality is that, for many, these difficulties do not just go away and the role of society is to remain sensitive to their needs, recognizing both the potential long-term impact and for individual change. Effectively, there is a need for a population or epidemiological approach to the management of DLI. Although originally advocated as being relevant to the field of speech and language science more than 10 years ago (Lubker & Tomblin, 1998) it has attracted relatively little attention. Such an approach is likely to lead to a better understanding of risk at the level of the individual and prevents over-reliance in judging continuities from the most extreme clinical cases. What is most needed now is consolidation of our understanding of the concept of risk, replicated across well-designed prospective studies and then effectively translated for doctors, therapists and educationalists so that they can provide information to parents anxious about their child's early development. This will allow them to know how best to address the needs of their child and weigh up the risk of long-term sequelae to early difficulties. What we do not need is professionals giving inappropriate advice – of either the 'they'll grow out of it' or the 'DLI condemns the child to lifelong difficulties' variety. We need better ways of incorporating risk into our models of identification of the children whose difficulties are most likely to persist.

References

Bishop, D.V.M. & Edmundson, A. (1987) Language impaired four year olds: Distinguishing transient from persistent impairment. *Journal of Speech and Hearing Disorders, 52*, 156–173.

Bishop, D.V.M., North, T. & Donlan, C. (1995) Genetic basis of Specific Language Impairment: Evidence from a twin study. *Developmental Medicine and Child Neurology 37*, 56–71.

Brimer, M.A. & Dunn, L.M. (1962) *English Picture Vocabulary Test*. Bristol, United Kingdom: Evaluation Enterprises.

Campbell, F.A., Pungello, E.P., Miller-Johnson, S., Burchinal, M. & Ramey, C.T. (2001) The development of cognitive and academic abilities: Growth curves from an early childhood educational experiment. *Developmental Psychology, 37*, 231–242.

Catts, H.W., Fey, M.E., Zhang, X. & Tomblin, J.B. (2001) Estimating the risk of future reading difficulties in kindergarten children: A research-based model and its clinical implementation. *Language, Speech and Hearing Services in Schools, 32*, 38–50.

Clegg, J., Hollis, C., Mawhood, L. & Rutter, M. (2005) Developmental language disorders

– a follow-up in later adult life. Cognitive, language and psychosocial outcomes. *Journal of Child Psychology and Psychiatry and Allied Disciplines*, 46, 128–149.

Conti-Ramsden, G. & Botting, N. (1999) Characteristics of children attending language units in England: A national study of 7-year-olds. *International Journal of Language and Communication Disorders*, 34, 359–366.

Conti-Ramsden, G., Durkin, K., Simkin, Z. & Knox, E. (2009) Specific language impairment and school outcomes. I: Identifying and explaining variability at the end of compulsory education. *International Journal of Language and Communication Disorders*, 44, 15–35.

Department for Education (2010) *SEN in England*. Nottingham: Department for Education.

Durkin, K., Simkin, Z., Knox, E. & Conti-Ramsden, G. (2009) Specific language impairment and school outcomes. II: Educational context, student satisfaction and post-compulsory progress. *International Journal of Language and Communication Disorders*, 44, 36–55.

Estella, P.-M. Ma, Threats, T.T. & Worrall, Linda E. (2008) An introduction to the International Classification of Functioning, Disability and Health (ICF) for speech-language pathology: Its past, present and future. *International Journal of Speech-Language Pathology*, 10, 2–8.

Hart, B. & Risley, T. (1995) *Meaningful Differences in the Everyday Experiences of Young American Children*. Baltimore: Paul Brookes.

Hayiou-Thomas, M.E., Harlaar, N., Dale, P.S. & Plomin, R. (2010) Preschool speech, language skills, and reading at 7, 9, and 10 years: Etiology of the relationship. *Journal of Speech Language and Hearing Research*, 53, 311–332.

Haynes, C. & Naidoo, S. (1991) *Children with Specific Speech and Language Impairment*. Clinics in Developmental Medicine 119. Cambridge: MacKeith Press.

Im-Bolterm, N. & Cohen, N.J. (2007) Language impairment and psychiatric comorbidities language, communication, and literacy: Pathologies and treatments. *Pediatric Clinics of North America*, 54, 525–542.

Johnson, C.J., Beitchman, J.H. & Brownlie, E.B. (2010) Twenty-year follow-up of children with and without speech-language impairments: Family, educational, occupational, and quality of life outcomes. *American Journal of Speech-Language Pathology*, 9, 51–65.

Law, J., Boyle, J., Harris, F., Harkness, A. & Nye, C. (1998) Screening for speech and language delay: A systematic review of the literature. *Health Technology Assessment*, 2, 1–184.

Law, J., Garrett, Z. & Nye, C. (2004) The effectiveness of speech and language therapy interventions for children with primary speech and language delay or disorder. *Journal of Speech, Language, and Hearing Research*, 47, 924–943.

Law, J., Rush, R., Schoon, I. & Parsons, S. (2009) Modelling developmental language difficulties from school entry into adulthood: Literacy, mental health and employment outcomes. *Journal of Speech, Language, and Hearing Research*, 52, 1401–1416.

Law, J., Rush, R., Schoon, I. & Parsons, S. (submitted) The relationship between gender, receptive language and literacy from school entry through to adulthood: Findings from the BCS70 birth cohort.

Lubker, B.B. & Tomblin, J.B. (1998) Epidemiology: Informing clinical practice and research on language disorders in children. *Topics in Language Disorders, 19*, 1–26.

Nelson, H.D., Nygren, P., Walker, M. & Panoscha, R. (2006) Screening for speech and language delay in preschool children: Systematic evidence review for the US Preventive Services Task Force. *Pediatrics, 117*, 298–319.

Nelson, J.R., Benner, G.H., Neil, S. & Stage, S. (2006) The interrelationship amongst language skills, externalising behaviour and academic fluency and their impact on the academic skills of children with emotional disturbance. *Journal of Emotional and Behaviour Disorders, 14*, 209–216.

Osborn, A.F., Butler, N.R. & Morris, A.C. (1984) *The Social Life of Britain's Five-Year-Olds*. London: Routledge & Kegan Paul.

Parsons, S., Schoon, I., Rush, R. & Law, J. (2009) Long-term outcomes for children with early language problems: Beating the odds. *Children and Society*. DOI:10.1111/j.1099-0860.2009.00274.x

Plomin, R. & Kovas,Y. (2005) Generalist genes and learning disabilities. *Psychological Bulletin, 131*, 592–617.

Reilly, S., Wake, M., Bavin, E.L., Prior, M., Williams, J., Bretherton, L., Eadie, P., Barrett,Y. & Ukoumunne, O.C. (2007) Predicting language at 2 years of age: A prospective community study. *Pediatrics, 120*, 1441–1449.

Reilly, S., Wake, M., Ukoumunne, O.C., Bavin, E., Prior, M., Cini, E., Conway, L., Eadie, P. & Bretherton, L. (2010) Predicting language outcomes at 4 years of age: Findings from early language in Victoria Study. *Pediatrics, 126*, 1530–1537. DOI: 10.1542/peds.2010-0254

Schoon, I. (2006) *Risk and Resilience: Adaptations in Changing Times*. Cambridge: Cambridge University Press.

Schoon, I., Parsons, S., Rush, R. & Law, J. (2010a) Children's language and ability and literacy development: A twenty-nine year follow-up study. *Pediatrics* published online 8 February 2010. DOI: 10.1542/peds.2008-2111

Shonkoff, J.P. (2004) Closing the gap between what we know and what we do. Ounce of Prevention Fund. http://www.buildinitiative.org/pdf/shonkoffweb.pdf

Tallal, P., Hirsch, L.S., Realpe-Bonilla, T., Miller, S., Brzustowicz, L.M., Bartlett, C. & Flax, J.F. (2001) Familial aggregation in specific language impairment. *Journal of Speech, Language, and Hearing Research, 44*, 1172–1182.

Tomblin, J.B., Records, N., Buckwalter, P., Zhang, X., Smith, E. & O'Brien, M. (1997) Prevalence of specific language impairment in kindergarten children. *Journal of Speech Language, and Hearing Research, 4*, 1245–1269.

Tomblin, J.B., Hammer, C.S. & Zhang, X. (1998) The association of parental tobacco use and SLI. *International Journal of Language and Communication Disorders, 33*, 357–368.

Whitehouse, H.J., Watt, E.A., Line, E.A. & Bishop, D.V.M. (2010) Adult psychosocial outcomes of children with specific language impairment, pragmatic language impairment and autism. *International Journal of Language and Communication Disorders*, 44, 511–528.

Zhang, X. & Tomblin, J.B. (2000) The association of intervention receipt with speech-language profiles and social-demographic variables. *American Journal of Speech-Language Pathology*, 9, 345–357.

Zubrick, S.R., Taylor, C.L., Rice, M.L. & Slegers, D.W. (2007) Late language emergence at 24 months: An epidemiological study of prevalence, predictors, and covariates. *Journal of Speech, Language, and Hearing Research*, 50, 1562–1592.

3 Autism Spectrum Disorder

Greg Pasco
University of Cambridge, UK

Vicky Slonims
Guy's Hospital, London, UK

Introduction

Most neuro-developmental problems in children are likely to be identified in the first instance by medical professionals even though the difficulty may relate to development and learning rather than illness. However, unlike most medical problems, the first professional to mention a problem relating to an autism spectrum disorder (ASD) to the family will vary depending on the initial presentation of the problem. It may be a speech and language therapist following a referral for language delay, a psychologist for a child presenting with behavioural problems, an occupational therapist for problems with motor coordination or a health visitor or general practitioner if parents are concerned about less specific development difficulties. Historically, the diagnosis of autism was made by a psychiatrist, but current best practice with younger children (e.g. National Initiative for Autism: Screening and Assessment, 2003) involves a multidisciplinary team including paediatricians and allied health professionals. In spite of the medical diagnosis the care and management of children with ASD is generally the responsibility of a mix of health and educational support, with school-based therapy being the norm. Later in childhood social services teams may become involved.

'Autism spectrum disorder' is widely used as an umbrella term covering a number of more specific variants, including autism, pervasive developmental disorder (PDD), Asperger syndrome, high-functioning autism (HFA) and atypical autism. Some professionals, parents and people with autism prefer the term 'autism spectrum condition' (ASC) as this does not carry the negative connotations of a disorder. On the whole, the use of the term 'spectrum' highlights the wide range of strengths and difficulties associated with autism, and the heterogeneity within the population of people with ASD.

In the past, estimates of the percentage of individuals with significant learning disabilities were high, but recognition of the broader autism spectrum has meant that more individuals with average cognitive abilities have been identified. Baird et al. (2006) estimate that 55% of people with ASD have intellectual disability. The absence of learning disability and the development of language in the first few years of life are considered to be good predictors of outcome for children with ASD, although clinicians recognize that children may learn language at any time up to 6 years of age and still acquire adequate verbal skills to meet basic needs.

Diagnosis and co-morbidity

ASDs are considered by those who work in this field as being uniquely complex. This might be viewed as a rather 'precious' notion but in some ways it is warranted. The diagnosis is based on descriptions and observations of behaviours and abilities relating to language and communication, social functioning, play and imagination. Problems with acquiring and using language, social anxiety and difficulties with attention are generally considered to be features of autism. Therefore the diagnosis of an ASD will take precedence over other possible co-morbid and associated conditions, such as developmental language disorder, language delay, ADD/ADHD and psychiatric/mental health problems. An additional diagnosis of this sort will only be given when their presentation is over and above that typically expected in ASD.

The lack of 'norms' for behaviours such as social competence, social imagination and non-verbal communication can mean that diagnosis is subject to the particular views and expertise of individual professionals. Even widely used assessment tools such as the Autism Diagnostic Observation Schedule (ADOS: Lord et al., 2000) do not provide exact measurement, though they have improved the reliability of assessments. Diagnostic decisions are the result of careful examination of a range of factors and a collation of information from different sources. Given the highly variable presentation of symptoms between individuals and the fact that every person will change significantly over time, the process of diagnosis is complex and prognosis can be very uncertain.

There has been increasing concern that children and adults with ASD often do not receive appropriate treatment for co-morbid physical and mental health problems. Seventy per cent of 10- to 14-year-olds with an ASD may have at least one co-occurring mental health problem, including anxiety, depression and obsessive compulsive disorder (Simonoff et al., 2008), and nearly half of young people with ASD experience their first episode of mental health problems before the age of 5 (Madders, 2010). Melville et al. (2008) concluded that, whilst the prevalence of mental health problems in the population of adults with autism and intellectual disability was not higher than for people with intellectual disability as a whole, recovery rates from problem behaviours were significantly lower. A recent report by the UK National Autistic Society (NAS) (Madders, 2010) identifies a lack of knowledge about ASD amongst Child and Adolescent Mental Health Service (CAMHS) professionals, leading to inadequate and inappropriate provision, excessive delays in accessing services and in some cases refusal to treat young people with ASD.

Furthermore, many people with ASD do not receive routine investigation for biomedical conditions, including gastrointestinal problems such as abdominal pain, constipation and reflux, which may lead to distress, 'challenging behaviour' and self-injury (Buie et al., 2010). Shavelle, Strauss and Pickett (2001) report higher death rates amongst children and adults with ASD compared to the general population, particularly in relation to causes such as seizures and accidents relating to suffocation and drowning. Those with autism and severe learning disability were also found to be at elevated risk of death from respiratory disease.

Family and financial issues

Like many disabilities, autism has a direct impact on the whole family, and the timing and sensitivity with which information about the diagnosis is presented can have long-lasting effects on parental acceptance of the diagnosis, coping strategies and relationships with professionals. Furthermore, the pervasive nature of the condition can mean that consequences are more widespread than for less complex disabilities. Even today, when the nature and range of the autism spectrum are much more widely understood than, for instance, a decade ago, parents often feel that they have to battle in order to get a clear and concrete diagnosis. Apart from the issue of waiting times for appointments, parents often feel frustrated because non-specialist professionals are unwilling or unable to mention autism, even though they suspect that this will be the eventual diagnosis. The gap between parents' first concerns about their child's development and eventual diagnosis can be several years (Howlin & Ashgarian, 1999) and this delay can exacerbate stress within the family, particularly in the absence of intervention. However, even those parents who felt that they had to fight to have their child diagnosed report that it can still be devastating to receive the formal diagnosis, partly because it is a confirmation that their child has a lifelong condition. Eventually, the majority of parents acknowledge that receiving the diagnosis gave them a sense of relief, as it meant that they, and others, could accept that the emotional and behavioural difficulties experienced by their child were not due to poor parenting. Sadly for many, early diagnosis is not synonymous with early intervention, which can lead to further frustration.

Siblings are often particularly affected by the presence of a child in the family with an ASD. Issues relating to the direct relationship between the child with ASD and their non-autistic siblings might arise from difficulties with playing creatively and sharing toys, lack of flexibility and insistence on certain routines, aggression and poor socio-emotional regulation on the part of the child with an ASD (Kaminsky & Dewey, 2001). Additionally, siblings may feel that the needs of their brother or sister with ASD dominate within the family, and that this child receives a disproportionate amount of parents' time and attention. Being a sibling of a child with ASD can also disrupt relationships with friends, as it may not be possible for other children to visit the family home, for example. Finally, many siblings also have to cope with a degree of social isolation if the family is unable to visit local amenities, parks and other public spaces due to the embarrassing or inappropriate behaviour of the child with ASD, the likelihood that they may run off, or the degree of distress that a busy, noisy or unpredictable public environment might cause for that child (Orsmond & Seltzer, 2007).

Hastings (2003) reports that parents of children with autism do not differ from each other in terms of their experience of stress and depression, though mothers express more anxiety than fathers. Stress in mothers of children with disabilities appears to be affected by the psychological wellbeing of all family members, whereas fathers' stress is affected more by other factors. Whilst it is recognized that children with ASDs may present a greater challenge for parents because of emotional and behavioural difficulties, a second study (Herring et al., 2006) compared toddlers with developmental delays with and without a diagnosis of PDD and found that emotional and behavioural problems were associated with parent-reported mental health problems and perceived family dysfunction independently of diagnosis, degree of delay or gender. In this study fathers reported significantly less stress in relation to parenting their child than mothers.

One further issue relating to the families of people with ASD stems from the fact that autism is now recognized as primarily a genetic condition (Abrahams & Geschwind, 2008). The implication of this is that many first-degree relatives of people with ASD will be affected in some way by difficulties associated with autism. This is not to say that parents and siblings will necessarily be diagnosed with an ASD, although 'multiplex' families are not as rare as was once suspected (Muhle, Trentacoste & Rapin, 2004), but that often family members will exhibit a number of autistic traits. Whilst the broader autism phenotype (BAP) is extremely heterogeneous and difficult to define, individuals with these milder, sub-clinical forms of autism may nevertheless have difficulties with social relationships, emotional regulation and stereotyped behaviours that impact on social, academic and employment experiences. Of course, some autistic traits, such as attention to detail, honesty and persistence can be very beneficial to an individual in all aspects of life.

In their study of the economic impact of autism, Knapp, Romeo and Beecham (2009) noted the high proportion of the overall financial cost that falls directly on the family, in the form of out-of-pocket expenses, lost income and employment opportunities and payment for informal care. In a recent paper from the Preschool Autism Communication Trial (PACT) Byford et al. (in press) found that families with very young children with core autism accessed a wide range of hospital and community services and the average total cost of these services over six months was £2581 per child, though there was substantial variation. The inclusion of 'out-of-pocket' family expenses (costs paid for by the parents or relatives) and productivity losses (loss of income) increased this total to just over £3000.

Green et al. found an 'unusual combination' (2005, p.25) of high educational status and low economic activity rate amongst parents of children with ASD in contrast to parents of children with mental health problems and other developmental disabilities. The authors speculate that this probably reflects the relatively heavy caring responsibilities for parents of children with ASD. Fifty-six per cent of the families with a child with ASD were in receipt of disability benefit, in contrast to 31% and 27% for families with a child with a conduct disorder and those with a hyperkinetic disorder, respectively. Knapp et al. (2009) indicate that a very large proportion of the costs required to support the needs of people with autism and their families fall to the public sector, particularly health services, social care agencies, education and housing budgets, demonstrating the impact of this complex and heterogeneous disorder.

In the past few years it has become increasingly apparent that autism spectrum disorders are fairly common and that significant resources are being allocated to the needs of these individuals, often without adequate strategic planning. Based on a prevalence rate of 1% Byford et al. (in press) estimate the total burden on services of preschool children with autism to be approximately

£109 million per annum and the wider societal costs to be approximately £130 million per annum. Knapp et al. (2009) estimate that autism costs the UK economy around £28.2 billion per year (£25.5 billion for adults and £2.7 billion for children). Of the cost for adults, 59% is accounted for by services, 36% by lost employment for the individual with autism, and the remainder by family expenses.

Education and social contexts

One factor that adds complexity to the picture is that much of the disability in ASD is invisible. Whilst recognizing that most people could identify a child who has autism and a severe learning disability, many individuals with ASD experience difficulties that are much less apparent to others until they react in a way that appears to be unpredictable or unreasonable. Most typically developing 3- to 4-year-old children have a sophisticated level of emotional and social competence with communication skills that allow them to apply local rules (i.e. behave differently at school and at home), to imagine what other people might think or feel and engage in complex conversations and repair situations arising from misunderstandings or mistakes. Self-conscious emotions such as pride, shame, embarrassment and guilt and an interest in how others evaluate them have a powerful effect on behaviour and compliance with social rules. The strategy of asking a child to stand or sit in a specific spot after a minor misdemeanour is a powerful reminder of how much a typically developing child would want to avoid such humiliation. This is the level of competence achieved by most children before they start formal schooling. Apart from the increasing expectations of sophistication with age, such basic skills are therefore never taught directly.

Whilst many people know that children with ASD have difficulty in these areas they are still unable to consider fully how these difficulties limit the child's ability to participate in the social milieu of the school. Staff and parents often indicate that, whilst they understand the diagnosis, they still wish the child would participate more at playtime, or perhaps behave better during music classes, school trips, etc. In particular, the presentation of the child with Asperger syndrome who may be reading well in advance of chronological age but has the social maturity of an 18-month-old consistently stretches the understanding of many.

The focus for education professionals is on the specific difficulties that ASD might present for a child in an educational setting. Schools are required by law to modify their input by making 'reasonable adjustments' to ensure that a child can achieve their potential (Department for Education, 2006). There is recognition that autism is likely to impact upon learning, though the degree to which this is the case varies. The government-led Inclusion Development Programme (IDP) for teachers in mainstream schools in the UK identifies how ASD affects the six curriculum areas in the Early Years Foundation Stage (Department for Children, Schools and Families, 2009a) (see box below).

Personal, social and emotional development: This is a core deficit area as most children with ASD find it difficult to form good relationships with adults and peers. They may be immature in their self-help skills and be highly reactive and emotional at times.

Communication, language and literacy: Some children with ASD need to use augmentative methods of communication, such as visual support materials including photographs or symbols.

Problem-solving, reasoning and numeracy: Some areas of the curriculum can be particular strengths, whereas others may be more challenging because they tend to involve problem-solving and reasoning or flexible thinking, social understanding and verbal reasoning.

Knowledge and understanding of the world: Children with ASD may lack curiosity – a bedrock of general teaching strategy – and may need persuasion to investigate new objects and ideas. They often have difficulty generalizing knowledge and concepts including social knowledge, which may mean that their behaviour is not appropriate in each context. Problems may arise because children have difficulty in seeing things from another's point of view or appreciating the cultures and beliefs of others.

Physical development: Many children with ASD have both fine and gross motor difficulties, though some are very agile.

Creative development: Although some children with ASD have strengths in art or music, many have difficulty generating ideas, expressing feelings and engaging in creative and flexible social imagination.

For primary and secondary school level provision (5–11 years of age) the IDP (Department for Children, Schools and Families, 2009b) makes recommendations to teachers in the areas of: Social and emotional understanding; Communication and language; Flexibility of thought and behaviour; Sensory perception and responses; Curriculum priorities; and Inclusive practice.

The IDP aims to explain the challenges experienced in these areas by children with ASD and to assist teachers in working with others to support them. The aim is to achieve a successful collaboration of universal and specialist services such as speech and language therapy, specialist teachers, outreach support teams and area SENCOs. One specific challenge is that most pupil support is provided within the context of lessons. However, this may not be a problematic environment for the pupil with Asperger syndrome, for whom unstructured times such as lunch and playtime are more stressful. Many children with ASD have phobias about things that are commonplace and difficult to avoid. Others experience significant levels of anxiety, which may result in 'challenging behaviour'. This might be expressed in school, although many children contain their anxiety until they get home, resulting in a discrepancy between school and family regarding the nature and extent of the problem. As children with ASD are not typically susceptible to the modifying influence of peer group behaviour, teachers are often confronted by problems of general compliance, a tendency to prefer rules that may result in the 'policing' of other children and the need to manage idiosyncratic ways or ideas.

Teaching staff are also required to adjust their systems to support children in situations outside of the classroom. Staff who are required to support individuals with ASD need significant additional training to manage emotional and behaviour outbursts. They require an understanding that a child with ASD may be unable to 'repair' situations that have gone awry and fail to show appropriate degrees of remorse or humility. Particular approaches may be recommended by autism outreach services, including visual timetables which can assist in reducing anxiety around special events and changes to routines, and Social Stories (Gray, 2010) which can help a child to learn about the social expectations of their behaviour.

Whilst the evidence base for such approaches lacks rigour, beneficial effects have been indicated from a number of case series (Research Autism, 2011).

It is important to note that children will not necessarily progress sequentially through the stages of a developmentally structured curriculum. Teachers of children with ASD are required to revise much of their knowledge about the progression of learning and adjust to the uneven pattern of skills that can occur in these children. For example, many children with ASD achieve well in early mathematical skills but struggle with later tasks that tap verbal reasoning and mathematical concepts. Literacy may be easily achieved but problems may occur with creative writing, making inferences and extrapolating subtle nuances from literature. For other children the form of teaching rather than the content may present a problem. Strategies which for most children add interest and improve motivation can be a problem for a child with ASD. For example, many children do well in science but become unstuck later in school when they are required by the curriculum to work collaboratively in small groups or to use technology to search for information which needs to be digested and synthesized into a cohesive report. Other subjects require perspective-taking and generalization of knowledge from one topic to another (Department for Children, Schools and Families, 2009b).

Typically, children with ASD have difficulty in shifting their attention from one activity to another and focusing on tasks that are not immediately of interest to them; repetition of instructions may not help, as it requires additional focus on verbal information. More able children can process verbal information rapidly and may become impatient if others need information repeated or if they are required to practise skills repeatedly. Some children listen adequately but do not then go on to comply with an instruction because they have not inferred its meaning adequately, do not think it applies to them or simply do not wish to do it and are not persuaded by the usual influence of group dynamics or intangible social rewards.

Many children with profound autism are educated in special schools but a significant number are taught in mainstream settings. These children may need a highly modified curriculum with direct teaching of basic skills such as tolerating other children in close proximity, learning to offer toys and negotiating swapping, learning to take turns with other children and participating in a group. For many such children the classroom environment can be very stressful and it may be necessary to provide frequent opportunities for breaks involving calming or physical activities. For the approximately 25% of individuals with autism who do not develop speech, assessment for augmentative or alternative communication is required. A commonly used approach is the Picture Exchange Communication Schedule (Frost & Bondy, 2002) which, by means of behaviour modification techniques, aims to teach non-verbal children how to make person-directed requests for desired objects and activities using symbols.

Adolescence, transition and higher education

Transition between schools and other services can often be a difficult and sometimes traumatic experience for people on the autism spectrum. The change from primary to secondary education is particularly challenging for many children with ASD. In primary school, children tend to have just one teacher each year and the majority of lessons take place in the same classroom alongside the same group of children. Whilst the social demands increase as children move up through the school, these may be relatively easy to manage in the comparatively structured environment of the primary school. By contrast, the secondary school environment can be bewildering for even the most able child with Asperger syndrome, with different teachers and classes for each subject, and the expectation that students will take responsibility for having the right books and equipment for each class and will know how to navigate their way around the school building. Secondary schools tend to have more pupils than primary schools, and may therefore be busy, noisy and chaotic at certain times of the day, posing a challenge to the sensory sensitivities of many young people with ASD.

All individuals in the UK who have been assessed as needing state-provided assistance for special educational needs (including ASDs) will be assessed in school at the age of 14 years. The resulting Transition Plan aims to collate information from as many sources as possible to plan for the young person's transition to adult life. The plan should be flexible in recognition that it is not possible to predict a young person's needs at this early stage. It is tied in to legislation from education, health and social government departments.

Unfortunately, many young people with ASD, particularly those with Asperger syndrome, report that they become the victims of bullying at secondary school. Research findings suggest that between 60% and 90% of children with Asperger syndrome or HFA are victims of bullying (Batten et al., 2006; Little, 2002). Although many children with ASD genuinely experience bullying, some perceive bullying when it does not occur because of a failure to read the social situation accurately. The child's attempts to resolve conflict may exacerbate the problem further and many children with ASD are not skilled at asking for support from others, and their attempts to resolve matters may actually make things worse. As the peer group increases in social sophistication, the child with ASD can become more vulnerable to manipulation by other children because they wish to participate in social contexts but lack the guile and wisdom to recognize the risks of certain actions – carrying cigarettes on behalf of another student at secondary school, for example. Many children with ASD have a strong sense of justice and correctness, which can lead to arguments with authority figures when they feel that they or a peer have been maligned. The need for routine and difficulties arising from literal thinking are also common. Sadly, depression, suicidal ideation, low self-esteem, school refusal, self-harm and social isolation are all common aspects of the adolescent experience of people with ASD (Ghaziuddin, Ghaziuddin & Greden, 2002).

The overall picture is that many young people with ASDs who do not have an additional significant learning disability can and do succeed academically and leave school with sufficient qualifications to apply for a place at university. The requirement is for teaching and therapy staff to assist the child to develop skills where feasible but also to accommodate to aspects of the child's learning style that cannot be altered. Since imagination is not an essential life skill in itself, the aim is to help a child who lacks it to pass subjects such as English Literature to the best of their ability.

In higher education the opportunity to focus on a relatively narrow topic that may be of special interest gives many young people with ASD the chance to demonstrate their ability to the full. However, in spite of increasing levels of support for students with Asperger syndrome at many higher education institutions, it is not uncommon for students with ASD to drop out of their course during the first year, because of the difficulty in coping with the lack of structure and the increasingly complex and intangible rules of independent adult life. Even those that complete their degree may end up struggling to get and keep a job, or at least one that is at the level at which they are qualified, as people with ASD typically struggle to cope with the complexities of office politics and many even find themselves being ostracized by colleagues because they are too diligent or hard-working.

Adulthood

It is estimated that there are around 400,000 adults with autism in England, many of whom require specialized support. Yet a National Audit Office report found that most NHS organizations and local authorities do not record the number of people with autism in their area and three-quarters do not have a specific commissioning strategy for adults with autism (National Audit Office, 2009). In their study evaluating the economic costs of autism in the UK, Knapp et al. (2009) estimate that 35% of adults with ASD and intellectual disability live in private households either with parents, relatives, partners or alone; with 7% in supported accommodation and 58% in residential care settings or hospital. For adults with ASD without intellectual disability, they estimate that

79% live in private households, 5% in supported accommodation and 16% in residential care. This suggests that, in spite of the intellectual competence of many adults with ASD, a significant proportion struggle to live independently although many continue to live with their family.

Barnard et al. (2001) indicate that just 12% of individuals with ASD without intellectual disability have full-time jobs, whilst across the whole spectrum the figure is 6%. These levels of employment are much lower than those for the overall population of individuals with disabilities. Specialist supported employment services for people with ASD can be effective. For example, between 1995 and 2003 the NAS Prospects Employment Consultancy assisted 67% of their clients to find work with a job retention rate of 68% (Howlin, Alcock & Burkin, 2005). However, some researchers suggest that a number of individuals with learning disabilities, including autism, and their families do not consider employment and independent living as achievable or desirable but would view access to opportunities for purposeful occupation and social inclusion as a priority (Clegg, Murphy, Almack & Harvey, 2008).

There has been a growing awareness of the need to investigate the extent to which the needs of adults with ASD are recognized and addressed within the forensic and criminal justice system (Paterson, 2007). In a case control study of adults with ASD conducted in Denmark, Mourisden, Rich, Isager and Nedergaard (2008) report that people with diagnoses of autism or atypical autism were less likely to be convicted of crimes than those in the general population, whereas there was no significant difference in rates of criminality between those with a diagnosis of Asperger syndrome and those without an ASD diagnosis. Despite the overall underrepresentation of people with ASD in the forensic population, there are certain features of autism that might lead to particular forms of criminality. For example, arson is a relatively overrepresented offence amongst people with ASD compared to those without an ASD (Haskins & Silva, 2006; Mourisden et al., 2008), behaviour that may stem from an obsessive and narrow interest in fire. Similarly, the proportion of offences involving inappropriate sexual behaviour committed by adults with Asperger syndrome appears to be relatively high (Haskins & Silva, 2006; Mourisden et al., 2008), which may relate to difficulties understanding social rules and sanctions, interpreting ambiguous information and inferring another person's thoughts and feelings.

In March 2010, the UK Government produced its first strategy specifically addressing the needs of adults with autism (Department of Health, 2010). Key actions from the strategy include:

1 **Improved training of frontline professionals in autism** by ensuring it is included in the training of all medical, community care and public sector professionals.

2 **Developing local autism teams**. These are intended to remove a problem that has occurred because adults with ASD who have an IQ above 70 have not qualified for support from the learning disability team and those who do not have a significant mental illness were not helped by mental health teams.

3 **Better planning and commissioning of services**, involving people with autism and their parents/carers. The recommendation is for local government 'Joint Strategic Needs Assessments (JSNAs)', which are planning tools to include autism. In addition, to develop local autism partnership boards bringing together organizations, services and stakeholders locally.

4 **Improved access to diagnosis and post-diagnostic support** in recognition that adults struggle to find suitable diagnostic services. The recommendations are to appoint a lead professional to develop a local diagnostic service for adults with suspected autism and to use the National Institute for Health and Clinical Excellence (NICE) to develope model care pathways ensuring that a diagnosis of autism will trigger a community care assessment and the provision of appropriate support.

5 **Leadership at national, regional and local levels** is necessary for delivery of the policy and review of the strategy to make sure that it is working.

Conclusion

Children and adults with autism spectrum disorder are cherished family members, classmates, students, colleagues, partners and friends, and they contribute meaningfully to many aspects of the social, educational and vocational spheres that they inhabit. However, the complex nature of the condition means that people with ASD, their family members and the professionals that work with them are faced with a wide array of challenges in virtually all aspects of daily life.

Individuals with ASDs range from those with profound, complex and challenging needs who require therapy and teaching outside the usual sphere of health and educational provision to those with Asperger syndrome who have the potential to contribute to society in unique ways, especially in a world where technology can allow people to circumvent the demands of direct social engagement. The challenge is for service providers to recognize and provide individually tailored support that takes into account the range and changing needs of people who may not be best equipped to describe their difficulties and ask for help.

References

Abrahams, B.S. & Geschwind, D.H. (2008) Advances in autism genetics: On the threshold of a new neurobiology. *Nature Reviews. Genetics, 9,* 341–355. DOI: 10.1038/nrg2346

Baird, G., Simonoff, E., Pickles, A., Chandler, S., Loucas, T., Meldrum, D. & Charman, T. (2006) Prevalence of disorders of the autism spectrum in a population cohort of children in South Thames: The Special Needs and Autism (SNAP) project. *Lancet, 368,* 210–215. DOI: 10.1016/S0140-6736(06)69041-7

Barnard, J., Harvey, V., Potter, D. & Prior, A. (2001) *Ignored or Ineligible? The Reality for Adults with Autism Spectrum Disorders.* London: National Autistic Society. http://www.nas.org.uk/12441

Batten, A., Corbett, C., Rosenblatt, M., Withers, L. & Yuille, R. (2006). *Make School Make Sense: Autism and Education, the Reality for Families Today.* London: National Autistic Society. http://www.autism.org.uk/18766

Buie, T., Fuchs, G.J., Furuta, G.T., Kooros, K., Levy, J., Lewis, J.D., Wershil, B.K. & Winter, H. (2010) Recommendations for evaluation and treatment of common gastrointestinal problems in children with ASDs. *Pediatrics, 125,* S19–S25. DOI: 10.1542/peds.2009-1878D

Byford, S., Barrett, B., Sharac, J., Hudry, K., Leadbitter, K., Temple, K., Aldred, C., Slonims, V., Green, J. & the PACT consortium (in press) Service and wider societal costs of pre-school children with autism in the UK. *Journal of Autism and Developmental Disorders.*

Clegg, J., Murphy, E., Almack, K. & Harvey, A. (2008) Tensions around inclusion: Reframing the moral horizon. *Journal of Applied Research in Intellectual Disabilities, 21,* 81–94. DOI: 10.1111/j.1468-3148.2007.00371.x

Department for Children, Schools and Families (2009a) *Inclusion Development Programme (IDP) – Supporting Children on the Autism Spectrum: Guidance for Practitioners in the Early Years Foundation Stage.* Nottingham: DCSF Publications. http://nationalstrategies. standards.dcsf.gov.uk/node/173893?uc+force_uj

Department for Children, Schools and Families (2009b) *Inclusion Development Programme: Primary and Secondary – Supporting Children on the Autism Spectrum.* Nottingham: DCSF Publications. http://nationalstrategies.standards.dcsf.gov.uk/node/173574?uc+force_uj

Department for Education (2006) *Implementing the Disability Discrimination Act in Schools and Early Years Settings*. DFES publications http://www.education.gov.uk/publications/standard/publicationdetail/page1/DFES%200160%202006

Department of Health (2010) *'Fulfilling and Rewarding Lives'. The Strategy for Adults with Autism in England*. Published to D of H website: www.dh.gov.uk/publications

Frost, L.A. & Bondy, A.S. (2002) *The Picture Exchange Communication System. Training Manual*, 2nd edition. Newark, Delaware: Pyramid Educational Consultants.

Ghaziuddin, M., Ghaziuddin, N. & Greden, J. (2002) Depression in persons with autism: Implications for research and clinical care. *Journal of Autism and Developmental Disorders, 32(4)*, 299–306. DOI: 10.1023/A:1016330802348

Gray, C. (2010) *The New Social Story Book*. Arlington, TX: Future Horizons.

Green, H., McGinnity, A., Meltzer, H., Ford, T. & Goodman, R. (2005). *Mental Health of Children and Young People in Great Britain, 2004. Summary Report*. London: Stationery Office. http://www.statistics.gov.uk/downloads/theme_health/summary report.pdf

Haskins, B.G. & Silva, J.A. (2006) Asperger's disorder and criminal behaviour: Forensic–psychiatric considerations. *Journal of the American Academy of Psychiatry and the Law, 34*, 374–384. http://jaapl.org/content/vol34/issue3/index.dtl

Hastings, R.P. (2003) Child behaviour problems and partner mental health as correlates of stress in mothers and fathers of children with autism. *Journal of Intellectual Disability Research, 47(4–5)*, 231–237. DOI: 10.1046/j.1365-2788.2003.00485.x

Herring, S., Gray, K., Taffe, J., Tonge, B., Sweeney, D. & Einfeld, S. (2006) Behaviour and emotional problems in toddlers with pervasive developmental disorders and developmental delay: Associations with parental mental health and family functioning. *Journal of Intellectual Disability Research, 50*, 874–882. DOI: 10.1111/j.1365-2788.2006.00904.x

Howlin, P., Alcock, J. & Burkin, C. (2005) An 8 year follow up of a specialist supported employment service for high-ability adults with autism or Asperger syndrome. *Autism, 9(5)*, 533–549. DOI: 10.1177/1362361305057871

Howlin, P. & Ashgarian, A. (1999) The diagnosis of autism and Asperger syndrome: Findings from a survey of 770 families. *Developmental Medicine and Child Neurology, 41*, 834–839. DOI: 10.1111/j.1469-8749.1999.tb00550.x

Kaminsky, L. & Dewey, D. (2001) Sibling relationships of children with autism. *Journal of Autism and Developmental Disorders, 31(4)*, 399–410. DOI: 10.1023/A:1010664603039

Knapp, M., Romeo, R. & Beecham, J. (2009) Economic cost of autism in the UK. *Journal of Autism and Developmental Disorders, 13(3)*, 317–336. DOI: 10.1177/1362361309104246

Little, L. (2002).Middle class mothers' perceptions of peer and sibling victimization among children with Asperger's syndrome and non-verbal learning disorders. *Issues in Comprehensive Pediatric Nursing, 25(1)*, 43–57. DOI: 10.1080/014608602753504847

Lord, C., Risi, S., Lambrecht, L., Cook, E.H., Leventhal, B.L., DiLavore, P.C., Pickles, A. & Rutter, M. (2000) The Autism Diagnostic Observation Schedule-Generic: A standard measure of social and communication deficits associated with the spectrum of autism. *Journal of Autism and Developmental Disorders, 30(3)*, 205–223. DOI: 10.1023/A:1005592401947

Madders, T. (2010) *You Need To Know*. London: National Autistic Society. http://www.nas.org.uk/26192

Melville, C.A., Cooper, S., Morrison, J., Smiley, E., Allan, L., Jackson, A., Finlayson, J. & Mantry, D. (2008) The prevalence and incidence of mental ill-health in adults with autism and intellectual disabilities. *Journal of Autism and Developmental Disorders, 38*, 1676–1688. DOI: 10.1007/s10803-008-0549-7

Mouridsen, S.E., Rich, B., Isager, T. & Nedergaard, N.J. (2008) Pervasive developmental disorders and criminal behaviour: A case control study. *International Journal of Offender Therapy and Comparative Criminology, 52*, 196–205. DOI: 10.1177/0306624X07302056

Muhle, R., Trentacoste, S.V. & Rapin, I. (2004) The genetics of autism. *Pediatrics, 113(5)*, e472–e486. DOI: 10.1542/peds.113.5.e472

National Audit Office (2009) *Supporting People with Autism Through Adulthood*. London: The Stationery Office. http://www.nao.org.uk/publications/0809/autism.aspx

National Initiative for Autism: Screening and Assessment. (2003) *National Autism Plan for Children* (NAPC). London: National Autistic Society. http://www.nas.org.uk/14956

Orsmond, G.I. & Seltzer, M.M. (2007) Siblings of individuals with autism or Down syndrome: Effects on adult lives. *Journal of Intellectual Disability Research, 51(9)*, 682–696. DOI: 10.1111/j.1365-2788.2007.00954.x

Paterson, P. (2007) How well do young offenders with Asperger syndrome cope in custody? *British Journal of Learning Disabilities, 36*, 54–58. DOI: 10.1111/j.1468-3156.2007.00466.x

Research Autism (2011) http://www.researchautism.net/pages/welcome/home.ikml. Retrieved on 21 January 2011.

Shavelle, R.M., Strauss, D.J. & Pickett, J. (2001) Causes of death in autism. *Journal of Autism and Developmental Disorders, 31*, 569–576. DOI: 10.1023/A:1013247011483

Simonoff, E., Pickles, A., Charman, T., Chandler, S., Loucas, T. & Baird, G. (2008) Psychiatric disorders in children with autism spectrum disorders: Prevalence, comorbidity, and associated factors in a population-derived sample. *Journal of the American Academy of Child and Adolescent Psychiatry, 47(8)*, 921–929. DOI: 10.1097/CHI.0b013e318179964f

4 Developmental Speech Disorders

Barbara Dodd
City University London, UK

Introduction

Children produce their first word at around 12 months and begin talking in simple sentences by 2 years (Cattell, 2000). Initially, all young children make errors when pronouncing words (e.g. [pun] *spoon*; [ti] *key*; [su] *shoe*). Most children of a particular age make the same mistakes, with different error patterns characterizing specific age bands. In English, for example, *splash* is usually initially pronounced [bæt], followed by [pæs] and [plæs] before it is said correctly. Children exposed to the same language tend to follow the same sequence of error patterns that resolve at similar ages (Grunwell, 1997; Preisser, Hodson & Paden, 1988). Their speech comes to accurately match adult-target production by around 5 years.

This is not, however, true for all children. The most common diagnosis made by paediatric clinicians is speech sound disorder (SSD). An incidence survey of a speech-language pathology service in England (Broomfield & Dodd, 2004), reported that 6.4% of all children are treated for SSD. Children's errors make their speech difficult to understand, resulting in communication breakdowns that place them at risk for social and academic, particularly literacy, failure (Gillon, 2004). One way of considering developmental speech disorder is in terms of the World Health Organization's (2011) international classification of functioning, disability and health: body function and structures (nature of impairment); activities (effect on independent living) and participation (impact on quality of life).

The nature of speech impairment

Relatively few cases of speech impairment have an organic aetiology affecting input (e.g. deafness) or output (e.g. motor disorders) (Dodd & McIntosh, 2008). Although about 10% of children with SSD have mislearned how to articulate a speech sound (e.g. a lisp), most children's SSD is a linguistic (i.e. phonological) impairment (Gierut, 1998). Each language has its own phonological system. Children must learn the rules (constraints) governing how a specific set of speech sounds can be combined to make up words in their native language. For example, /ts/ occurs word finally in English (*cats*) but not word initially as in Asian languages (*tsunami*). Research suggests that many children with a SSD have an incomplete knowledge of the phonological system (how speech sounds can be put together to make up words) as opposed to difficulty articulating speech sounds (Gierut, 1998; Baker, 2010). For example, at around 3 years of age children often pronounce both *brush* and *bus* as 'but', despite being able to articulate both 'sh' and 's'.

Children with a phonological impairment are a heterogeneous group. They differ in the number and type of errors made, coping strategies and response to intervention. While there is consensus about the need to subgroup this large, diverse population, to advance research and clinical practice, how that classification is best done remains controversial. Shriberg and his colleagues (e.g. Shriberg et al., 2010) argue for classification based on aetiological factors. Stackhouse and Wells (1997) proposed a psycholinguistic model that would allow identification of underlying deficits. Kamhi (2005) suggested the need to consider the communication profile of children referred for assessment of SSD. Another way of classifying phonological disorders is in terms of the type of error patterns characterizing speech matched with psycholinguistic profiles (Dodd, 1995, 2005).

This approach was adopted in Broomfield and Dodd's (2004) incidence study of 320 children with speech difficulties. Four subgroups of SSD were identified:

1 **Articulation disorder** (12.5% of total sample): an inability to produce a perceptually acceptable version of phones due either to a physiological condition (e.g. dysarthria) or mislearning of the sounds' motor program (e.g. lisp).

2 **Phonological delay** (57.5%): all errors can be accounted for by phonological error patterns (e.g. cluster reduction, fronting) that occur during typical speech development at a younger chronological age.

3 **Consistent atypical phonological disorder** (20.6%): use of one or more error patterns (usually in addition to some age-appropriate and/ or delayed error patterns) that are atypical of normal development in

English (e.g. backing, favoured sound, initial consonant deletion). The criterion often used for identification of an atypical error pattern is occurrence in at least five different lexical items in a picture-naming task of 50 words.

4 Inconsistent speech disorder (9.4%): production of the same words and phonological features differently within the same context, providing evidence of multiple error types. This speech characteristic is thought to indicate persistent, pervasive speech processing difficulties (Grunwell, 1982; Forrest, Elbert & Dinnsen, 2000). No children who met the criteria for Childhood Apraxia of Speech (oro-motor signs, inconsistent errors, poorer performance in imitation than spontaneous production) were identified in this sample.

Each of these four types of speech difficulty is associated with a different profile of communication difficulties and associated abilities (see Table 4.1). Age of referral differs between the groups, reflecting parental and school concern. The effect of treatment (or lack of it) at specific ages also differs according to group. Consequently, as for many broad diagnostic categories of communication disorder, there is variation in the consequences of speech disorder on communication, and its impact on children and their families.

Table 4.1 Characteristics of subtypes of SSD (see Dodd, 1995, 2005).

Functional articulation disorder (in isolation)
Case history: Close relative with same articulation of same sound(s) *Intelligibility:* Intelligible *Other aspects of language:* Performs within normal limits (WNL) on standardized tests of vocabulary, receptive and expressive language *Psycholinguistic abilities:* Performs no differently from typically developing (TD) controls on measures of input, output, consistency of production, cognitive abilities *Literacy:* Reading accuracy and comprehension WNL; good non-word spelling and phonological awareness (PA) *Response to intervention:* Rapid response to van Riper's approach to articulation therapy, most successful at 6+ years *Cont. overleaf*

Phonological delay
Case history: > 4 episodes of otitis media with effusion, family history of SSD   *Intelligibility:* Mild to moderate impairment   *Other aspects of language:* Associated with articulation and expressive language delay   *Psycholinguistic abilities:* Performance at the bottom end of the normal range   *Literacy:* Make fewer phonologically plausible spelling errors; otherwise WNL; including PA   *Response to intervention:* Responds well to phonological contrast and whole language; do best in therapy when 5 years, slowly improve spontaneously on waiting lists

Consistent atypical phonological disorder
Case history: Family history of SSD   *Intelligibility:* Moderate to severe impairment   *Other aspects of language:* Receptive language WNL; poor performance on measures of expressive language perhaps due to phonological disorder   *Psycholinguistic abilities:* Poor performance on executive function tasks (rule derivation, cognitive flexibility, cross-modal integration); input and output speech tasks WNL   *Literacy:* Poor performance on PA, reading and spelling of real and non-words   *Response to intervention:* Rapid response to phonological contrast; need early treatment as no spontaneous change on waiting list, disorder becomes more severe

Inconsistent speech disorder
Case history: Perinatal difficulties (e.g. resuscitation at birth)   *Intelligibility:* Severe impairment   *Other aspects of language:* Receptive language WNL; assessing expressive language problematic but some children may have associated word-finding difficulties   *Psycholinguistic abilities* Performance on executive function tasks WNL; real word input and output speech tasks WNL. Poor performance on non-word repetition, sentence repetition tasks and receptive non-word discrimination. Difficulty learning new words and non-verbal sequences of skilled fine movements   *Literacy:* PA (apart from syllable counting) and reading comprehension WNL, spelling of multisyllabic real and non-words poor   *Response to intervention:* Responds well to core vocabulary intervention at 3 years

Factors affecting the lives of children with speech disorder

Speech disorder affects children's ability to communicate their wants and needs. Not being able to make themselves understood may limit children's engagement in leisure and educational activities, curtail their social development, and place them at risk for teasing and bullying. Children who cannot speak for themselves may be disempowered, and that affects family dynamics. Some children become socially withdrawn, others develop behaviour disorders, many experience academic failure. This section begins by reviewing research on the short- and long-term consequences of speech difficulty, followed by an exploration of factors influencing the impact of speech disorders on children's lives, including the effect of intervention.

Short-term consequences

Most literature on the short-term consequences of developmental speech disorder focuses on literacy and school performance. It is estimated that around 3.8% of all children have speech difficulties that persist into primary school (Shriberg et al., 1999). Extensive research indicates that many, but not all, of these children will be identified as having spoken and written language impairments that place their academic success at risk (e.g. Leitao, Hogben & Fletcher, 1997; Lewis, Ekelman & Aram, 1989; Gierut, 1998; Gillon, 2004). Surface speech errors may allow identification of those children with speech difficulties who will later develop literacy difficulties. Investigation of the relationship between type of SSD, phonological awareness (PA) and literacy abilities indicated that children who consistently made errors atypical of normal development performed poorly on measures of PA and literacy (Harris, Botting, Myers & Dodd, in press; Preston & Edwards, 2010). In contrast, children with delayed phonology perform similarly to typically developing controls. Children who make inconsistent speech errors have difficulty with spelling, but not reading (Holm, Farrier & Dodd, 2007). Children who make disordered speech errors have difficulty acquiring literacy compared to those with delayed phonology, or articulation (motor speech) disorders (Dodd, McCormack & Woodyatt, 1995; Leitao & Fletcher, 2004).

Children with speech difficulties are at risk for behavioural and social difficulties in primary and secondary school (e.g. Cantwell & Baker, 1987; Silva, Justin, McGee & Williams, 1984). Even 3- to 5-year-olds are vulnerable to social rejection. Odom et al. (2006) investigated whether peers in preschool classrooms socially accepted children with a range of disabilities. The study included 80 children, attending 16 preschools. One measure used was a peer rating assessment where the typically developing children sorted pictures of children in their class into three boxes: one with a happy face, one with a neutral face, and one with a sad face. In addition, an observational assessment recorded social behaviour including talking, sharing and calling by name as well as negative behaviors such as hitting, negative remarks, and crying.

The children with disabilities who were socially accepted displayed some of the following characteristics: good social skills, ability to make friendships; appropriate positive affect; adequate communication skills, use of pretend play, perceived dependence, following class rules and routines and interacting with peers. The children with disabilities who were socially rejected (actively excluded from peer group activity) had behaviour characterized by social withdrawal and problems with conflict and aggression. Odom et al. (2006) concluded that lack of an effective system of communication was strongly associated with social rejection.

In a study of older children, Botting and Conti-Ramsden (2000) initially recruited 242 children with speech and language impairments, aged 6;6–7;9 years, who attended 118 language units. One year later, 214 of the children were reassessed. Performance on the Rutter Behavioural Scale (Rutter, 1967) indicated that around 40% fell over the clinical threshold for behavioural difficulties at both assessments. Fewer children with expressive difficulties, however, were identified as having emotional and social difficulties than those with more complex expressive–receptive communication impairments, and the number of children with difficulties reduced over time. Botting and Conti-Ramsden (2000) suggested that children with poor speech/expressive language difficulties may have fewer behavioural difficulties because they make faster progress in the early school years than children with receptive–expressive and receptive difficulties who are at most risk of increasing behavioural problems as they grow older.

Longer-term consequences

Behavioural and social difficulties (Clegg, Hollis & Rutter, 1999) as well as impaired literacy (Dodd et al., 1995) may persist after speech and language difficulties have resolved, either spontaneously or as a result of intervention. There is evidence that adults with a history of speech difficulties do less well on speech, language and socioeconomic success measures than adults without a history of communication difficulty (Felsenfeld, Broen & McGue, 1992, 1994). Lewis's (2007, p.3) review indicated that 'they required more remedial services throughout their academic careers and completed fewer years of formal education' than a control group. While there was no group difference on measures of non-verbal reasoning skills and job satisfaction, adults with a history of speech difficulty 'occupied jobs requiring fewer skills than the adults without histories' (Lewis, 2007, p.3).

Broomfield and Dodd (2005) argued that one reason why people with communication disorders are overrepresented in lower socioeconomic groups is that the consequences of communication disorder are associated with fewer employment opportunities, resulting in downward social mobility. As Lewis (2007, p.1) noted: 'The importance of [spoken and written] communication and information processing skills and technologies in the work place will continue to increase in the future; and the individual who has a communication disorder will thus be at a disadvantage.'

Factors affecting impact of speech impairment are covered below.

Family context

Harrison and McLeod (2010) identified risk and protective factors for speech and language impairment in early childhood in a sample of 4983 children. One factor that lessened the chance of persistent communication difficulties was higher levels of maternal wellbeing, although parental support for children's learning at home was associated with attendance at speech and language therapy, perhaps reflecting set 'therapy homework'. Only having an older sibling was a risk factor for the measure of concern about expressive speech and language, and for attending speech-language therapy. These data provide evidence for the clinical observation that older siblings may 'talk for' younger children, particularly if they have impaired speech (see below).

Children exposed to languages other than English at home were less likely to be referred for speech and language therapy and their parents did not express concern about their communication development, although their performance on the measure of English vocabulary was poor in comparison to monolinguals, probably because testing occurred only in the children's second language (see Hemsley, Holm & Dodd, 2006). Harrison and McLeod (2010) concluded that decisions about children's need for therapy should include consideration of the child's family context as well as the results of communication assessment, biological and psychosocial factors.

Temperament and response to impairment

One study that considered the effect of child temperament on 'increased severity of speech delay' (Hauner, Shriberg, Kwiatkowski & Allen, 2005, p.635) reported that low approachability and sociability, negative mood and low task persistence were associated with severity of speech impairment. In Harrison and McLeod's (2010) study, the reported characteristics of children's temperament predicted speech and language impairment in terms of parent-rated concern, use of speech-language pathology services, and low receptive vocabulary. In contrast, children who were reported to be persistent and able to stay on task were less likely to elicit parental concern. Although Harrison and McLeod concluded that children who were reported to be less sociable had a higher risk of speech and language impairment, it seems plausible that having impaired communication might result in a degree of social withdrawal (see above).

Intelligibility

Studies (e.g. Lass, Ruscello, Harkins & Blankenship, 1993) measuring peer perceptions of the non-speech characteristics (e.g. honesty, strength, physical attractiveness, wisdom) of normal speakers and those with different types of speech disorders (dysarthria, stuttering, voice disorders) all judge normal speakers more positively. It might be argued that the more unintelligible a child's speech is, the greater the negative impact the impairment has on their lives. Some types of speech disorders are less harshly judged than others (e.g. voice disorders are more favourably perceived than dysarthria, Lass et al., 1993). However, Freeby and Madison (1989) reported that gliding /r/ to [w] can lead to the speaker being judged less favourably on intelligence and personality factors by peers. Even mild speech impairment can, then, lead to social disadvantage.

Age

While most children are referred for assessment of a speech difficulty when they are 3 or 4 years of age (Broomfield & Dodd, 2004), the age of referral differs according to type of speech disorder. The youngest to be referred, primarily between 3–4 years, were children with inconsistent speech disorder, perhaps because parents often report that they find their children's speech unintelligible. Referral of children with consistent atypical disorder and delay was more evenly spread between 3 and 6 years, with a slight trend for children with delay to be older than those with disorder. Children with an articulation disorder due to mislearning of the production of specific speech sounds (e.g. a lisp, w/r substitution) were most often referred between 7 and 11 years.

It is puzzling that assessment and intervention services begin so late, given that first words are uttered at around 12 months. Further, early intervention may benefit children later identified as having speech disorder, by minimizing the disadvantage that accrues with persistence of speech impairment (but see Intervention: quality and timing, below). Broomfield and Dodd (2005) reported that the earlier intervention is provided for phonological disorder, the better the outcome, indicating that it may be easier to shape a developing system than one that is well established.

While parental report can be used to identify early language difficulties (e.g. McArthur Communication Development Index, Fenson et al., 1993), parents are often unaware of how children pronounce words. Dodd et al. (1995) reported that parents use contextual cues to seek meaning in their young children's utterances rather than listening to how words are pronounced. While diagnosing atypical speech development at 2 years is problematic, one recent study demonstrated that qualitative analysis of error types at 2 years predicted performance on a standardized speech assessment one year later (McIntosh & Dodd, 2008). Children who made many atypical errors at 2 years were diagnosed as phonologically disordered at 3 years. These findings provide initial evidence that direct formal assessment of 2-year-old phonology is possible, allowing exploration of earlier intervention that may reduce the number of children with persistent speech difficulties.

Persistence of speech disorder

Lewis et al. (2006) identified factors that predicted the long-term outcomes for children with early speech difficulties. Speech and language therapists referred 185 3- to 7-year-old children with speech impairment, with 38 being reassessed four years later. Thorough assessment included standardized tests, parental questionnaires and direct testing of siblings to determine family history. Factor analyses suggested that 'articulation/ phonology' and 'semantic/

syntactic' impairments were two distinct constructs with different implications for academic development. Nevertheless, deficits in both domains did co-occur and predicted the poorest outcomes. Children who had difficulties with 'syntax/semantics' did less well than children with 'articulation/phonology' impairment. While the factors identified were claimed to predict the communication status of family members, school-age outcomes and the persistence of speech difficulty, the numbers were small.

Other studies have investigated the effect of subgroups of speech disorder on spontaneous recovery from phonological disorder. Dodd, Hua and Shatford (2000) measured change in per cent consonants correct, performance on phonological awareness tasks and number and type of error patterns used by 39 children on a waiting list for therapy (mean length of waiting list time 12 (+/– 4.9) months). The groups did not differ on any measure when they were first assessed at the time of referral. When reassessed around 12 months later, the delayed group performed better than children with disordered phonology on all measures. These findings indicate that children with delayed phonological development make significant spontaneous progress while on the waiting list for therapy compared to children with disordered phonology.

Impact of intervention: Quality and timing

There is now considerable evidence that intervention for speech impairment can have a positive outcome (e.g. Law, Garret & Nye, 2004). What is, perhaps, more critical for development of quality intervention is the emerging consensus that there are different types of speech disorder that require specific and different treatment approaches (Williams, McLeod & McCauley, 2010; Tyler, 2011). For example, Bernstein-Ratner (2006) argued that development of evidence-based practice is dependent upon research studies establishing whether (and why, theoretically) one therapy approach is better than another for a well-defined diagnostic category of communication disorder.

Broomfield and Dodd's (2005) randomized control trial of children with speech impairment differentially diagnosed children into four subgroups providing therapy that targeted speech sounds in isolation for articulation disorder, phonological contrasts for delay and consistent disorder, and whole words for children with inconsistent disorder. The findings showed that those (n=212) randomly assigned to receive six months of intervention made major gains in comparison to the no-treatment control group (n=101). The treated group showed a z-score increase of .61 on a standard assessment measure (per cent consonants correct: PCC) compared to the group receiving no treatment, whose z-score increase was .02. Children in the no-treatment group, irrespective of type of speech disorder, made very little progress. The extent of improvement in PCC in the treated group, however, varied across subgroups. Children with phonological delay made most change in therapy (z-score increase .66). Those with inconsistency made the least change (z-score increase .37), although this increase in accuracy was positive given that therapy focused on consistency rather than accuracy. A number of factors affected intervention outcome.

1 **Age**: children with an articulation disorder did best in therapy when over 6 years of age, while those with phonological delay did best when over 4 years. Children with phonological disorders need to be treated at a younger age. Those children who make consistent atypical errors suffer increasing severity of impairment if not treated at 4 years of age and those with inconsistent disorder make more progress in therapy at 3 years than when they are 4 years old.

2 **Gender:** the data indicated that girls with a phonological delay do better than boys in therapy. More importantly, girls who make consistent atypical errors do worse than boys when treatment is withheld. Further research is needed to verify these findings, as they have important implications for service delivery.

3 **Case history:** two case factors associated with slow response to therapy and limited spontaneous development while awaiting therapy were (i) late language onset and (ii) family history of communication disorders. Factors associated with positive therapy outcome were adverse perinatal histories and intermittent hearing loss.

The literature reflects a focus on impairment-based therapy in planning intervention for speech disorder. If such intervention allowed the acquisition of age-appropriate, intelligible speech with no associated literacy difficulties, it would still be too narrow an approach to intervention planning because speech impairment affects the lives of children and their families, and continues to do so even when the speech difficulty has been resolved. Nevertheless, intervention is key in minimizing the effects of speech impairment.

Participation: Impact on quality of life

The United Nations Convention on the Rights of the Child (2008) recognizes the need for children to participate and be heard. McLeod, Daniel and Barr (2006) emphasized the importance of listening to children with communication disorders. They reported a study of five children whose speech was unintelligible. When questioned about how they felt about their speech, parents or siblings often responded for these children. To provide them with the opportunity to express their own feelings, McLeod et al. (2006) encouraged children to draw pictures of themselves talking to someone, with their family, and doing something enjoyable. The drawings were interpreted as indicating that children with speech disorder are often aware and unhappy about their lack of intelligibility, enjoying activities that are often non-verbal and solitary (e.g. computer games). Control data are needed to extend knowledge of the usefulness of McLeod et al.'s (2006) conclusion that clinicians might routinely ask children with communication disorder to make drawings of how they feel.

Another way of collecting information about children's response to their speech disorder is by using a questionnaire (Speech Participation and Activity of Children, SPAA-C) developed by participants at the Speech Pathology Australia in 2003 (McLeod, 2004). The questionnaire has six sections requesting information:

- The child (non-verbal response by marking one of five symbols (e.g. unhappy face) is asked questions such as 'How do you feel about the way you talk?').

- Friends and siblings provide a verbal response to questions like 'Is there anything your friend/sibling has trouble with?'

- Parents are asked to describe their child, their difficulties and the response elicited by their unintelligible speech (e.g. 'What does your child do when he/she isn't understood?' 'How do other people react to your child?').

- Teachers and others are asked about the child's participation (does s/he participate in class activities/volunteer information in class), and consequences of disorder (e.g. Is s/he teased at school? How does this child react to conflict?).

The SPAA-C (McLeod, 2004) has been used in research case studies (e.g. Holm & Crosbie, 2006) to describe children's reactions to their speech difficulties. A recent larger-scale study (McCormack, McLeod, McAllister & Harrison, 2010) sought to understand the experience of having a speech impairment for children and their communication partners. Thirteen preschool children with mild to severe speech impairment and 21 family members and teachers were interviewed. Two themes emerged: the frustration caused by living with speech impairment for children and their communication partners and the strategies used to overcome the problems, such as intervention, home practice and alternative communication. It is not clear, however, how information gained through use of the questionnaire changes clinical practice for children with speech disorder.

One interesting use of the SPAA-C was made by Barr, McLeod and Daniel (2008), who interviewed the siblings of children with speech and/or language difficulties. Previous research has indicated that siblings of children with a disability may feel distress, guilt and anxiety but also jealousy and the need to overachieve (e.g. Naylor & Prescott, 2004). Barr et al.'s (2008) investigation used the SPAA-C to conduct semi-structured interviews of the siblings, aged 5 to 14 years of age, of six communication-disordered children aged 5–8 years, with moderate to severe difficulties. The findings suggested that children with communication disorder and their siblings often had a close relationship, with siblings taking on the role of protector and interpreter, and acknowledging their caring role. Siblings reported that they were aware that they received less parental attention and sometimes felt resentment and jealousy as well as concern.

Case study (Leahy & Dodd, 1989)

A's speech was unintelligible when she was 3;9 years old. Her parents often had difficulty understanding her, asking her elder sister, C, to 'translate'. An audio recording of a family conversation at mealtime illustrated the dangers of being dependent on an elder sibling for communication.

A: [Unintelligible utterance].
Mother: *What did A say?*
C: *She says she doesn't want any ice-cream, she wants to go to bed.*
A: *Oooh* [protest].

Clinical implications

All textbooks on intervention for children with speech impairments acknowledge the need to tailor therapy to the child. This axiom is non-specific and interpreted in widely different ways. It can be taken to mean making therapy materials and sessions age- and gender-appropriate. Another interpretation (Stackhouse & Wells, 1997) concerns the need to identify a particular child's strengths and weaknesses and plan therapy to address the latter using the former. Students are currently encouraged to explore the evidence base for intervention that has been shown to be useful for a specific diagnostic category, often finding little information.

One implicit assumption, which is often overlooked, is that the child is part of a wider world that involves home, school and community. Research published very recently by McLeod and her colleagues is beginning to address the issues of how children feel about being speech disordered and the impact of speech disorder on families and a child's peers. How those research results should change clinical practice seems to have received little attention.

Clinical research suggests that there is a need to acknowledge that children have a specific problem, and that not being understood creates huge difficulties, at home and at school. It is also important that children are told what will happen in each therapy session and why it will help to make them more intelligible. Children and their carers may attend speech and language therapy without knowing why they are there or what is expected of them (Hand, 2006). Perhaps a first step in addressing the issue of how speech impairment affects children's lives and their participation in the community is recognizing their need to know about their difficulty.

Case study (Ripich & Panagos, 1985)

A researcher (R) interviewed a child (C1) about why he came to see a speech language therapist and what happened in the therapy session.

R: *What do you usually do in therapy?*

C1: *Well, I'm supposed to make the bad r sounds, and Mrs Smith is supposed to make the good r sounds.*

R: *Don't you ever make the good r sounds?*

C1: *No! I'm supposed to make the bad rs.*

Future research directions

Lewis (2007, p.6) argued that: 'Well-designed longitudinal, prospective studies with an appropriate matched control group are needed to assess the functional significance of early speech-sound disorders at school age, adolescence and adulthood.' She stressed the importance of investigating the different trajectories of outcomes for subgroups of children with speech impairments as different subgroups of impairment are associated with different long-term outcomes. Further, emerging research indicates children require specific intervention approaches to achieve their life potential.

Children with speech impairments are also frequently identified as having other co-morbid conditions, particularly language impairment and ADHD. Research on communication disorders, however, has rarely examined the effect of co-morbid conditions on the outcome of therapy. Rather, studies contributing to the knowledge base have focused on building understanding of 'pure' cases, explicitly excluding children with co-morbid diagnoses.

The concept of evidence-based practice is now widely accepted. There are a number of barriers, however, to its implementation: lack of research evidence (e.g. for typical clinical caseloads where co-morbidity is common); poor quality evidence (e.g. meta-analyses of studies evaluating different amounts and types of intervention for different diagnostic populations); and inappropriate research methodologies and evaluation criteria borrowed uncritically from medicine. An alternative approach would be to extend basic research to better understand the nature of speech disorders, and ensure that clinical trials evaluating intervention seek to consider factors inherent to the child, the family and the society that impact on the outcome of intervention.

References

Baker, E. (2010) Minimal pair intervention. In A.L. Williams, S. McCleod & R. McCauley (Eds) *Interventions for Speech Sound Disorders in Children*, pp.41–72. Baltimore: Brookes.

Barr, J., McLeod, S. & Daniel, G. (2008) Siblings of children with speech impairment: Cavalry on the hill. *Language, Speech and Hearing Services in Schools, 39(1)*, 21–32.

Bernstein-Ratner, N. (2006) Evidence-based practice: An examination of its ramifications for the practice. *Language, Speech and Hearing Services in Schools, 37(4)*, 257–267.

Broomfield, J. & Dodd, B. (2004) The nature of referred subtypes of primary speech disability. *Child Language Teaching and Therapy, 20(2)*, 135–151.

Broomfield, J. & Dodd, B. (2005) Clinical effectiveness. In B. Dodd (Ed.) *Differential Diagnosis and Treatment of Children with Speech Disorder*, pp.211–229. London: Whurr.

Botting, N. & Conti-Ramsden, G. (2000) Social and behavioral difficulties in children with SLI. *Child Language Teaching and Therapy, 16(2)*, 105–120.

Cantwell, D.P. & Baker, L. (1987) Clinical significance of childhood communication disorders: Perspectives from a longitudinal study. *Journal of Child Neurology, 2(4)*, 257–264.

Cattell, R. (2000) *Children's Language. Consensus and Controversy*. London: Cassell.

Clegg, J., Hollis, C. & Rutter, M. (1999) Life sentence: What happens to children with developmental language disorders in later life? *Bulletin of the Royal College of Speech Language Therapists, 571*, 16–18.

Dodd, B. (1995) *Differential Diagnosis and Treatment of Children with Speech Disorder.* London: Whurr.

Dodd, B. (2005). *Differential Diagnosis and Treatment of Children with Speech Disorder,* 2nd edition. London: Whurr.

Dodd, B., Hua, Z. & Shatford, C. (2000) Does speech disorder spontaneously resolve? In I. Barriere, G. Morgan, S. Chiat & B. Woll (Eds) *Current Research in Language and Communication Science*, pp.3–10. London: City University.

Dodd, B., McCormack, P. & Woodyatt, G. (1995) Training parents of children with Down syndrome as agents of therapy. In B. Dodd (Ed.) *Differential Diagnosis and Treatment of Children with Speech Disorder*, pp.249–261. London: Whurr.

Dodd, B. & McIntosh, B. (2008) The input processing, cognitive linguistic and oro-motor skills of children with speech difficulty. *International Journal of Speech Language Pathology*, *10*, 169–178.

Felsenfeld, S., Broen, P.A. & McGue, M. (1994) A 28-year follow-up of adults with a history of moderate phonological disorder: Educational and occupational results. *Journal of Speech and Hearing Research*, *37(6)*, 1341–1353.

Felsenfeld, S., Broen, P. & McGue, M. (1992) A 28-year follow-up of adults with a history of moderate phonological disorder: Linguistic and personality results. *Journal of Speech and Hearing Research*, *35*, 1114–1125.

Fenson, L., Dale, P., Resnick, J., Thal, D., Bates, E., Hartung, J., Pethick, S. & Reilly, J. (1993) *MacArthur Communicative Development Inventories (CDI).* San Diego, CA: Singular Publishing.

Forrest. K., Elbert, M. & Dinnsen, D. (2000) The effect of substitution patterns on phonological treatment outcomes. *Clinical Linguistics and Phonetics*, *14*, 519–531.

Freeby, N. & Madison, C.L. (1989) Children's perceptions of peers with articulation disorders. *Child Study Journal*, *19(2)*, 133–144.

Gierut, J.A. (1998) Treatment efficacy: Functional phonological disorders in children. *Journal of Speech, Language and Hearing Research*, *41(1)*, S85–S100.

Gillon, G. (2004) *Phonological Awareness: From Research to Practice.* New York: Guilford Press.

Grunwell, P. (1982) *Clinical Phonology.* London: Croom-Helm.

Grunwell, P. (1997) Developmental phonological disability: Order in disorder. In B. Hodson & M. Edwards (Eds) *Perspectives in Applied Phonology,* pp.61–104. Aspen: Gaithersberg.

Hand, L. (2006) Clinicians as 'information givers': What communication access are clients given to speech-language pathology services? *Topics in Language Disorders, 26(3)*, 240–266.

Harris, J., Botting, N., Myers, L. & Dodd, B. (in press) The relationship between speech impairment, phonological awareness and literacy. *Australian Journal of Learning Disabilities.*

Harrison, L. & McLeod, S. (2010) Risk and protective factors associated with speech and language impairment in a nationally representative sample of 4- to 5-year-old children. *Journal of Speech, Language, and Hearing Research, 53,* 508–529.

Hauner, K.K.Y., Shriberg, L.D., Kwiatkowski, J. & Allen, C.T. (2005) A subtype of speech delay associated with developmental psychosocial involvement. *Journal of Speech, Language, and Hearing Research, 48,* 635–650.

Hemsley, G., Holm, A. & Dodd, B. (2006) Diverse but not different: The lexical skills of two primary age bilingual groups in comparison to monolingual peers. *International Journal of Bilingualism, 10,* 453–476.

Holm, A. & Crosbie, S. (2006) Introducing Jarrod: A child with a phonological impairment. *Advances in Speech-Language Pathology, 8(3),* 164–175.

Holm, A., Farrier, F. & Dodd, B. (2007) The phonological awareness, reading accuracy and spelling ability of children with inconsistent phonological disorder. *International Journal of Language and Communication Disorders, 42,* 467–486.

Kamhi, A. (2005) Summary, reflections, and future directions. In A. Kamhi & K. Pollock (Eds) *Phonological Disorders in Children: Clinical Decision Making in Assessment and Intervention.* Baltimore: Brookes.

Lass, N., Ruscello, D., Harkins, K. & Blankenship, B. (1993) A comparative study of adolescents' perceptions of normal-speaking and dysarthric children. *Journal of Communication Disorders, 26(1),* 3–12.

Law, J., Garret, Z. and Nye, C. (2004) The effect of treatment for children with developmental speech and language delay/disorder: A meta-analysis. *Journal of Speech, Language, and Hearing Research, 47,* 924–943.

Leahy, J. & Dodd, B. (1987) The development of disordered phonology: A case study. *Language and Cognitive Processes, 2(2),* 115–132.

Leitao, S. & Fletcher, J. (2004) Literacy outcomes for students with speech impairment: Long-term follow-up. *International Journal of Language and Communication Disorders, 39(2),* 245–256.

Leitao, S., Hogben, J. & Fletcher, J. (1997) Phonological processing skills in speech and language impaired children. *European Journal of Disorders of Communication, 32,* 73–93.

Lewis, B. (2007) Short- and long-term outcomes for children with speech sound disorders. *Encyclopedia of Language and Literacy Development,* pp.1–6. London, Ontario: Canadian Language and Literacy Research Network. Retrieved 29 October 2010 from http://www.literacyencyclopedia.ca/pdfs/topic.php?topId=23

Lewis, B., Ekelman, B. & Aram, D. (1989) Familial phonological disorders. *Journal of Speech and Hearing Research, 35,* 819–831.

Lewis, B., Freebairn, L., Hansen, A., Stein, C., Shriberg, L., Iyengar, S. & Taylor, G. (2006) Dimensions of early speech sound disorders: A factor analytic study. *Journal of Communication Disorders, 39,* 139–157.

McCormack, J., McLeod, S., McAllister, L. & Harrison, J. (2010) Speech problem, your listening problem, and my frustration: The experience of living with childhood speech impairment. *Language, Speech, and Hearing Services in Schools, 41,* 379–392.

McIntosh, B. & Dodd, B. (2008) Two-year-olds' phonological acquisition: Normative data. *International Journal of Speech Language Pathology, 10,* 460–469.

McLeod, S. (2004) Speech pathologists' application of the ICF to children with speech impairment. *Advances in Speech-Language Pathology, 6(1),* 75–81.

McLeod, S., Daniel, G. & Barr, J. (2006) Using children's drawings to lsten to how children feel about their speech. Poster presented at the 2006 Speech Pathology Australia National Conference, Perth.

Naylor, A. & Prescott, P. (2004) Invisible children? The need for support groups for siblings of disabled children. *British Journal of Special Education, 31,* 199–296.

Odom, S.L., Zercher, C., Shouming, L., Marquart, J.M., Sandall, S. & Brown, W.H. (2006) Social acceptance and rejection of preschool children with disabilities: A mixed-method analysis. *Journal of Educational Psychology, 98(4),* 807–823.

Preisser, D., Hodson, B. & Paden, E. (1988) Developmental phonology: 18–29 months. *Journal of Speech and Hearing Disorders, 53,* 125–130.

Preston, J. & Edwards, M.-L. (2010) Phonological awareness and types of speech errors in preschoolers with SSD. *Journal of Speech, Language and Hearing Research, 53,* 44–60.

Ripich, D.N. & Panagos, J.M. (1985) Accessing children's knowledge of sociolinguistic rules of speech therapy lessons. *Journal of Speech and Hearing Disorders, 50,* 335–346.

Rutter, M. (1967) A children's behaviour questionnaire for completion by teachers: Preliminary findings. *Child Psychology and Psychiatry, 8,* 1–11.

Shriberg, L., Fourakis, M., Hall, S., Karlsson,H., Lohmeier, H., McSweeny, J., Potter, N., Scheer-Cohen, N., Strand, E., Tilkens, C. & Wilson, D. (2010) Extensions to the speech disorders classification system (SDCS). *Clinical Linguistics and Phonetics, 24(10),* 795–824.

Shriberg, L.D., Tomblin, J.B. & McSweeny, J.L. (1999). Prevalence of speech delay in 6-year-old children and comorbidity with language impairment. *Journal of Speech, Language, and Hearing Research, 42(6),* 1461–1481.

Silva, P.A., Justin, C., McGee, R. and Williams, S.M. (1984) Some developmental and behavioural characteristics of seven-year-old children with delayed speech development. *British Journal of Disorders of Communication, 19,* 147–154.

Stackhouse, J. & Wells, B. (1995) *Children's Speech and Literacy Difficulties. A Psycholinguistic Framework.* London: Whurr.

Tyler, A. (2011) Speech sound disorders in children: Exploring subtypes. *Topics in Language Disorder,* Special Issue.

United Nations Convention on the Rights of the Child (2008) Retrieved on 12 November 2010 from http://www.unicef.org/crc/

World Health Organization (2011) International Classification of Functioning. Retrieved on 5 January 2011 from http://www.who.int/icidh/

Williams, A.L., McLeod, S. & McCauley, R. (2010) *Interventions for Speech Sound Disorders in Children*. Baltimore: Brookes.

5 Children with Learning Disabilities

Celia Harding

City University London, UK

Introduction

This chapter seeks to give an overview of the challenges associated with language acquisition and language use for children and young people who have learning disabilities. It will explore the additional issues that are associated with learning disabilities and the impact on communication opportunities.

There is no widely accepted definition of 'Learning Disability' (LD), and within this field there is ongoing debate as to what LD actually means. In the past, labels have included terms such as 'mental retardation', 'mentally defective' and 'mental handicap'. People within the disability movement prefer the term 'learning disability'. This is the term which shall be used throughout this chapter.

The World Health Organization (2006) ICD-10 defines learning disability as 'A condition of arrested or incomplete development of the mind'. Aspects of learning disability include a reduced level of intellectual functioning and adaptive behaviour as well as deficits in psychological and emotional functioning. There are also likely to be increased health needs as well as the need to make adjustments within familiar environments to ensure participation is maximized. In the UK, the view is that there is a continuum of LD focusing on psychological and social adaptation. The shift is away from labelling and categorization of an LD to identifying what the special educational needs are, as well as targeting the child's strengths. Children who have an IQ of 70 upwards are included within mainstream school settings should the parents feel that the school could meet their child's needs.

Until 1971, children who had an IQ below 50 did not have access to teaching from education professionals and were therefore the responsibility of health carers. In 1971, the Education Act transferred responsibility for educating these children to the Educational Authorities. Education Authorities used the terms 'Moderate Learning Difficulties' (MLD), 'Severe Learning Difficulties' (SLD) and 'Profound and Multiple Learning Difficulties' (PMLD) to describe the range of children with learning needs, and educational settings were set up to meet these varying needs. The 1981 Education Act recognized the reluctance to 'label' disabled children, but sought to encourage identifying a child's individual strengths and needs with a view to enabling them to access a curriculum. Inevitably, a vital element of this process would be focusing on identifying communication strengths and needs.

What are the key differences between those with MLD and those with SLD?

Although there are differences between MLD and SLD, there are some core aspects that are central to disability as a whole. People with LD have difficulties with academic achievement and progress. Discrepancies may exist between a person's potential for learning and what he or she actually learns, so, for example, one common area of discussion is that a child may have a certain level of cognition and receptive language skills, but may be using language and communication skills of a lower competence in relation to cognition and receptive function (Grove & Dockrell, 2000; Harding et al., 2010). It is likely that they will show an uneven pattern of development (language development, physical development, academic development and/or perceptual development). People with LD may also have language processing deficits due to limited attention skills, slower speed of processing, limited phonological working memory, limited visuo-spatial working memory and difficulties with executive function.

Problems in maintaining attention appear to be inherent to LD. Some attention deficits may be linked to particular syndromes and are more likely when there is an organic dysfunction. As a result, many people with LD may have difficulties with selecting information, filtering distractions, sustaining attention, habituation, transfer and general language processing skills. Children with learning difficulties and additional physical difficulties have been identified as having reduced joint attention behaviours and are therefore at risk of not acquiring language to their full potential (Cress & Marvin, 2004).The development of joint attention and attention skills generally during social interaction is important for social competence, language learning and the development of receptive skills (Striano, Chen, Cleveland & Bradshaw, 2006).

Verbal memory is also an area of difficulty in many individuals with LD (Merrill, Lookadoo, Rilea & Abbeduto, 2003). This is a skill necessary for rehearsal of information, and is well developed by the time a child reaches 7 years of age. People with LD do not easily show spontaneous rehearsal skills. Metacognitive skills include recall, self-monitoring, reality testing, generalization, coordinating and controlling learning, inventiveness and flexibility of thinking. Children with LD tend to have difficulties with information adaption and may also find generalization of newly learned language skills challenging (Merrill et al., 2003).

Children with learning difficulties and communication delay tend to find using language in social settings difficult, and because of this they are at risk of reduced social interaction experiences. Peer interactions often need to be mediated in order to become sustained and interactive. To achieve this, developing appropriate environmental cues during the interactive process is a necessary part of intervention. This can include adult and peer modelling of target social vocabulary and skills as well as use of specific cues such as a communication book that has a static prompt to support a child. Peer learning opportunities can help promote more confident social interaction, and therefore help develop initiation skills as well as maximizing communicative competence (Harding, 2007).

Beyond cognitive levels alone, there are differences between those who have SLD and those with MLD. Children with SLD frequently show evidence in a developmental profile or clinical examination of some form of brain pathology. This is less common in MLD. SLD is usually a result of organic pathology and it is likely that the child may have other physical impairments, whereas MLD is most commonly due to a combination of genetic and environmental factors (Emerson & Hatton, 2004). Children with SLD generally find tasks such as reading and writing harder to acquire. Children who have SLD are less likely to lead independent lives, whereas children who have MLD can adjust and, later on, can cope within the adult world of work in more practical tasks. MLD is more common in lower socioeconomic groupings, where SLD is more evenly distributed across all social groups.

There may also be other sensory and health issues that may significantly impact on the potential to develop competent speech, language, communication and social skills. Hearing and vision are judged to be areas of risk, and estimates range from 5% to 60% with hearing impairment (Kerr et al., 2003), and an audit that found vision completely normal in <1% of population studied (Kerr et al., 2003). Epilepsy is another risk area and Kerr et al. (2003) found that 34% of the people studied had an active problem with fits, 17% were in remission and anticonvulsant medication was prescribed for 28%. Mental health difficulties tend to have a higher prevalence rate within the LD population. Excluding challenging behaviours, prevalence rates are between 25% and 40% compared with 25% within the normal population. Emerson (2003) carried out a study on 10,438 children who were non-learning disabled and compared them to a matched age group of peers with LDs. Within the LD group, 39% had a psychiatric disorder, whereas only 8% had any specific emotional and mental health issues in the non-learning-disabled group.

Estimations are that up to 50–90% of people with LD are likely to have some form of language and/or communication difficulty. About 80% of people with SLD fail to develop effective speech and/or language skills and are highly likely to require access to augmentative and alternative communication (AAC) to promote communication opportunities; 20% have no verbal skills but demonstrate some level of communicative intent; around 20% have no intentional communication skills (DoH, 2009).

Epidemiology/prevalence

Within the UK, the Department of Health estimates that there are approximately 210,000 people with severe learning disabilities (children, adults and older people) and that potentially there are around 1.2 million people with mild/moderate learning disabilities (DoH, 2009). The National Statistics Office suggests that about 2% of the UK population have some level of learning disability. It is recognized that there is no official statistic which accurately reflects this population.

MLD is more difficult to define; if it is on IQ alone, then 3% of the population have an IQ of two standard deviations below the mean. This ignores other influences, such as social competence, educational management and family support. These variables determine whether or not a person needs support in adult life.

Predicted figures for 2011 are 799,830 people with learning disabilities, including 625,199 20–59-year olds, and 174,631 people of 60 and over. It is also predicted that the number of people with LD will increase 11% in 2021. Looking specifically at the population of people with PMLD, there will be an increase to 5 in every 250,000 in 2026 (Emerson & Hatton, 2004). In terms of influences, there are a greater number of males compared to females who have a severe learning disability due to sex-linked genetic factors. Additionally, there are higher prevalence rates in some ethnic minority groups (DoH, 2009).

Interaction with infants and children with learning difficulties

It is important to be aware of the various interactive styles expected within disability, as this should influence the type of intervention that practitioners will implement. Pragmatic skills are an important framework on which to build other language and communication skills, particularly for children with LD. However, pragmatic competence is the outcome of an interaction of language factors, socio-emotional, cognitive and contextual factors that are set into motion early on during language acquisition and development. Children with LD may lack confidence and self-esteem, display learned passivity and initiate very little, and have difficulty generalizing and adapting skills (Basil, 1992). These difficulties will all interact and will affect conversational competence and therefore quality of life, potentially inhibiting development in this area.

Parents and carers are going to be influenced by the language and communication behaviour of children with language and learning needs. Children who are less likely to initiate communication may influence parents and carers to adopt a more directive and instructional style of communication. With infants who have Down syndrome, syllabic babbling appears to be delayed. There are many factors that could contribute to this, such as hypotonia, hearing impairment, ill health and maturational delay, but the delayed babbling in conjunction with carers feeling unsure about which communication style to adopt to support their child may impact on the development of effective social communication (Rondal & Buckley, 2003).

Mothers of children with LD may be more concerned to try to teach language explicitly and these children may require more intensive, focused interactions to help them develop language. For example, directives were used by mothers of children with LD to help them engage in object play and compliance, whereas mothers of normally developing children used them to encourage attention and exploration. The strategy seemed effective for the children with LDs, who were more likely to engage in appropriate play following a maternal directive (Maurer & Sherrod, 1987). Adapting communication by focusing on a child's lead, supporting attention and focusing on key vocabulary can have benefits for language learning.

Case study on Karl, aged 6 years and 2 months

General health and sensory information

Description: Is described as having profound and multiple learning disabilities (PMLD) and 'challenging behaviour'. No specific difficulties with hearing and vision.

Present educational placements: Attends a school for children who have severe learning disabilities for four days a week, and a mainstream school with full-time support one day a week.

Attention and listening: Is supported by use of touch, simplified language, repetition and gesture. Attention can also be sustained by use of objects and sometimes by use of photographic material.

Understanding skills: Responds to simple instructions, e.g. 'Close the door' in familiar contexts. Responds to own [name] by turning and vocalizing and/or smiling. Can identify [familiar people] on command. Anticipates in familiar routines. Recognizes familiar objects such as his [cup/spoon/ball/shoe/coat] and will eye-point to a specific item if asked; needs time to process the information, and minimal peripheral distraction. Has recognition of photographs of the mentioned items. Has shown some understanding of high-frequency symbols within the class such as [drink/more]. Can sometimes imitate simple posting and gross motor actions, e.g. [waving/clapping]. Informal assessment indicates a receptive language performance of around 15 months.

Expressive skills: Uses vocalization to gain attention. Can point, using his whole hand, to objects and photographs of everyday objects. Can use some gestures: [hugs / facial expression and sign attempt for *sad* / touches self for *me* / *hello* and *goodbye*, waving]. Informal assessment indicates an expressive performance of 8–12 months.

Intervention: Photographs were selected to build on Karl's existing abilities with using objects communicatively. Karl had also demonstrated some emerging abilities with gesture and signs.

Evidence: Reduced complexity of language and pacing of communication interactions helps processing and comprehension

(Iverson, Longobardi & Caseli, 2003); use of signing to support communication attempts (Iverson et al., 2005); use of gesture supports vocabulary learning (Zampini & D'Odorico, 2009); tactile cues can reinforce concept learning when introducing AAC (Blairs & Slater, 2007); word learning is strengthened with AAC support (Brady, 2000); use of AAC will help empowerment, participation, development and opportunities to learn from modelling (Basil, 1992).

Outcomes: *Spontaneous communication included*: Spontaneous reaching; spontaneous use of waving to indicate [hello/bye] when people greet him; spontaneous use of [hug] gesture to indicate contentment; spontaneous use of the [more] sign on hearing the word in classroom tasks; spontaneous ability to select one out of two photographs/symbols from: [cup/spoon/plate/more/bye/ball/car/book/teddy/dolly/bubbles/train].

Comprehension: Karl was able to respond more frequently to his [name]. Karl also responded more frequently to verbal output from others in the classroom, usually by pointing to a photograph or by signing [more].

Social interaction: There was an indication that Karl showed increased use of eye contact to engage others within a communicative context.

Behaviour: Karl appeared to show fewer signs of stress, such as crying and shouting during mealtimes, after the intervention. He also demonstrated fewer food refusals.

Peer relationships have been studied in both integrated and segregated settings (Midlarsky, Hannah, Shvill & Johnson, 2008). In integrated settings, children with learning disabilities may adapt their behaviour positively in line with the models provided by peers, but equally they may experience problems with peer interactions due to their limited vocabulary skills.When non-disabled children interact with children with disabilities they are likely to either take over and dominate, or withdraw, particularly if the child with an intellectual impairment cannot communicate effectively, does not seem to know the appropriate strategies for social interchange and if there are associated behavioural problems (Midlarsky et al., 2008). The quality of interactions can be improved by teaching relevant skills to people with learning disabilities and ensuring that communication opportunities are encouraged as well as by training more able peers (Harding, 2007; Midlarsky et al., 2008).

Specific areas of risk in language and communication development

Speech development and difficulties with speech production are prevalent in LD populations related to level of disability and to syndrome. Much research in this area has focused on people who have Down syndrome, although the themes of difficulties in communicating with others are pertinent to all children with disabilities. Children with LD seem to follow the normal pattern of phonological acquisition overall, though with more inconsistencies. It has been estimated that 70–90% of people with moderate to severe LDs have severe difficulties in speech production. About 80% of people with severe to profound LD fail to develop effective speech and language (Rondal & Buckley, 2003; Emerson & Hatton, 2004).

Unintelligibility from children who have LD and problems making themselves understood is reported by parents to be a major problem. The evidence for oral motor work to improve speech and intelligibility for children with LD really needs further appropriate neurolinguistic research, as the evidence base is weak and at present there is no constructive evidence to support its value (Clarke, 2003).Work on speech for children who have LD needs to be integrated alongside other strategies, particularly AAC approaches, to promote interactive and language learning opportunities.

The long-term development of vocabulary and syntax is another area of concern for practitioners who work with children and young people with LD. It is known that the pattern of acquisition in the development of language with learning disabled children is similar to typically developing children: social words, object names, followed by relational words, but development may never progress to full grammatical competence, and the range of vocabulary learned will not be as extensive. Development appears to be greatest in the preschool years, then slows down, but may show an increase during early adult years. The majority of adults with moderate to severe intellectual impairments use short utterances, single propositions, with reduced and unstable grammatical morphology.

Receptive and expressive vocabularies are often smaller than would be predicted from maturational age and more dominated by concrete, basic category terms. Use of simplified language can aid processing skills and facilitate greater interaction and opportunities to use vocabulary. Many people with learning disabilities will use AAC to support their understanding as well as their expressive skills, and visual signing and symbol supports can be of great benefit in supporting vocabulary resourcing skills (Harding et al., 2010).

Case study on Abdi, aged 2 years and 11 months

General health and sensory information

Abdi was born prematurely at 32 weeks. Somali and English are spoken in the home. Abdi's mother became concerned when he was approximately 22 months when he appeared to regress after being ill with a cold. His sight, hearing and general health are good.

Present educational placements: Attends a nursery for children from the local community.

Attention and listening: Abdi does not come and sit on verbal command and requires the use of tactile support and a strong visual presentation of items to gain his attention.

Receptive language: Abdi requires tactile and visual support to help his understanding. He demonstrates the ability to use objects functionally, has an awareness of object permanence and can interpret some natural gestures such as [Give me]. Anticipation of familiar songs and events is evident. Abdi's receptive function currently appears to be around 12–15 months age equivalent.

Expressive language: Abdi does not use any words or sounds with intent. He will initiate contact by reaching for an adult's hand and can shake hands for [hello] after a model. He will reach to indicate [more] and will sometimes wave [bye]. Abdi's expressive skills currently appear to be below the 12-month level.

Summary: Abdi has severe difficulties in all areas of his communication. His difficulties are such that he will find accessing a nursery curriculum challenging without additional language support to enable him to learn and interact.

Cont. overleaf

Intervention: Photograph exchange for [drink]. (*Adult to visually model, use hand over hand prompting.*)

Use structure with two to three motivating tasks to develop an understanding and anticipation within a consistent work routine. (*Adult to use visually motivating items to encourage Abdi to sit and physical prompting as well as natural gesture.*)

Develop and encourage consistent reaching skills to enhance requesting skills and motivation in sharing as well as developing a gesture with meaning. (*Adult to visually model, use hand over hand prompting.*)

Develop opportunities to encourage sounds to be used with intent in rough and tumble games. (*Adult to reward sound produced through another turn, i.e. tactile feedback.*)

Evidence: Reduced complexity of language and pacing of communication interactions helps processing and comprehension (Iverson, Goldin-Meadow et al, 2003); use of signing to support communication attempts (Iverson et al., 2005); use of gesture supports vocabulary learning (Zampini & D'Odorico, 2009); use of peer modelling has some language learning benefits (Harding, 2007); use of symbols has a permanence that supports communication attempts; tactile cues can reinforce concept learning when introducing AAC (Blairs & Slater, 2007); word learning is strengthened with AAC support (Brady, 2000); use of AAC will help empowerment, participation, development and opportunities to learn from modelling (Basil, 1992).

Outcomes: Abdi was able to spontaneously take a single photograph of a [drink] from his communication book by week 4.

Abdi was scanning and reaching to request within 2 weeks of implementation. By 4 weeks he was observed hesitating before reaching, thereby demonstrating that he was thinking about the choice offered to him.

There are some syndrome-specific associations with the risk of speech, language and communication delay. Children with Fragile X and Down syndrome may be at risk of delayed lexical development and may show particular difficulties with lexical retrieval. Additionally, there may be problems with jargon, perseveration, and repetition as well as morphosyntactic acquisition. With Williams syndrome, children may appear to achieve first words without having understood, or appeared to understand, the use of pointing or referential gestures. They may also have difficulties understanding figurative language, and this therefore can impact on vocabulary learning (Annaz et al., 2009). Deficits in both comprehension and use of linguistic rules for children with Williams syndrome have been reported (Karmiloff-Smith, Brown, Grive & Paterson, 2003). However, children with Down syndrome can develop vocabulary understanding and use (through sign, gesture and vocal attempts) when adults interacting with them use signing, gesture and targeted vocabulary in a play context (Zampini & D'Odorico, 2009).

Comprehension of grammatical structures with children who have LD has been shown to be similar to that of typically developing children, showing reliance on word order and semantic information for the decoding of complex sentences. There are particular difficulties for children who have an LD in comprehending more complicated language where there is an interrelationship between language processing, working memory and tacit memory (Merrill et al., 2003). Early multi-word combinations may emerge at later maturational age than would be predicted, and it is suggested that difficulties in this area are partly attributed to memory as well as comprehension level.

The impact of LD on communication quality

The reality is that, due to difficulties with language and communication acquisition, many children who have a learning disability will probably need some form of AAC support, either for receptive language, expressive skills or as a means of supporting both. AAC is described as a form of support that attempts to compensate for communication difficulties experienced by children with learning needs.

Typically, AAC approaches cover a wide range of skills, from using natural gaze and objects, through to using more complex signing systems or electronic support. AAC is usually divided into 'unaided' and 'aided' systems. 'Unaided' communication involves face-to-face interaction with the sender of the message generating communication using speech, word approximations, objects, signs and symbols, and so on. 'Aided communication' tends to be where all types of linguistic 'utterances' (letters, words/graphic symbols) have to be selected from a display. Examples include communication boards, communication books and electronic aids such as voice output communication aids.

Some positive outcomes have been identified in the literature in relation to AAC use. Tactile cues and verbal as well as visual feedback when teaching a child to use an AAC system can support learning how to use the system as independently as possible (Blairs & Slater, 2007). Object naming has been found to improve with AAC support (Brady, 2000). Signing is a productive support for both receptive and expressive skills as atypical cerebral organization may impair some auditory processing skills and memory, whereas visual–spatial skills may be a strength and support development (Iverson et al., 2003; Iverson & Goldin-Meadow, 2005). Use of early sign with infants and young children with Down syndrome appears to facilitate development of language overall (Rondal & Buckley, 2003; Iverson & Goldin-Meadow, 2005), and parents of children with Down syndrome tend to simplify their spoken language and use more gestures and pointing during interactions to support their children (Iverson et al., 2003). Many children who have Down syndrome progress from using sign and speech to speech, sometimes backed up by sign to help intelligibility. Zampini and D'Odorico (2009) stress that use of gesture can support the comprehension of vocabulary and therefore competent expressive use later.

Inclusion and reducing risk for children with LD and their carers

Infants and children who have learning difficulties are at risk of exclusion from a range of social and educational environments due to language acquisition difficulties and environmental challenges that impact on consistent use of communication strategies. Clinically, children who are introduced to AAC are at risk of impoverished outcomes in terms of their language and communication development, particularly in the area of vocabulary knowledge and acquisition (Grove & Dockrell, 2000). This can in turn lead to reduced social and educational achievements. Cognitive and linguistic limitations are argued as having an impact on capacity for language development and retention. Input limitations have been suggested as a counter-argument, in that the AAC used by those caring for and teaching those with an LD appears to be very limited (Grove & Dockrell, 2000). Teachers tend to use one sign per spoken clause inconsistently throughout the day, and consistent home use by families is rare. This may impair a child's opportunity to learn to develop more complicated utterances and/or AAC combinations and therefore their abilities to link ideas using their communication may be limited (Grove & Dockrell,

2000). Using an AAC strategy can also slow down the pace of an interaction, can be effortful, slow with limited options for topics and topic expansion, and this needs to be considered for all children who use AAC. Natural speech can be up to 150–250 words per minute but aided rates of interaction are usually less than 15 words per minute.

Practitioners are aware that having a child with an LD, especially one with associated health problems, physical difficulties and communication difficulties, is likely to cause increased psychological stress (Sloper & Turner, 1993). Parents may feel challenged to interact and communicate with a child when other care aspects may take up a considerable amount of time and effort. Consequently, it may be perceived to be an additional burden by parents to undertake any goals that have been suggested by health care and/or education professionals. Therefore, the need to embed communication goals within functional contexts is essential.

Research that targets coping with disability yields some additional information about parents and families and this information is important when thinking about interaction and communication development. Parents who care for children with disabilities mention that their quality of life is reduced, and that undertaking the additional care aspects for that child impacts on the family health and the maintenance of social-emotional networks. Maintaining a stable and predictable routine is a challenge, especially if there are other siblings in the family and, overall, parents talk of feeling disempowered (Sloper & Turner, 1993). For families of children with Down syndrome, the feeling was that their coping strategies were challenged and that family relationships were strained. Mothers were particularly concerned with the child developing behavioural problems. These concerns were less with mothers who had some employment responsibilities (Sloper, Knussen, Turner & Cunningham, 1991; Sloper & Turner, 1993). A child's social and communication competence, as well as behaviour problems, have a correlation with parental levels of stress (Dyson, 2003). Mothers who have learning difficulties themselves are at high risk of depression from social isolation. Given the level of stress that parents experience, ensuring that communication strategies are integrated into the child's daily experience is vital and ensures that the strategies are more likely to be used.

Certain vulnerabilities are exposed in families of a child who has a disability, particularly at times of transition between life stages. A lack of predictability in the disabled child's life course means that preparing for change is made difficult. Uncertainty in transitions is a source of stress for parents. This relates to the services on offer, the emotional maturation of the child, if new people will be able to communicate effectively with their child and the changing of needs to suit a new environment. Consequently, practitioners working with families need to prepare well and link with the teams children will be moving on into, as well as providing relevant information in an accessible format (such as a clear communication passport that highlights a child's preferred method of communication and level of understanding).

There is a correlation between communication difficulties and challenging behaviour. Challenging behaviour is more likely amongst children with more severe intellectual disabilities and those who are non-verbal or experience particular difficulty with reception and expression of language (Borthwick-Duffy, 1994). Therefore, the need to embed appropriate receptive and expressive language strategies into functional contexts is crucial to reduce deprived communication opportunities for vulnerable children.

Summary

It is important to be aware of the key characteristics of speech, language and communication difficulties that may arise within the population of infants, children and young people who have learning difficulties. There are a number of specific issues that could help drive forward research and intervention underpinning speech and language therapy intervention for this group. These are: philosophy of intervention; clinical characteristics of children who have specific difficulties; intervention strategies; the process of intervention; and how AAC supports language and communication development.

Practitioners working with children who have an LD should have a strong philosophy underlying intervention. Much intervention will be looking at interpretation of a person's needs and facilitating the right communication environment that can meet those needs. This stems from looking at what the child can attempt to do and therefore what they can communicate, then providing the opportunities to enable the child to fulfil these opportunities. Responding to children in a specific way using relevant strategies to make the interaction meaningful can assist a child.

If children are responded to and interacted with within a communicative context pitched at their receptive level of functioning, they are likely to attempt to communicate again. Where possible, the client will need to be fully involved in the goal-setting process as well as the evaluation of any strategies implemented. In addition, training will be needed for carers or significant others.

Intervention will use the communication strengths identified by the speech and language therapist in collaboration with others involved in that child's education and care. Any sensory and/or physical needs as well as the environment the child will be interacting in need to be accommodated in goal-setting. The evidence underpinning selected goals is another important part of the therapy process. Consideration needs to be given to the child's diagnosis (and hence some hypothesis about how he or she will progress), and whether their level of cognition and receptive function is at the right level to support the intervention, be it AAC or verbal. Research really needs to explore the process of developing receptive and expressive support for children with LD so that clinicians can make appropriate choices of support for children that have meaning both for the child and their carers and educators.

Some clear and rigorous distinction also needs to be made between those children with more profound needs who will require changes in the environment to support their communication attempts and those who will make progress and be able to initiate and interact using a range of strategies (Harding et al., 2010). Research into differentiating such interventions and considering key aspects of an approach is important. However, there also need to be further surveys of AAC use in disability provisions, alongside a more robust review of training programmes for key users to enable practitioners to understand better the challenges of implementing speech, language and communication opportunities for infants, children and young people with learning difficulties.

Issues regarding AAC need serious consideration by clinicians, researchers and those who care for children with learning disabilities. There are a number of key aspects that need further exploration. Firstly, there are not enough studies that actually explore the rationale underpinning which type of AAC support to use; and there needs to be further research that actually examines a clear series of steps related to which support to use linked to the interaction between a child's level of cognition, receptive function and their expressive needs. Secondly, consideration needs to be given to how training is provided to parents, carers and educators, and how it can engage people so that AAC can be used at an appropriate level to support and develop a child's capacity to participate.

References

Annaz, A., van Herwegen, J., Thomas, M., Fishman, R., Karmiloff-Smith, A. & Runblad, G. (2009) Comprehension of metaphor and metonymy in children with Williams syndrome. *International Journal of Language and Communication Disorders, 44(6)*, 962–978.

Basil, C. (1992) Social interaction and learned helplessness in severely disabled children. *AAC, 8*, 188–199.

Blairs, S. & Slater, S. (2007) The clinical application of deep touch pressure with a man with autism presenting with severe anxiety and challenging behaviour. *British Journal of Learning Disabilities, 35*, 214–220.

Borthwick-Duffy, S.A. (1994) Epidemiology and prevalence of psychopathology in people with mental retardation. *Journal of Consulting and Clinical Psychology, 62*, 17–27.

Brady, N.C. (2000) Improved comprehension of object names following voice output communication aid use: Two case studies. *AAC, 16(3)*, 197–204.

Clarke, H.M. (2003) Neuromusculature treatments for speech and swallowing: A tutorial. *American Journal of Speech-Language Pathology, 12*, 400–415.

Cress, C.J. & Marvin, C.A. (2004) Common questions about early AAC services in early intervention. *Augmentative and Alternative Communication, 19(4)*, 254–272.

Department of Health (2009) *Valuing People Now: Making it Happen for Everyone.* London: Department of Health Publications.

Dyson, L.L. (2003) Children with learning disability within the family context: A comparison with siblings in global self-concept, academic self-perception and social competence. *Learning Disabilities Research and Practice, 18(1)*, 1–9.

Emerson, E. (2003) The prevalence of psychiatric disorders in children and adolescents with and without intellectual disabilities. *Journal of Intellectual Disability Research, 47*, 51–58.

Emerson, E. & Hatton, C. (2004) *Estimating Future Need/Demand for Supports for Adults with Learning Disabilities in England.* Institute for Health Research at Lancaster University.

Grove, N. & Dockrell, J. (2000) The analysis of multi-sign combinations in children with intellectual impairments. *Journal of Speech, Language, and Hearing Research, 43*, 309–323.

Harding, C. (2007) Involving adult service users with learning disability in the training of speech and language therapy students: A pilot project. *International Journal of Teaching in Higher Education, 20(2)*, 205–211.

Harding, C., Lindsay, G., O'Brien, A., Dipper, L. & Wright, J. (2010) Implementing AAC to children with profound and multiple learning disabilities: A study in rationale underpinning intervention. *Journal of Research in Special Educational Needs, 11(2)*, 120–129. DOI: 10.1111/j.1471 – 3802.2010 01184

Iverson, J.M. & Goldin-Meadow, S. (2005) Gesture paves the way for language development. *American Psychological Society, 16*, 367–471.

Iverson, J.M., Longobardi, E. & Caseli, M.C. (2003) Relationship between gestures and words in children with Down's syndrome and typical developing children in the early stages of communicative development. *International Journal of Language and Communication Disorders, 38*, 179–197.

Karmiloff-Smith, A., Brown, J., Grive, S. & Paterson, S. (2003) Dethroning the myth: Cognitive dissociations and innate modularity in Williams syndrome. *Developmental Neuropsychology, 23*, 227–242.

Kerr, A.M., McCulloch, D., Oliver, K., McLean, B., Coleman, E., Law, T., Beaton, P., Wallace, S., Newell, E., Eccles, T. & Prescott, R.J. (2003) Medical needs of people with intellectual disability require regular reassessment and the provision of client and carer-held reports. *Journal of Intellectual Disability Research, 47*, 134–145.

Maurer, H. & Sherrod, K. (1987) Context of directives given to young children with DS and nonretarded children: Development over two years. *American Journal of Mental Deficiency, 91*, 579–590.

Merrill, E.C., Lookadoo, R., Rilea, S. & Abbeduto, L. (2003) Memory, language and comprehension, and mental retardation. In E.C. Merrill, R. Lookadoo, S. Rilea & L. Abbeduto (Eds) *Language and Communication in Mental Retardation*, pp.151–189. Elsevier.

Midlarsky, E., Hannah, M.E., Shvill, E. & Johnson, A. (2008) Siblings of children with mental retardation: The role of helping. *International Review of Research on Mental Retardation, 35*, 291–317.

Rondal, J. & Buckley, S. (2003) *Speech and Language Intervention in Down Syndrome.* London: Whurr.

Sloper, P., Knussen C., Turner, S. & Cunningham, C. (1991) Factors related to stress and satisfaction with life in families of children with Down's syndrome. *Journal of Child Psychology and Psychiatry, 32(4)*, 655–676.

Sloper, P. & Turner, S. (1993) Risk and resistance factors in the adaption of parents of children with severe learning disability. *Journal of Child Psychology and Psychiatry, 34(2)*, 167–188.

Striano, T., Chen, X., Cleveland, A. & Bradshaw, S. (2006) Joint attention social cues influence infant learning. *European Journal of Developmental Psychology, 3*, 289–299.

Sudhalter, V., Maranion, M. & Brookes, P. (1992) Expressive semantic deficit in the productive language of males with Fragile X syndrome. *American Journal of Medical Genetics, 38*, 65–71.

World Health Organization (2006) *ICF: International Classification of Functioning, Disability and Health.* Geneva: WHO.

Zampini, L. & D'Odorico, L. (2009) Communicative gestures and vocabulary in 36-month-old children with Down's syndrome. *International Journal of Language and Communication Disorders, 44(6)*, 1063–1074.

6 Stuttering

Mark Onslow
University of Sydney, Australia

Marilyn Langevin
University of Alberta, Canada

The nature of stuttering

Causal theory

The cause of stuttering is unknown and there are many causal theories, which are overviewed comprehensively by Packman and Attanasio (2004). At the time of writing, the dominant causal explanation for stuttering is that it is a problem with the neural processing underpinning speech (Packman & Attanasio, 2004). Packman and Attanasio argue that such an explanation has the greatest explanatory power of any class of causal theory in terms of parsimony and capacity to explain what is known of the disorder. The compelling nature of this prospect has been bolstered by Chang, Erickson, Ambrose, Hasegawa-Johnson and Ludlow's (2008) finding that brain anomalies found for adults in the left perisylvian white matter exist in children, and by the Cykowski, Fox, Ingham, Ingham and Robin (2010) imaging findings that suggested a hypothesis connecting stuttering onset and development with myelogenesis of perisylvian areas.

Epidemiology of stuttering

Some caveats

Ideally, knowledge of the circumstances surrounding the onset of stuttering and its nature at onset and early development would be obtained from prospective cohorts of large numbers of children with apparently normally developing speech and language. From that cohort, children would be identified as they begin to stutter, and studied subsequently. Another problem that we have with our knowledge of the onset of stuttering is that it has not been informed by such an ideal method. Instead, our knowledge of the matter comes mostly from parent report after the event of stuttering onset, often many years later (see Yairi, 1997).

Incidence and prevalence

There has been a long-standing belief that the lifetime incidence of stuttering – the risk of ever stuttering during life – is around 5% (for an overview see Bloodstein & Bernstein Ratner, 2008). However, that consensus seems somewhat at odds with a review by those authors of reports where adults recalled ever having stuttered. Bloodstein and Bernstein Ratner concluded that:

> it would seem that a plausible figure for the lifetime incidence of all those who at one time either consider themselves or are considered by their parents to be stutterers is at least as high as 10 percent. (p.91)

Again, the caveat here is the absence of longitudinal data derived from a community-ascertained cohort, with the appearance of stuttering in participants subsequent to their recruitment into the study. Recently, however, a preliminary prospective community-ascertained cohort study reported cumulative incidences of 8.5% and 12.2% at 36 and 48 months respectively (Onslow & Menzies, 2010; Reilly et al., 2009). An analysis of a review of nine studies (n=44,129) (Bloodstein & Bernstein Ratner, 2008, Table 3.3) shows a mean adult lifetime recall of 7.3% of ever having stuttered.

The prevalence of stuttering – the proportion of the population affected at any one time – is generally accepted to be around 1% based on many studies (for an overview see Bloodstein & Bernstein Ratner, 2008). However, the caveat to that consensus is that the bulk of reports supporting it are cross-sectional and have not involved detailed and expert diagnosis of the presence and absence of stuttering. Again, ideally, the prevalence of stuttering would be known from sound epidemiological methods involving prospective community-ascertained cohorts.

Onset of stuttering

With the foregoing caveats in mind, there seems to be strong agreement that the onset of stuttering mostly occurs at some time during the first few years of life. That agreement is based on the results of many retrospective studies of the matter based on parent recall (for an overview see Bloodstein & Bernstein Ratner, 2008), and prospective studies based on parent interviews reasonably soon after onset. Yairi (1983) reported that all of a group of 22 stuttering children appeared to have begun to stutter by 36 months of age. This report is broadly consistent with the Jones, Onslow, Harrison and Packman (2000) report of 250 children who received treatment, with a mean age of 46.4 months (SD=9.4 months) at the first treatment session, and a mean period from reported onset to treatment of 12.4 months (SD=7.9 months). It is likely, though, that if there are a number of cases of early stuttering that do appear subsequent to the preschool years, as suggested by Andrews and Harris (1964), they would be missed by studies such as those that focus on preschool children.

Stuttering can appear quite suddenly, with reports of Yairi (1983) and Yairi and Ambrose (1992) suggesting that half of cases begin within one week, and one third of cases begin stuttering during a single day. The Reilly et al. (2009) report, involving parent interview soon after onset, reported 49.6% of cases beginning during one to three days, and 37.2% during a single day. A case study by Wyatt (1969) contains a clear account of sudden early onset of stuttering. Stuttering is not insidious in its development, with evidence of severe stuttering at onset associated with superfluous behaviours (Conture & Kelly, 1991; Yairi, 1983; Yairi, Ambrose & Niermann, 1993; Yairi & Lewis, 1984).

Development of stuttering

Again with the caveat that research methods have not been ideal, there seems to be a consensus that, as a general rule, stuttering becomes more severe soon after onset and its topography changes to include fixed postures and superfluous behaviours (Bloodstein & Bernstein Ratner, 2008), or greater proportions of those types of stuttering moments if they were present at onset (see above). A comparison of data from O'Brian, Packman, Onslow and O'Brian (2004) and Jones, Onslow, Packman and Gebski (2006) provides some support for the contention that stuttering may progressively worsen across age groups. The former study measured stuttering severity in 90 affected adults and the latter in 54 children treated in clinics. In light of reasons to believe that interclinic consistency may be questionable for %SS scores (Kully & Boberg, 1988; Cordes & Ingham, 1994), this comparison is bolstered by the fact that measures in the two studies were made by the same research team. The mean %SS scores for the adults and the children, respectively, were 9.0 and 6.6.

It seems fairly self-evident that stuttering becomes increasingly intractable quite soon after onset. It is obvious that the treatment of children is much quicker and effortless, with more durable effects, when they are in the preschool years than when they are adults. Presumably this is due to the loss of plasticity within the speech motor system as neural networks for speech become established (Wohlert & Smith, 2002). This is consistent with the result of comparisons of an identical treatment with preschool and school-age children, using similar methods. Preschoolers attain 92% reductions (Rousseau, Packman, Onslow, Harrison & Jones, 2007), 97% reductions (Onslow, Andrews & Lincoln, 1994) and 99% reductions post-treatment. However, with school-age children 80% reduction (Lincoln, Onslow, Lewis & Wilson, 1996) and 81% reduction (Koushik, Shenker & Onslow, 2009) has been attained. Although these are likely overestimates of effect size because of non-randomized trial designs (Kunz & Oxman, 1998), the comparison between the two seems suggestive. It is not clear exactly at what age this intractability becomes a clinical problem, or whether it occurs at around the same age or period post onset for all children. However, it does appear to be veridical.

Natural recovery from stuttering

It is well known that many children recover naturally from early stuttering. Regardless, it is currently not possible to predict whether an individual child will recover spontaneously or will require treatment (Packman, Onslow & Attanasio, 2003). For this reason, the general consensus is for treatment to occur at some time during the preschool years.

Again, the bulk of research that has addressed this issue has not been methodologically ideal. However, there have been three studies that have studied large cohorts of children prospectively.

The first large prospective data set concerning the onset and course of stuttering came from the so-called '1000 family study', which was conducted in England between 1946 and 1962 (Andrews & Harris, 1964). The findings of that study indicated that 79% of children who started stuttering during the preschool years subsequently recovered. Another large-scale longitudinal study of the topic was of 1021 preschool children conducted in Denmark (Mansson, 2000). The first speech and language evaluation occurred around the children's third birthday, and the children were re-evaluated two years and four years later. At the second assessment, at around 5 years of age, 71% no longer stuttered, while at the third assessment, at around 9 years of age, 85% no longer stuttered.

Another large-scale prospective study of natural recovery from early stuttering is from the United States. This is the Illinois Early Childhood Stuttering Project (for an overview, see Yairi & Ambrose, 2005). Yairi and colleagues recruited, from the general population, children who had started to stutter during the previous 12 months. Estimates of natural recovery from this project are ranging at present from 75% to 89%. A recent report of 84 children who were followed for at least four years after the onset of stuttering (Yairi & Ambrose, 1999) indicated that 74% of them recovered naturally.

Reported time to natural recovery varies widely, ranging from a few months to a number of years (Andrews & Harris, 1964; Yairi & Ambrose 1999). For clinical purposes, though, it is difficult to interpret those research findings because subjects were recruited from the general population rather than from speech clinics, and were not recruited prior to stuttering onset. Parents do not typically bring their children to the clinic immediately following onset, and may not do so until the child has been stuttering for some time. The Jones et al. (2000) study of 250 cases, for example, had a mean period from reported onset to the start of treatment of 12.4 months. However, many children experience bouts of stuttering for shorter periods than 12 months (see Andrews & Harris, 1964; Yairi & Ambrose, 1992), and those children may never present to a speech clinic. Consequently, recovery rates for children whose parents bring them to speech clinics because of stuttering are likely to be much lower than population recovery rates.

It is interesting to consider the Andrews and Harris (1964) data with the notion that a transient case of stuttering may not present to a clinic. The original data for this study contains 16 cases where stuttering is reported to have occurred for less than 6 months, leaving 27 children who stuttered for more than 6 months (pp.30–31). In the event that none of those transient cases presented to a speech clinic, the Andrews and Harris recovery rate may tell a different story. Of the remaining 27 children in the sample, 14 were reported to have onset at 5 years or younger, and of those, seven were reported to have recovered (p.32). This gives a recovery estimate of 50% of stuttering children who present to a clinic during the preschool years. Arguably, then, the best interpretation of published, large-scale prospective studies of natural recovery is that the natural recovery rate of clinical populations will be much lower than the 75% mark that is emerging from studies of nonclinical populations.

The impact of stuttering

Speech rate

Not surprisingly, many of the problem speech behaviours of stuttering are time-consuming, notoriously those involving fixed postures. Depending on how it is measured, normal adult speech rate is in the range of 200–250 syllables per minute, and stuttering greatly reduces this verbal information transfer rate. According to a comprehensive study of the matter (Johnson, 1933), those who stutter appear on average to speak at three-quarters the rate of those who do not stutter. In view of the skewed distribution of stuttering severity in the population of those with the disorder (see above), it might be reasonable to assert that moderate to severe cases of stuttering would have half the verbal transfer rate of non-stuttering speakers. In the case of severe stuttering, with speech rate below 50 syllables per minute, verbal transfer rate would be less than a quarter of normal values. In other words, during an adult life without control of stuttered speech, those affected could well have half or less the verbal output of their non-stuttering peers. This is one of the self-evident facts of stuttering that is seldom stated explicitly: those affected cannot say as much as their peers, or take longer to say it. Most likely, the former would be expected to be the case.

Language and phonology

Children

Another issue about which there is lack of clarity at present is the association between stuttering and language and phonology in children. Much research has been directed to this topic in children, driven predominantly by various theoretical positions about the cause and development of stuttering (see Packman & Attanasio, 2004). Arguably, Reilly et al. (2009) found that advanced vocabulary development was one of the predictors of stuttering onset by 36 months, suggesting the intuitive prospect that the origins of stuttering are precipitated by bursts of language development. A study by Bonelli, Dixon, Ratner and Onslow (2000) of stuttering prior to successful treatment of preschoolers found many of the children to have advanced language for their ages. Consistent with this notion is that stuttering moments during early childhood seem to coincide with the initiation of clauses, and that stuttered utterances are generally longer and more grammatically complex than non-stuttered utterances (Bloodstein & Bernstein Ratner, 2008; Buhr & Zebrowski, 2009; Melnick & Conture, 2000; Reichels, Buhr, Conture & Ntourou, 2010). As argued by Bonelli et al. (2000):

> In light of notions such as 'bucket' theory of language and phonological development (Crystal, 1987) it might even be surprising if speech and language processing was unaffected during a period when a child learned to offset such a potentially troublesome disorder as stuttering. Trading relationships among components of the language production system in children are well-known (Camarata, 1988) and extend to trade-offs between language length and complexity and fluency (Ratner, 1997; Tetnowski, 1998).

In any event, reviews of this literature by Nippold (1990, 2001, 2004) have yielded equivocal results. An early report by Andrews et al. (1983) found that children who stutter often present with co-morbid language or phonology impairments, and this was replicated by some subsequent studies indicating that language levels of stuttering preschoolers are below their control peers (e.g. Anderson & Conture, 2000; Silverman & Ratner, 2002; Ryan, 1992). Yet others have reported that there are no such differences (e.g. Bajaj, 2007; Reilly et al., 2009; Watkins & Yairi, 1997; Watkins, Yairi & Ambrose, 1999). On the face of it, a report by Arndt and Healy (2001) provided compelling data from a large cohort of clinicians who provided information on 467 school-age stuttering children, of which 44% were said to also have a language or phonological disorder. However, Nippold (2004) provided a caveat to such caseload information with evidence that children are more likely to be referred for stuttering treatment if they have such concomitant language or phonological disorders. In other words, clinical caseloads not only are likely to underestimate the population rate of natural recovery (see above), but they are likely to overestimate the population rate of clustering of stuttering with language and phonological disorders. Another methodological problem with this body of research is that, considering the social problems that school-age children who stutter may have (see below), they may well be reticent in a test situation, leading to underestimates of their language abilities (Bajaj, 2007).

Adults

While the association between language and stuttering has been explored a great deal with children, the topic has been largely overlooked in the case of adults who stutter. This is somewhat surprising, considering that stuttered speech quantitatively reduces speech output (see above) and this might be expected to be associated with some qualitative language compromises. The possibility that this may be so was shown in two preliminary studies. Packman, Hand, Cream and Onslow (2001) found that the complexity of spoken language of 10 adult stuttering participants was 30% lower than that of matched controls. Spencer, Packman, Onslow and Ferguson (2005) used a systemic functional grammar analysis to show that two participants, before a treatment that controlled their stuttering, may have been using modality in such a fashion to reduce the chance of conversational engagement from a speaking partner. Subsequently, Spencer, Packman, Onslow and Ferguson (2009) studied 10 stuttering adults and 10 matched controls. They replicated previous findings that the stuttering participants' language was significantly less complex than the control group, and that the former group used linguistic modality significantly less than controls.

Stuttering and social anxiety

The preschool years

It is obvious that the complaints of those who stutter are not constrained to the speech perturbations of their disorder. The modern psychological concept of anxiety involves an expectation of some harmful occurrence (see Menzies, Onslow & Packman, 1999). As noted by those authors, such cognitions may or may not be associated with physiological arousal. It is clear that they may not (Dietrich & Roaman, 2001). Negative conditioning experiences associated with stuttering during early childhood are implicated in the development of speech-related social anxiety. The critical period of early social development for those who stutter during childhood is often distressing and dysfunctional. There is evidence that such negative conditioning may occur during the early years of stuttering.

It is known that stuttering evokes negative peer reactions (Ezrati-Vinacour, Platzky & Yairi, 2001) and disturbs peer interactions (Langevin, Packman & Onslow, 2009) during the preschool years. In the former study, 80 children aged 3–7 years watched two puppets, one of which stuttered and one of which did not. When asked which puppet they would prefer as a friend, the non-stuttering puppet was chosen by 46.7 % of 3-year-olds, 68.8% of 4-year-olds and 87.5% of 5-year-olds. The Langevin et al. report provides video evidence of peers reacting to stuttering with confusion, and interrupting, ignoring and walking away from stuttering children. Stuttering children were also observed to have difficulty leading peers in play, participating in pretend play, resolving conflicts, participating in problem-solving discussions and providing explanations. There is ample documentation of the distressing effects of early stuttering on affected children (Yairi, 1983; Langevin et al., 2009; Packman et al., 2003). Packman et al. (2003) provide examples of parental reports of stuttering in preschoolers. Parents describe interactions where their children are ignored by peers when they attempt to speak or attempt to enter a play situation, are left mid-utterance, are chosen less as playmates and are actively excluded and teased. At the end of the preschool years, there is evidence that these early conditioning experiences promote negative attitudes to speech and communication (Vanryckeghem, Brutten & Hernandez, 2005).

Although credible, it is not clear to what extent these reports reflect the experiences of children who begin to stutter as a group. It may be that the majority of stuttering children have no such experiences shortly after onset. It may be the case that such parental reports underestimate the extent of the problem, because negative peer reactions to stuttering may be subtle. It is unlikely, for example, that such reactions will always be verbal, such as comments along the lines of 'you talk funny'. A negative reaction can be face-pulling, or simply walking away from the child during a stutter. It is also the case that the negative reactions may occur out of the sight and hearing of playground supervisors. Nor will it necessarily be apparent to a busy preschool teacher that peers are excluding a child who stutters from play activities. However, the indirect and anecdotal evidence that preschool children are teased because of their stuttering is consistent with findings in relation to preschooler communication more generally. These findings indicate that preschoolers are well tuned to communication ability, that they behave as if they know who talks well and who does not, and that they prefer to interact with children who are communicatively competent (Hadley & Rice, 1991).

In general, though, there have been few direct studies of social and emotional factors in preschoolers who stutter. It is not clear why this is the case when so much research has been directed at preschoolers with other communication disorders (see Guralnick, Connor, Hammond, Gottman & Kinnish, 1996).

One possible explanation for this anomaly is the quite recent emergence of evidence that stuttering can be treated soon after onset during the preschool years (see Clinical implications, below).

The school years

The earliest signs of any cognitive ill effects of stuttering have been directly measured at the threshold of the school years, in 6- and 7-year-olds, in terms of negative attitudes to communication (DeNil & Brutten, 1991; Vanryckeghem & Brutten, 1997). They worsen progressively during the school years, whereas attitudes to communication in control children become healthier (DeNil & Brutten, 1991). Elevated trait anxiety has been measured with this age group (Davis, Shisca & Howell, 2007). Indeed, virtually every affected adult reports that stuttering had adverse effects on school life (Hayhow, Cray & Enderby, 2002). The majority report immediate negative emotional effects from this, and 46% report some long-term effects on functioning (Hugh-Jones & Smith, 1999). These effects are obviously related to, but not limited to, bullying. School-age children who stutter are more likely to be bullied than their peers. For example, Langevin, Bortnick, Hammer and Wiebe (1998) reported that 81% of children with stuttering problems were bullied during their time at school, with 56% reporting being bullied about their stuttering once a week or more often. Blood and Blood (2004) reported that 43% of stuttering adolescents compared to 11% of controls reported experiencing bullying during the past week. Further, children and adolescents who stutter are perceived negatively by peers (Langevin & Hagler, 2004; Langevin, 2009; Langevin, Kleitman, Packman & Onslow, 2009), and are rejected by peers more often than those who do not stutter (Davis, Howell & Cooke, 2002).

Adulthood and adolescence

General anxiety

The following statements about anxiety and social phobia are supported by much research and overviewed by Iverach, Menzies, O'Brian, Packman & Onslow (2011) and Menzies et al. (1999). Unusual levels of social anxiety are reported for those who stutter. Extreme differences have been reported, with around half the scores of stuttering clients on a scale of social discomfort being clients in the range of psychiatric anxiety conditions. There are no differences in anxiety levels between a stuttering group and a social phobia group. These findings have been linked directly to the presence of stuttering and are reflected in trait anxiety scores and state anxiety scores in communication situations. Two-thirds of adults seeking treatment for stuttering are diagnosed with one or more mental health disorders, most of which are anxiety related. However, elevated anxiety levels appear not to be constrained to those seeking treatment. Adolescents are known to have higher anxiety scores than controls; however, frank clinical pathology has not been demonstrated with this age group. The majority of those who stutter report speech-related social anxiety, and this is confirmed by the management strategies of their clinicians. Population studies reflect higher state anxiety scores for stuttering compared to control samples. Stuttering varies under conditions intuitively associated with state anxiety, such as the size of an audience and status of conversational partner. Anxiety-related responses to speaking situations distinguish between stuttering and control groups independently of speech.

The Unhelpful Thoughts and Beliefs About Stuttering scale (Iverach et al., 2010; St Clare et al., 2009) is a clinical tool for assessing intrusive and negative thoughts about stuttering. It documents 66 such thoughts that are reported commonly by adults who stutter. Examples are 'people will doubt my ability because I stutter', 'no one will like me if I stutter', 'people who stutter are boring', and 'everyone will laugh at me or they will think I am dumb'. Those who stutter have been found to score higher on the Fear of Negative Evaluation scale than controls, and to specifically fear social situations but not situations involving physical threat (Messenger, Onslow, Packman & Menzies, 2004).

Social phobia

The following statements also are supported by much research and overviewed by Iverach et al. (2011) and Menzies et al. (1999). Social phobia, or social anxiety disorder, is a debilitating psychiatric condition involving social anxiety. DSM-IV diagnostic criteria include extreme distress in social situations, social isolation, and failure to participate in normal occupational, social and interpersonal relationships. Social phobia involves pervasive and excessive fear of humiliation, embarrassment and negative evaluation in social or performance-based situations. Those harm expectancies are clearly excessive and irrational in light of the actual threat.

A DSM-IV diagnosis of social phobia is warranted for a clinically significant portion of those who stutter and seek treatment; debilitating distress and maladaptive social isolation is clearly excessive for the social threat posed by their stuttering. The psychiatric literature contains many such case reports. Diagnosis of social phobia is reported for between 40% and 60% of cohorts of those who stutter and seek speech rehabilitation. A cohort of stuttering participants seeking treatment had a 16- to 34-fold increased risk of social phobia compared to an age- and gender-matched community control group. Additionally, those who stutter are at risk also for other anxiety-related mood and personality disorders.

Occupational and educational consequences of stuttering

Ruben (2000) has made the observation that in the United States at the start of the 20th century, 80% of occupations relied on manual skills, with only 20% of work requiring communication abilities. In 1950 the number of so-called 'white-collar' workers had risen to 38%, and at the start of this century 62% of the United States' workforce had occupations that depended on communication abilities. A further change during the previous century was that those whose occupations did not rely directly on communication skill nonetheless needed communication skills to function in the workplace. Not surprisingly, then, there are many recent reports showing that those who stutter suffer deleterious occupational consequences. Those who stutter seem to think this to be the case (Klein & Hood, 2004). In arguably the classic study of the topic, Hurst and Cooper (1983) surveyed 644 employers and reported the common perception that those who stutter are less employable and less likely to be promoted. These findings of adverse affects of stuttering on occupation are commonly replicated (Crichton-Smith, 2002; Hayhow et al., 2002). Craig and Calver (1991) reported evidence that control of stuttered speech was associated with upgrading in occupational level and promotion prospects. A report by O'Brian, Jones, Onslow, Packman and Menzies (2011) showed a significant, negative, linear relationship between stuttering and educational completion. Those who do not complete high school have stuttering six times more severe than those who complete a postgraduate degree.

Clinical implications

Preschool children

Efficacious early intervention for stuttering shortly after onset during the preschool years is critical because of the effects of the chronic condition as described above. Using an arguably clinically usable definition of a clinical trial (Onslow, Jones, O'Brian, Menzies & Packman 2008), trials of three treatment styles have been published. There have been two non-randomized trials of a treatment known as Palin Parent Child Interaction Therapy, which is based on multifactorial causal theory (see Causal theory) (Millard, Edwards & Cook, 2009; Millard, Nicholas & Cook, 2008). Additionally, there have been three non-randomized trials of a treatment based on non-programmed syllable-timed speech (Trajkovski, Andrews, O'Brian, Onslow & Packman, 2006; Trajkovski et al., 2009; Trajkovski et al., in press). However, as stated previously, it is difficult to interpret evidence from non-randomized clinical trials because of its tendency to overestimate the effect size for the treatment (Kunz & Oxman, 1998).

The prominent evidence base for early intervention is clinical trials of a treatment model of verbal response contingent stimulation known as the Lidcombe Program. This is a behavioural treatment that is administered by parents under the direction of a speech pathologist. Several non-randomized Phase I and Phase II trials of this treatment have been published (for an overview, see Onslow et al., 2008). Randomized, controlled clinical laboratory experiments (Harris, Onslow, Packman, Harrison & Menzies, 2002; Harrison, Onslow & Menzies, 2004) and randomized controlled trials of the treatment in standard and telehealth formats have also been published (Jones et al., 2005; Lewis, Packman, Onslow, Simpson & Jones, 2008) and these trials have been replicated by independent groups (Franken, Kielstra-Van der Schalka & Boelens, 2005; Lattermann, Euler & Neumann, 2008). A meta-analysis of methodologically stringent sources of randomized clinical evidence established the odds ratio for the treatment as 7:5 (Onslow, Jones, Menzies, O'Brian & Packman, in press).

Speech rehabilitation for adults

Speech restructuring treatment (Onslow & Menzies, 2010) is best practice stuttering control for adults. Clients are trained to use a new speech pattern to reduce or eliminate stuttering while sounding as natural as possible. During speech restructuring, clients learn to speak initially with a slow, drawling speech pattern that is stutter free. The speech pattern is then shaped toward stutter-free speech that is natural sounding. The treatment is typically administered over one to three weeks with an intensive group format, followed by regular one-to-one visits with a clinician, but non-intensive versions are starting to appear in clinical trials. As early as the end of the 1970s there was sufficient clinical research for a meta-analysis of the efficacy of speech restructuring treatment compared to others and a conclusion that it is more efficacious than other treatments (Andrews, Guitar & Howie, 1980). Clinically significant control of stuttered speech with a natural-sounding speech pattern is attainable. Virtually all recent published clinical trials for chronic stuttering have incorporated variants of speech restructuring (for an overview, see Onslow et al., 2008).

Social anxiety treatments for adults

Cognitive Behaviour Therapy (CBT) is the most efficacious intervention available for treating social anxiety and has been evaluated extensively in non-stuttering populations. A variety of researchers have included various CBT procedures in their stuttering treatment packages for more than 30 years. A CBT intervention for chronic stuttering has been developed based on cognitive models of the disorder (Clark & Wells, 1995) and research findings about stuttering and anxiety described above. The CBT programme comprises 10 weekly sessions of individual treatment totalling 15 hours. The components are: (1) a psycho-education component exploring the role of cognition in driving anxiety, as well as the problems of safety behaviours, avoidance, emotion-based reasoning and biased attention; (2) exposure and behavioural experiments; (3) rational restructuring; and (4) attentional training. The components are based on standard procedures in the social phobia treatment literature. Importantly, each of the components is tailored to the specific needs of individual clients who stutter. Phase I and Phase II trials of internet-driven and face-to-face versions of the treatment have been completed and a successful Phase III randomized controlled trial has been published (Helgadottir, Menzies, Onslow, Packman & O'Brian, 2009a, 2009b; McColl, Onslow, Packman & Menzies, 2001; Menzies, O'Brian, Onslow, Packman, St Clare & Block, 2008).

Conclusions

Scientific research has generated much information about stuttering that is potentially pertinent to its evidence-based management. The severity of stuttering is skewed so that more mild and mild to moderate cases will be encountered than will be moderate to severe or severe cases. Stuttering generally begins during the early years of life, sometimes suddenly and severely, and may generally be milder than stuttering of adult life. There is support for the contention that the topography of stuttering is dominated at onset by repeated movements, with fixed postures and superfluous behaviours figuring at some later time.

There seems little doubt that stuttering is quite tractable during the preschool years soon after onset, but that a chronic version of the disorder begins to develop at some time during the school years. Many cases of early stuttering will experience natural recovery; however, the exact proportion of such recoveries that might be expected from clinic populations is unknown. Further, many of those recoveries may occur later than the preschool years, past the time when clinicians may judge that stuttering treatment should have begun.

The extent to which stuttering children have co-morbid language or phonological disorders has not been resolved by any means. Nor has the issue of whether adults who stutter make any qualitative changes to their language behaviour to offset their reduced speech rate. The first issue has not been resolved because of a confusing literature, and the latter has not been resolved for want of research.

It is not at all clear how stuttering affects preschool children socially and cognitively, and this obviously requires much research. It is clear, though, that school-age children suffer considerably from the disorder, notably from teasing and bullying at school. Apart from the fact that adults who stutter cannot say as much as unaffected adults, there are two other clearly documented effects on this age group. The first is the occupational limitations that it poses, and the second is speech-related social anxiety, and often psychiatric illness. On balance, it appears that these effects seem more likely than not to occur in cases that come to a speech clinic.

References

Anderson, J.D. & Conture, E.G. (2000) Language abilities of children who stutter: A preliminary study. *Journal of Fluency Disorders, 25,* 283–304.

Andrews, G., Craig, A., Feyer, A.M., Hoddinott, S., Howie, P. & Neilson, M. (1983) Stuttering: A review of research findings and theories circa 1982. *Journal of Speech and Hearing Disorders, 48,* 226–246.

Andrews, G., Guitar, B. & Howie, P. (1980) Meta-analysis of the effects of stuttering treatment. *Journal of Speech and Hearing Disorders, 45,* 287–307.

Andrews, G. & Harris, M. (1964) *The Syndrome of Stuttering.* London: Heinemann.

Arndt, J. & Healy E.C. (2001) Concomitant disorders in school-age children who stutter. *Language, Speech and Hearing Services in the Schools, 32,* 68–78.

Bajaj, A. (2007) Analysis of oral narratives of children who stutter and their fluent peers: Kindergarten through second grade. *Clinical Linguistics and Phonetics, 21,* 227–245.

Blood, G.W. & Blood, I.M. (2004) Bullying in adolescents who stutter: Communicative competence and self-esteem. *Contemporary Issues in Communication Science and Disorders, 31,* 69–79.

Bloodstein, O. & Bernstein Ratner, N. (2008) *A Handbook on Stuttering,* 6th edition. Clifton Park, NY: Delmar.

Bonelli, P., Dixon, M., Ratner, N.B. & Onslow, M. (2000) Child and parent speech and language following the Lidcombe Program of Early Stuttering Intervention. *Clinical Linguistics and Phonetics, 14,* 427–446.

Buhr, A. & Zebrowski, P. (2009) Sentence position and syntactic complexity of stuttering in early childhood: A longitudinal study. *Journal of Fluency Disorders, 34,* 155–172.

Chang, S.E., Erickson, K.I., Ambrose, N.G., Hasegawa-Johnson, M.A. & Ludlow, C.L. (2008) Brain anatomy differences in childhood stuttering. *Neuroimage, 39,* 1333–1344.

Clark, D.M. & Wells, A. (1995) A cognitive model of social phobia. In R. Heimberg, M. Liebowitz, D.A. Hope & F.R. Schneier (Eds) *Social Phobia: Diagnosis, Assessment, and Treatment,* pp.69–93. New York: Guilford Press.

Conture, E. & Kelly, E. (1991) Young stutterers' nonspeech behaviors during stuttering. *Journal of Speech and Hearing Research, 34,* 1041–1056.

Cordes, A.K. & Ingham, R.J. (1994) The reliability of observational data: II. Issues in the identification and measurement of stuttering events. *Journal of Speech and Hearing Research, 37,* 279–294.

Craig, A.R. & Calver, P. (1991) Following up on treated stutterers: Studies of perceptions of job status. *Journal of Speech and Hearing Research, 34,* 279–284.

Crichton-Smith, I. (2002) Communicating in the real world: Accounts from people who stammer. *Journal of Fluency Disorders, 27,* 333–352.

Cykowski, M.D., Fox, P.T., Ingham, R.J., Ingham, J.C. & Robin, D.A. (2010) A study of the reproducibility and etiology of diffusion anisotropy differences in developmental stuttering: A potential role for impaired myelination. *Neuroimage, 52(4),* 1495–1504.

Davis, S., Howell, P. & Cooke, F. (2002) Sociodynamic relationships between children who stutter and their non-stuttering classmates. *Journal of Child Psychology and Psychiatry, 43,* 939–947.

Davis, S., Shisca, D. & Howell, P. (2007) Anxiety in speakers who persist and recover from stuttering. *Journal of Communication Disorders, 40,* 398–417.

DeNil, L. & Brutten, G. (1991) Speech-associated attitudes of stuttering and nonstuttering children. *Journal of Speech and Hearing Research, 34,* 60–66.

Dietrich, S. & Roaman, M.H. (2001) Physiologic arousal and predictions of anxiety by people who stutter. *Journal of Fluency Disorders, 26,* 207–225.

Ezrati-Vinacour, R., Platzky, R. & Yairi, E. (2001) The young child's awareness of stuttering-like disfluency. *Journal of Speech, Language, and Hearing Research, 44,* 368–380.

Franken, M.C.J., Kielstra-Van der Schalka, C.J. & Boelens, H. (2005) Experimental treatment of early stuttering: A preliminary study. *Journal of Fluency Disorders, 30,* 189–199.

Guralnick, M.J. Connor, R.T., Hammond, M.A., Gottman, J.M. & Kinnish, K. (1996) The peer relations of preschool children with communication disorders. *Child Development, 67,* 471–489.

Hadley, P.A. & Rice, M.L. (1991) Conversational responsiveness of speech- and language-impaired preschoolers. *Journal of Speech and Hearing Research, 34,* 1308–1317.

Harris, V., Onslow, M., Packman, A., Harrison, E. & Menzies, R. (2002) An experimental investigation of the impact of the Lidcombe Program on early stuttering. *Journal of Fluency Disorders, 27,* 203–214.

Harrison, E., Onslow, M. & Menzies, R. (2004) Dismantling the Lidcombe Program of Early Stuttering Intervention: Verbal contingencies for stuttering and clinical measurement. *International Journal of Language and Communication Disorders, 39,* 257–267.

Hayhow, R., Cray, A.M. & Enderby, P. (2002) Stammering and therapy views of people who stammer. *Journal of Fluency Disorders, 27,* 1–16.

Helgadottir, F.D., Menzies, R., Onslow, M., Packman, A. & O'Brian, S. (2009a) Online CBT I: Bridging the gap between Eliza and modern online CBT treatment packages. *Behaviour Change, 26,* 245–253.

Helgadottir, F.D., Menzies, R., Onslow, M., Packman, A. & O'Brian, S. (2009b) Online CBT II: A Phase I trial of a standalone, online CBT treatment program for social anxiety in stuttering. *Behaviour Change, 26,* 254–270.

Hugh-Jones, S. & Smith, P.K. (1999) Self-reports of short- and long-term effects of bullying on children who stammer. *British Journal of Educational Psychology, 69,* 141–158.

Hurst, M.I. & Cooper, E.B. (1983) Employer attitudes toward stuttering. *Journal of Fluency Disorders, 8,* 1–12.

Iverach, L., Menzies, R., Jones, M., O'Brian, S., Packman, A. & Onslow, M. (2010) Further development and validation of the Unhelpful Thoughts and Beliefs About Stuttering (UTBAS) scales: Relationship to anxiety and social phobia among adults who stutter. *International Journal of Language and Communication Disorders.* DOI 10.3109/13682822.2010.495369

Iverach, L., Menzies, R., O'Brian, S., Packman, A. & Onslow, M. (2011) Anxiety and stuttering: Continuing to explore a complex relationship. *American Journal of Speech Language Pathology.* DOI: 10.1044/1058-0360(2011/10-0091)

Johnson, W. (1933) An interpretation of stuttering. *Quarterly Journal of Speech, 19,* 70–77.

Jones, M., Onslow, M., Harrison, E. & Packman, A. (2000) Treating stuttering in young children: Predicting treatment time in the Lidcombe Program. *Journal of Speech, Language, and Hearing Research, 43*, 1440–1450.

Jones, M., Onslow, M., Packman, A. & Gebski, V. (2006) Guidelines for statistical analysis of percentage of syllables stuttered data. *Journal of Speech, Language, and Hearing Research, 49*, 867–878.

Jones, M., Onslow, M., Packman, A., Williams, S., Ormond, T., Schwarz, I. et al. (2005) Randomised controlled trial of the Lidcombe Program of Early Stuttering Intervention. *British Medical Journal, 331*, 659–661.

Klein, J.F. & Hood, S.B. (2004) The impact of stuttering on employment opportunities and job performance. *Journal of Fluency Disorders, 29*, 255–273.

Koushik, S., Shenker, R. & Onslow, M. (2009) Follow-up of 6–10-year-old stuttering children after Lidcombe Program treatment: A Phase I trial. *Journal of Fluency Disorders, 34*, 279–290.

Kully, D. & Boberg, E. (1988) An investigation of interclinic agreement in the identification of fluent and stuttered syllables. *Journal of Fluency Disorders, 13*, 309–318.

Kunz, R. & Oxman, A. (1998) The unpredictability paradox: Review of empirical comparisons of randomised and non-randomised clinical trials. *British Medical Journal, 317*, 1185–1190.

Langevin, M. (2009) The Peer Attitudes Toward Children who Stutter Scale: Reliability, known groups validity, and negativity of elementary school-age children's attitudes. *Journal of Fluency Disorders, 34*, 72–86.

Langevin, M., Bortnick, K., Hammer, T. & Wiebe, E. (1998) Teasing/bullying experienced by children who stutter: Toward development of a questionnaire. *Contemporary Issues in Communication Sciences and Disorders, 25*, 12–24.

Langevin, M. & Hagler, P. (2004) Development of a scale to measure peer attitudes toward children who stutter. In A.K. Bothe (Ed.) *Evidence-based Treatment of Stuttering: Empirical Issues and Clinical Implications.* Mahwah, NJ: Lawrence Erlbaum Associates.

Langevin, M., Kleitman, S., Packman, A. & Onslow, M. (2009) The Peer Attitudes Toward Children who Stutter (PATCS) Scale: An evaluation of validity, reliability, and the negativity of attitudes. *International Journal of Language and Communication Disorders, 44*, 352–368.

Langevin, M., Packman, A. & Onslow, M. (2009) Peer responses to stuttering in the preschool setting. *American Journal of Speech-Language Pathology, 18*, 264–278.

Lattermann, C., Euler, H.A. & Neumann, K.A. (2008) Randomized control trial to investigate the impact of the Lidcombe Program on early stuttering in German-speaking preschoolers. *Journal of Fluency Disorders, 33*, 52–65.

Lewis, C., Packman, A., Onslow, M., Simpson, J.A. & Jones, M. (2008) A Phase II trial of telehealth delivery of the Lidcombe Program of Early Stuttering Intervention. *American Journal of Speech Language Pathology, 17*, 139–149.

Lincoln, M., Onslow, M., Lewis, C. & Wilson, L. (1996) A clinical trial of an operant treatment for school-age children who stutter. *American Journal of Speech-Language Pathology, 5*, 73–85.

Mansson, H. (2000) Childhood stuttering: Incidence and development. *Journal of Fluency Disorders, 25*, 47–57.

McColl, T., Onslow, M., Packman, A. & Menzies, R.G. (2001) A cognitive behavioural intervention for social anxiety in adults who stutter. *Proceedings of the 2001 Speech Pathology Australia National Conference*, Melbourne, Australia.

Melnick, K.S. & Conture, K.G. (2000) Relationship of length and grammatical complexity to the systematic and nonsystematic speech errors and stuttering of children who stutter. *Journal of Fluency Disorders, 25*, 21–45.

Menzies, R., O'Brian, S. Onslow, M., Packman, A., St Clare, T. & Block, S. (2008) An experimental clinical trial of a cognitive behavior therapy package for chronic stuttering. *Journal of Speech, Language, and Hearing Research, 51*, 1451–1464.

Menzies, R.G., Onslow, M. & Packman, A. (1999) Anxiety and stuttering: Exploring a complex relationship. *American Journal of Speech-Language Pathology, 8*, 3–10.

Messenger, M., Onslow, M., Packman, A. & Menzies, R. (2004) Social anxiety in stuttering: Measuring negative social expectancies. *Journal of Fluency Disorders, 29*, 201–212.

Millard, S.K., Edwards, S. & Cook, F.M. (2009) Parent-child interaction therapy: Adding to the evidence. *International Journal of Speech-Language Pathology, 11*, 61–76.

Millard, S.K., Nicholas, A. & Cook, F.M. (2008) Is Parent-Child Interaction Therapy effective in reducing stuttering? *Journal of Speech, Language, and Hearing Research, 51*, 636–650.

Nippold, M. (1990) Concomitant speech and language disorders in stuttering disorders: A critique of the literature. *Journal of Speech and Hearing Disorders, 55*, 51–60.

Nippold, M.A. (2001) Phonological disorders and stuttering in children: What is the frequency of co-occurrence? *Clinical Linguistics and Phonetics, 15*, 219–228.

Nippold, M.A. (2004) Phonological and language disorders in children who stutter: Impact on treatment recommendations. *Clinical Linguistics and Phonetics, 18*, 145–159.

O'Brian, S., Jones, M., Onslow, M., Packman, A. & Menzies, R. (2011) Stuttering severity and educational achievement. *Journal of Fluency Disorders*. DOI: 10.1016/j.jfludis.2011.02.006

O'Brian, S., Packman, A., Onslow, M. & O'Brian, N. (2004) Measurement of stuttering in adults: Comparison of stuttering rate and severity scaling methods. *Journal of Speech, Language, and Hearing Research, 47*, 1081–1087.

Onslow, M., Andrews, C. & Lincoln, M. (1994) A control-experimental trial of an operant treatment for early stuttering. *Journal of Speech and Hearing Research, 37*, 1244–1259.

Onslow, M., Jones, M., Menzies, R., O'Brian, S. & Packman, A. (in press). Stuttering. In P. Sturmey & M. Hersen (Eds) *Handbook of Evidence-Based Practice in Clinical Psychology*. Hoboken, NJ: Wiley.

Onslow, M., Jones, M., O'Brian, S., Menzies, R. & Packman, A. (2008) Defining, identifying, and evaluating clinical trials of stuttering treatments: A tutorial for clinicians. *American Journal of Speech Language Pathology*, *17*, 401–415.

Onslow, M. & Menzies, R. (2010) Speech restructuring. Accepted entry in www.commonlanguagepsychotherapy.org

Onslow, M., Packman, A., Ukoumunne, O., Bavin, E., Block, S., Cini, E., Conway, L., Eadie, P., Wake, M. & Reilly, S. (2010) Predictors of natural recovery from early stuttering. Manuscript in preparation.

Packman, A. & Attanasio, J.S. (2004) *Theoretical Issues in Stuttering*. London: Taylor & Francis.

Packman, A., Hand, L., Cream, A. & Onslow, M. (2001) An investigation of linguistic factors in the rhythm effect in stuttering. *Proceedings of the 4th International Speech Motor Conference*, Nijmegen, The Netherlands.

Packman, A., Onslow, M. & Attanasio, J. (2003) The timing of early intervention with the Lidcombe Program. In M. Onslow, A. Packman & E. Harrison (Eds) *The Lidcombe Program of Early Stuttering Intervention: A Clinician's Guide*. Austin, TX: Pro-Ed.

Reichels, C., Buhr, A., Conture, E. & Ntourou, K. (2010) Utterance complexity and stuttering on function words in preschool-age children who stutter. *Journal of Fluency Disorders*, *34*, 314–331.

Reilly, S., Onslow, M., Packman, A., Wake, M., Bavin, E.L., Prior, M. et al. (2009) Predicting stuttering onset by the age of 3 years: A prospective, community cohort study. *Pediatrics*, *123*, 270–277.

Rousseau, I., Packman, A., Onslow, M., Harrison, E. & Jones, M.I. (2007) An investigation of language and phonological development and the responsiveness of preschool age children to the Lidcombe Program. *Journal of Communication Disorders*, *40*, 382–397.

Ruben, R. (2000) Redefining the survival of the fittest: Communication disorders in the 21st century. *The Laryngoscope*, *110*, 241–245.

Ryan, B. (1992) Articulation, language, rate, and fluency characteristics of stuttering and nonstuttering children. *Journal of Speech and Hearing Research*, *35*, 333–342.

Silverman, S. & Ratner, N.B. (2002) Measuring lexical diversity in children who stutter: Application of *vocd*. *Journal of Fluency Disorders*, *27*, 289–304.

Spencer, E., Packman, A., Onslow, M. & Ferguson, A. (2005) A preliminary investigation of the impact of stuttering on language use. *Clinical Linguistics and Phonetics*, *19*, 191–201.

Spencer, E., Packman, A., Onslow, M. & Ferguson, A. (2009) The effect of stuttering on communication: A preliminary investigation. *Clinical Linguistics and Phonetics*, *23*, 473–488.

St Clare, T., Menzies, R., Onslow, M., Packman, A., Thompson, R. & Block, S. (2009) Unhelpful thoughts and beliefs linked to social anxiety in stuttering: Development of a measure. *International Journal of Language and Communication Disorders*, *44*, 338–351.

Trajkovski, N., Andrews, C., Onslow, M., Packman, A., O'Brian, S. & Menzies, R. (2009) Using syllable-timed speech to treat preschool children who stutter: A multiple baseline experiment. *Journal of Fluency Disorders, 34*, 1–10.

Trajkovski, N., Andrews, C., O'Brian, S., Onslow, M. & Packman, A. (2006) Treating stuttering in a preschool child with syllable timed speech: A case report. *Behaviour Change, 23*, 270–277.

Trajkovski, N., Andrews, C., Onslow, M., O'Brian, S., Packman, A. & Menzies, R. (in press) A Phase II trial of the Westmead Program: Syllable-timed speech treatment for preschool children who stutter. *International Journal of Speech-Language Pathology.*

Vanryckeghem, M. & Brutten, G.J. (1997) The speech-associated attitude of children who do and do not stutter and the differential effect of age. *American Journal of Speech-Language Pathology, 6*, 67–73.

Vanryckeghem, M., Brutten, G.J. & Hernandez, L.M. (2005) A comparative investigation of the speech-associated attitude of preschool and kindergarten children who do and do not stutter. *Journal of Fluency Disorders, 30*, 307–318.

Watkins, R.V. & Yairi, E. (1997) Language production abilities of children whose stuttering persisted or recovered. *Journal of Speech, Language, and Hearing Research, 40*, 385–399.

Watkins, R.V., Yairi, E. & Ambrose, N.G. (1999) Early childhood stuttering III: Initial status of expressive language abilities. *Journal of Speech, Language, and Hearing Research, 42*, 1125–1135.

Wohlert, A.B. & Smith, A. (2002) Developmental change in variability of lip muscle activity in speech. *Journal of Speech, Language, and Hearing Research, 45*, 1077–1087.

Wyatt, G.L. (1969) *Language, Learning and Communication Disorders in Children.* New York: The Free Press.

Yaruss, J.S., Quesal, R.W., Reeves, L., Molt, L.F., Kluetz, B., Caruso, A.J. et al. (2002) Speech treatment and support group experiences of people who participate in the National Stuttering Association. *Journal of Fluency Disorders, 27*, 115–134.

Yairi, E. (1983) The onset of stuttering in two- and three-year-old children: A preliminary report. *Journal of Speech and Hearing Disorders, 48*, 171–177.

Yairi, E. (1997) Disfluency characteristics of childhood stuttering. In R.F. Curlee & G.M. Siegel (Eds) *Nature and Treatment of Stuttering: New Directions,* 2nd edition. pp.49–78. Boston: Allyn & Bacon.

Yairi, E. & Ambrose, N. (1992) A longitudinal study of stuttering in children: A preliminary report. *Journal of Speech and Hearing Research, 35*, 755–760.

Yairi, E. & Ambrose, N. (1999) Early childhood stuttering I: Persistency and recovery rates. *Journal of Speech, Language, and Hearing Research, 5*, 1097–1112.

Yairi, E. & Ambrose, N.G. (2005) *Early Childhood Stuttering for Clinicians by Clinicians.* Austin, TX.: Pro-Ed.

Yairi, E., Ambrose, N. & Niermann, R. (1993) The early months of stuttering: A developmental study. *Journal of Speech and Hearing Research, 36*, 521–528.

Yairi, E. & Lewis, B. (1984) Disfluencies at the onset of stuttering. *Journal of Speech and Hearing Research, 27*, 154–159.

7 Deafness, Language and Communication

Ros Herman and Gary Morgan
City University London, UK

Introduction

Deafness may be present from birth or acquired[1] at any stage in the lifespan. This chapter will focus solely on the developmental communication issues surrounding individuals who are deaf from birth, or shortly thereafter.

Figures for the UK suggest that 2 in 1000 live births experience hearing impairment or 12,000 children per annum will have problems by the age of 7 or 8. Fifty per cent of hearing losses are bilateral and identified by 4–6 weeks of age, and families generally enter into intervention programmes between 8 and 20 weeks of age. Later screening relies on parental and professional concern. In London, ethnicity increases the incidence two- to threefold to around 4–12 per 1000. The prevalence is eight times higher in graduates of NICU/PICU, 40% of whom have some other systemic disorder.

Although the vast majority of deaf children have no intrinsic impairment in their language learning abilities (Parker & Rose, 1990; although see Mason et al., 2010 for the co-existence of specific language impairment in a minority of deaf children), the presence of a severe or profound degree of sensorineural hearing loss, experienced by approximately one third of prelingually deaf children (Davis et al., 1997), presents significant challenges to the perception and production of spoken language. This, in turn, has potentially far-reaching consequences for interaction with hearing people, educational attainment and

---

1 We do not propose to cover issues surrounding deafness acquired in adulthood, since communication is established by this stage in life and the role of communication intervention is less defined. This is not to deny the significant impact of acquired deafness on an individual's lifestyle: although much can be done in terms of amplification, assistive technology and use of hearing tactics, for many the psychosocial consequences of acquired deafness remain challenging (Kerr & Cowie, 1997).

social-cognitive development (Schick, de Villiers, de Villiers & Hoffmeister, 2007).

The use of the term 'deaf' to denote a group defined by their audiological profile is in the main widely accepted. For many within the Deaf community who use sign language (e.g. British Sign Language, BSL), the use of 'hearing impairment' carries negative connotations, as it defines a group of people primarily through the medical condition of deafness. An alternative viewpoint proposes use of the word 'Deaf' (written with an initial capital) to indicate affiliation to Deaf culture and the use of sign language (see Padden & Humphries, 1988, 2005; Lane, Hoffmeister & Bahan, 2000; Ladd, 2003, for further accounts of Deaf culture). Unlike the medical perspective, this perspective on 'culturally' Deaf people views deafness more positively, as a minority cultural and linguistic group rather than as a disabled group (Robinson & Adam, 2003). While this may seem to be a philosophical question, there are in fact significant consequences for communication development based on how deafness is defined by parents of deaf children and for professionals. While not denying the need for intervention for children who are born deaf, taking a more positive perspective on deafness can lead to better outcomes in terms of self-esteem and aspiration in deaf children and their families. An awareness of such terminology and of political divisions within the field of deafness relating to the use of signing is key for professionals working in this area. Having clarified our terms, for convenience, we will henceforth use the term 'deaf' to encapsulate both audiologically deaf and culturally Deaf individuals.

Important considerations in any discussion of people who are born deaf include the following: parental hearing status; mode of communication; co-morbidity of additional disabilities; age at which deafness was first identified; and benefit obtained from amplification. These are now discussed in turn.

Deaf children from deaf families represent a small minority of the deaf population (less than 10%; Mitchell & Karchmer, 2004). Parental hearing status is likely to impact on a number of areas, including principally a deaf child's preferred mode of communication, literacy skills and their social and emotional development. These children are likely to be raised in a home environment where sign language is used from birth. Sign languages have the same capabilities as any human language and are acquired naturally by children in deaf families, following the same broad trajectory as children acquiring any other language. Indeed, research on sign language acquisition among native signers has drawn parallels with hearing children exposed to a spoken language in terms of ages and stages of development (Mayberry & Squires, 2006; Morgan & Woll, 2002; Newport & Meier, 1985; Schick, 2003). The early establishment of a first language in sign among children in deaf families conveys advantages for the acquisition of a second language in the written form (Stuckless & Birch, 1966; Chamberlain & Mayberry, 2000), with obvious consequences for educational attainment. However, to date there is a lack of systematic evidence that for the majority of deaf children (born to hearing parents) sign bilingualism leads to better educational attainment (Spencer & Marschark, 2006).

Another area of difference for children born into deaf families is that deafness is accepted, since it is perceived to be the norm and this, along with easy communication within the home, sets the scene for a positive 'socialisation climate' (Meadow, 2005). Natural interaction between mother and child has positive benefits for a range of cognitive and socio-emotional developments (e.g. Moeller & Schick, 2006; Schick et al., 2007). Although there may still be issues relating to communicating with hearing speaking individuals, the availability of deaf role models can offer support in this area.

By contrast, deaf children of hearing parents will generally be exposed to spoken language, since this is the language used within the home. Although sign language may also be used, deaf children within hearing families rarely have early or optimal exposure to sign language since many hearing parents and professionals have poorly developed sign language skills (Calderon & Greenberg, 2000). A move towards bilingual education for deaf children in recent years has led to improvements in some areas, with deaf adults going into the homes shortly after identification of deafness to teach families sign language and act as language role models and mentors (Joint Committee on Infant Hearing, 2007; Swanwick & Gregory, 2007). An important consideration when working with people who are deaf is the likely co-morbidity of other conditions. It is estimated that up to 40% of deaf children have additional disabilities (McCracken, 2010), ranging from visual impairments to learning disabilities. Clearly, such conditions will compound the impact on language development.

Finally, within the population of deaf people is a further divide relating to changes in technology, which have had a significant impact on the lives of deaf people. For adults and children currently in the latter stages of their education or beyond, identification of deafness was typically late and amplification technology often inadequate, with major consequences for the development of spoken communication. Recent years have seen the introduction of newborn hearing screening (NHS Newborn Hearing Screening Programme, 2011; Bamford et al., 2009) and major developments in amplification technology, in particular the use of cochlear implants with younger children. Together, these offer better outcomes for deaf children because of improved access to spoken language and the opportunity for earlier intervention (Ackley & Decker, 2006), although research on early identified children is still in its infancy. It is crucial that future research evaluating the success of cochlear implants in young deaf children is not blinkered in its focus on speech to the exclusion of general social and pragmatic aspects of communicative development.

The remainder of this chapter seeks to review research and clinical evidence concerning the impact of deafness among deaf children and adults (in the main) from hearing families and existing interventions under the following headings: early communication skills; intelligible speech; communication with hearing people; and mental health issues. In addition, we include a brief account of the impact on literacy and education.

Impact of deafness on early communication skills and social-cognitive development

Marschark (2000) explains that those deaf children who are most competent socially tend to be those who actively participate in linguistic interactions with their parents from an early age. Good parent–child interaction allows deaf children to gain social knowledge, cognitive and problem-solving strategies, information about self and others, and a sense of being part of the environment (Marschark, 1993). Spencer, Erting and Marschark (2000) conclude that there is a need to explicitly focus on teaching socio-emotional skills to deaf children and to emphasize, beginning in early intervention, the powerful role parents and professionals can play in promoting social competence.

The study of hearing and deaf children's language and communicative development is inextricably linked with the overarching growth in their social cognitive skills. Children's expressive language (their first words) emerges from previous non-verbal interaction with adults, which in part fosters children's visual attention, turn-taking, labelling and language comprehension skills. All of this involves some ability on the part of the child to 'mindread' (Nurmsoo & Bloom, 2008; Liebal, Behne, Carpenter & Tomasello, 2009).

The issue of how deaf children of hearing parents enter into the mindreading game is complex. Several studies have demonstrated that deaf children of hearing parents as old as 10 years of age have persistent delays on Theory of

Mind tasks (e.g. Schick et al., 2007; Morgan & Kegl, 2006) while deaf children of deaf parents score age-appropriately on the same tasks (Woolfe, Want & Siegal, 2002). The origin of these delays can be traced back to the very early interaction deaf infants' experience with hearing parents. Part of this early atypical development is linked with difficulties in establishing good joint attention (Harris & Chasin, 2005). These missed interactions arise because hearing parents are not aware of how to adapt their communication for a child that needs to share his visual attention between the speaker (in order to know that communication is taking place and to receive speech-reading and signing/gestural cues) and the object being labelled. This fundamental difficulty in establishing connected communication leads to vocabulary learning delays and, perhaps more significantly, potential problems with interpreting intentional communication and the mindreading element of interpersonal communication. Even children whose hearing parents start using sign language when their child is as young as 2 years of age have been shown to have difficulty with standard Theory of Mind tasks compared to hearing children. In a longitudinal study of deaf children of hearing parents, Falkman, Roos and Hjelmquist (2007) found that over a two-year period there were no changes in children's low performance on standard Theory of Mind tasks, while hearing peers already performed at ceiling on the first testing occasion.

Currently there are very few studies of parent–child interaction in young deaf children with cochlear implants. What has been published paints a mixed picture. When the implant occurs early, one study found that children do not seem to show delays in Theory of Mind performance (Remmel & Peters, 2009), contrary to previous results from children implanted at a later age (Peterson, 2009). From only two studies it is not possible to draw any conclusions, but one thing that came out of both studies was that it was not age at implantation that was the most important factor in Theory of Mind performance but the time since implantation. This suggests that the more time a deaf child has to engage in successful and connected communication with parents around rich and abstract conversation topics, the better (Meristo, Hjelmquist & Morgan, in press).

There is now a growing body of knowledge about how early communication fosters later Theory of Mind development (e.g. Taumoepeau & Ruffman, 2008). This, coupled with what we observe as the significant differences in how hearing mothers talk and interact with their hearing or deaf toddlers (Moeller & Schick, 2006), can be used to design interventions aimed at effective social cognitive outcomes. We are now at a stage where an intervention aimed at early connected conversations and mental state talk in hearing mother–deaf child dyads can be attempted. It may be possible to adapt successful Theory of Mind training studies with typically developing individuals (e.g. Hale and Tager-Flusberg, 2003) for families with deaf children.

Impact of deafness on intelligible speech

Of relevance to today's deaf adults are the findings of numerous research studies completed a number of years ago which showed that, despite amplification and speech training, the speech of individuals with severe to profound deafness was on average only 20% intelligible (Ertmer, 2010). This is because the typical audiological configuration of sensorineural deafness impacts significantly on the perception and, hence, the production of spoken language.[2]

In general, because perception precedes production (Fletcher, Dagenais & Critz-Crosby, 1991), it follows that speech sounds that are more difficult to access auditorily are also more difficult to produce. Many studies have identified common features of the speech of deaf people (e.g. Hudgins and Numbers, 1942; Monsen, 1974) and find consonants to be affected more than vowels (Geffner & Rothman Freeman, 1980). Errors include omissions of word-final consonants (Subtelny, 1977); fronting/backing errors (Martin, Herman, Hirson & Pring, 2007); fricatives realized as plosives (Bernhardt, Gick, Bacsfalvi & Ashdown, 2003) and voicing errors (Gold, 1980; Fletcher et al., 1991). Reduction of consonant clusters and deletion of unstressed syllables have also been reported (Bernhardt et al., 2003). Whereas some of these errors are similar to those found in typically developing young hearing children, others are not, e.g. where consonants that are less visible on the lips are replaced by other sounds, such as glottal stops (Pantelemidou, Herman & Thomas, 2003).

Suprasegmental aspects of speech may also be affected among deaf speakers: voice quality may be compromised by excess laryngeal tension (Wirz, 2001); resonance may be hypernasal, hyponasal, mixed or cul-de-sac (Boone, 1966; Boone & McFarlane, 2000); deaf speakers may adopt a higher fundamental frequency compared to hearing speakers (Gilbert & Campbell, 1980) and exhibit

---

2   An understanding of speech acoustics and speech perception by deaf children and adults is essential to speech and language therapists who work in this area (see Hazan (2001) for further information).

difficulties with the use of intonation (Monsen, 1979; Gold, 1980; O'Halpin, 2001; Bernhardt et al., 2003); rate and rhythm of speech may be affected by the use of lengthened syllables, longer pauses between words and shortened voiced segments (Bernhardt et al., 2003).

More recently, studies have examined changes in speech intelligibility and speech perception as a result of cochlear implantation (Svirsky et al., 2000). Indeed, the advent of cochlear implantation in increasingly younger children has had a major impact on the potential for intelligible speech (Moeller et al., 2007). Children who have implants early may exhibit intelligible speech by the third year post-cochlear implantation and age-appropriate speech and language skills after 5 (Allen, Nikolopoulos, Tait & O'Donoghue, 1998, Nicholas & Geers, 2006; Peng, Spencer & Tomblin, 2004), although some variability in performance is also acknowledged (Nicholas & Geers, 2006).

However, not all deaf children are equally successful following cochlear implantation and others are simply not eligible for cochlear implants; hence, speech intelligibility continues to be a target for intervention. Interventions traditionally emphasize the use of residual hearing with amplification to develop auditory skills and consequently speech production skills (e.g. Erber, 1982; Hogan et al., 2008). In addition, there is some evidence that working on speech production can lead to changes in speech perception (Novelli-Olmsted & Ling, 1984; Massaro & Light, 2004).

In some cases, visual feedback has been used to develop speech production skills with deaf clients. Systems that use hand signals to provide information about the phonological features of speech include Cued Articulation (Passy, 1990) and Cued Speech (Cornett, 1967). There has been very little research into the use of Cued Articulation with deaf children (but see Fordham, 2003). Although the same is true for Cued Speech in the UK, there is a more extensive literature on the benefits of this method in other countries, suggesting its use conveys significant advantages for spoken language (Vieu et al., 1998), speechreading (Gregory, 1987), reading (Alegria, Dejean, Capouillez & Leybaert, 1990) and spelling (Leybaert & Charlier, 1996).

Computer-based visual displays such as electropalatography (EPG) have also been used to provide information about specific phonemes that are difficult to perceive auditorily and visually (Parsloe, 1988; Pantelemidou et al., 2003; Martin et al., 2007). Interestingly, Parsloe (1998) found that following an intervention programme using EPG to teach a profoundly deaf child to produce certain phonemes, the child also showed improvements in his speech perception skills. While speech is undeniably important for deaf children we repeat that intervention should not focus exclusively on this aspect to the expense of general social and pragmatic aspects of communicative development.

Impact of deafness on communication with hearing people

People who are born deaf experience much discrimination and lack of understanding in society at large, whether they communicate using spoken or sign language (Higgins, 1980). This may be attributed to negative attitudes towards people who have communication difficulties (Morgan, Herman & Woll, 2002) as well as the fact that profoundly deaf signers have considerable difficulty in communicating with hearing people (Bench, 1992; Gagne, Stelmacovich & Yovetich, 1991).

Speech that is of limited intelligibility has consequences for deaf children's interactions with others. Roberts and Rickards (1994) showed that deaf children in mainstream schooling were more likely to have hearing friends than those in specialist schooling, and that children with less severe hearing loss had more hearing friends than children with more severe hearing loss. However, placing a child who is deaf in a mainstream setting does not ensure that the child will be integrated (Antia & Kreimeyer, 1992). Among the reasons given for social segregation in integrated preschool settings were the low communicative competences of children who were deaf or hard of hearing (Lederberg, 1991; Nunes, Pretzlik & Olsson, 2001) and their limited understanding of how others think and feel (Bat-Chava, Martin & Kosciw, 2005). Hearing children who were friends with deaf peers reported friendships to involve prosocial functions (Nunes et al., 2001). Where communication is perceived as presenting an obstacle to friendship, deaf children are likely to be neglected (although not necessarily disliked) by their peers, and to feel correspondingly isolated (Nunes et al., 2001).

Easy communication between deaf and hearing children is important for friendships and also for successful learning in class. Stinson and Antia (1999) highlight barriers to classroom participation for deaf children. They include: fast rate of discussion; rapid turn-taking; frequent changes of topic; inclusion of many speakers in discussions; and instances where several students speak concurrently leading to unmanageable levels of noise. Overcoming these barriers requires skilled and sensitive management. Despite in-service training for teachers in mainstream schools who have deaf children in their class, there is no evaluation of whether this is adequate (Powers, 2002). Indeed, deaf students have reported that mainstream teachers lack deaf awareness (NDCS, 2001).

Many of the skills deaf children need to interact successfully with hearing peers are language based. In addition to speech intelligibility issues referred to above, prelingually deaf children and adults typically display poor mastery of English vocabulary and syntax and find learning the rules of social communication challenging (Crocker & Edwards, 2004). As most hearing people cannot sign, this frequently leads to the emergence of a 'shared handicap of communication' between deaf and hearing partners (Bouvet, 1990), causing both to be unsure and ineffective at communicating with each other. Common pragmatic difficulties identified by researchers include: failure by deaf children and adults to clarify misunderstandings, solve disagreements or lead conversations (Stinson, Liu, Saur & Long, 1996); inability to ask questions (Lederberg & Everhart, 2000; Nicholas & Geers, 2003) and difficulties explaining that they do not understand or in seeking clarification (Bench, 1992; Silvestre, Ramspott & Pareto, 2007; Wood, Wood, Griffiths & Howarth, 1986; Jeanes, Nienhuys & Rickards, 2000).

A compounding factor is that deaf children are not always made aware of the lack of clarity of their own communication. Often, a hearing parent or teacher will fail to signal the ineffectiveness of a message or may themselves repair it for the child (Beazley, 1992; Brackett, 1983; Wood et al., 1986), thereby denying deaf children the chance to develop the effectiveness of their interactions or take responsibility for their own communication. Reduced exposure to naturalistic, meaningful conversations (Akamatsu & Musselman, 1998; Carney & Moeller, 1998) and difficulty accessing incidental learning account for why these patterns of difficulties develop. Reduced quality and quantity of interactions means fewer opportunities for these behaviours to be modelled and fewer opportunities for the deaf child to apply the behaviours in natural settings (Brackett, 1983; Carney & Moeller, 1998; Jeanes et al., 2000).

Traditionally, speech and language therapy with deaf clients has focused on improving auditory perception, speechreading, speech production, vocal characteristics and understanding and use of language (spoken and, more recently, sign languages) (Carney & Moeller, 1998; Bench, 1992). Less consideration has been given to the everyday communication experiences of deaf children. Bench (1992) points out that, despite the large literature on the limited pragmatic abilities of many deaf people, little of it relates to intervention directed at functional communication skills. In their review of treatment efficacy in children with hearing loss, Carney and Moeller (1998) mention no studies that focus on either functional communication skills or social interaction. Given the potential implications of a deaf person's inability to interact with the hearing world, the need to develop therapy techniques to address this area becomes apparent.

A recent intervention developed by Threadgill and Schamroth (Schamroth & Threadgill, 2007) currently in use in the UK is the *smiLE* approach (Strategies and Measurable Interaction in Live English). This intervention focuses on developing deaf people's communication skills in real communication situations. The therapy involves filming deaf clients in interactions with hearing people and using the film to help them evaluate and consequently improve their own skills in group sessions, using role play and group feedback. Clients are taught a hierarchy of strategies to use to support their communication, ranging from improved speech intelligibility to gesture and written language. Two small-scale studies have shown this approach to be successful in developing the functional communication skills of deaf children (Alton, 2008) and young adults (Lawlor, 2009) in live interactions with hearing people. Further research is needed to investigate the long-term benefits and generalization of new skills.

Impact of deafness on educational achievement

Studies have shown that deaf children's reading develops at a slower rate and that they make approximately a third of the reading progress each school year when compared with their hearing peers (e.g. Allen, 1986; Kyle & Harris, 2010; Trybus & Karchmer, 1977). As a result, the severity of their reading delay increases as they progress through schooling, culminating in the average deaf school leaver having a reading age equivalent to that of a 9-year-old hearing child (e.g. Conrad, 1979; DiFrancesca, 1972; Wauters, Agnes, Tellings, van Bon & Mak, 2007). Higher levels of reading achievement have been reported in some studies of deaf children with cochlear implants (see Marschark, Rhoten & Fabich, 2007) and also in studies with selective populations of orally educated deaf children (e.g. Daneman, Nemeth, Stainton & Huelsmann, 1995; Gravenstede & Roy, 2009; Lewis, 1996). The main reason that deaf children experience such severe problems with learning to read is that written English is essentially derived from spoken English, to which deaf children typically have limited access. This can adversely affect the development of both 'bottom up' skills involved in reading, such as phonological and syntactical knowledge, and also 'top down' skills such as vocabulary, language and world knowledge (King & Quigley, 1985).

Deaf children are frequently reported to have weaker phonological skills in comparison with hearing peers, both in terms of phonological awareness and phonological coding (e.g. Harris & Beech, 1998; Leybaert & Alegria, 1993; Waters & Doehring, 1990). Despite lower levels of ability, there is some evidence that phonological skills are predictive of reading achievement in deaf children (Campbell & Wright, 1988; Dyer, McSweeney, Szczerbinski & Green, 2003; Harris & Beech, 1998). Phonic-based interventions have had some success in improving reading levels of poor deaf readers (Trezek & Malmegren, 2005; Trezek & Wang, 2006). These findings fit in with other recent evidence indicating that, for deaf and hearing children alike, phonological knowledge of the written language is essential if they are to become competent readers (e.g. Mayer, 2008). This phonological knowledge relies on the development of phonological representations that Leybaert (2005) argued are mainly based on visual (lip-reading, Cued Speech, finger-spelling and alphabetic script) rather than acoustic phonology.

Unfortunately, the consequences of poor literacy are that many deaf children leave school with fewer qualifications than their hearing peers (Gregory, Powers & Thoutenhoofd, 1998); deaf adults are four times more likely to be unemployed and, of those working, are three times more likely than hearing adults to be earning a lower wage (RNID, 2002).

Impact of deafness on mental health

Poor communication has consequences for emotional learning and mental wellbeing (Crocker & Edwards, 2004; Hindley, 2000). Deaf people who communicate poorly in the hearing world are more likely to be socially isolated (Bain, Scott & Steinberg, 2004; Steinberg, Sullivan & Loew, 1998), are at greater risk for psychological distress (Marschark, 1993) and have a greater overall prevalence of mental illness than the general population (Crocker & Edwards, 2004; Hindley, 2000).

Marschark (1993) notes that many social-emotional problems of deaf children and adults are rooted in early socialization and intertwined with impairments in hearing and language competence. While there is nothing inherent in a hearing deficit that causes social immaturity or inadequacy, there is evidence indicating that deaf children are relatively passive and less socially mature than their hearing peers (Carney & Moeller, 1998; Lemanek, Williamson, Gresham & Jensen, 1986; Meadow, 1980; White, 1982). This can often be related to distortions of parent–child interaction, limited early communication, reduced access to incidental learning and deprivation of social experiences (Hindley, 2000).

As described previously, deaf children of hearing parents have been shown to demonstrate significant delays in recognizing and labelling emotional states in themselves and others (abilities subsumed under the term Theory of Mind). Hindley (2004) stresses the importance of encouraging early conversation about thoughts and feelings to develop children's awareness of people's thoughts (metacognition). Because many deaf children miss out on these kinds of conversation and are vulnerable to delays in metacognition, Theory of Mind development and emotional functioning, this will put them at risk for emotional/social and behavioural problems in later life.

Some approaches have been developed to address emotional wellbeing, including the PATHS curriculum (Promoting Alternative Thinking Strategies) and the innovative 'Life and Deaf' project. PATHS seeks to develop deaf children's emotional literacy by teaching emotional vocabulary, social skills and improving self-confidence in problem-solving social situation issues. PATHS was evaluated by Greenberg and Kusche (1998) using primary-aged deaf schoolchildren and found to have lasting benefits. Another programme, 'Life and Deaf', was developed by UK speech and language therapists to encourage children to explore their identity through poetry in written English and BSL and aims in addition to develop their communication skills and self-esteem, although no formal evaluation has to date been carried out.

Conclusions

It is increasingly evident that early identification of deafness before the age of 6 months brings significantly better speech and language outcomes than when identification occurs beyond this age (Yoshinaga-Itano, 2009). There have also been encouraging reports in relation to early use of cochlear implants, although Woll (2008) highlights the need for long-term studies of the educational, communication and mental health outcomes for implanted and unimplanted deaf children. For older children and adults who have missed out on recent developments, the situation remains unchanged. However, while general improvements can be anticipated in future generations of deaf children, it seems likely that a significant number of deaf children will continue to exhibit speech and language difficulties, with consequences for communication and social relationships with hearing children, for mental health, for educational attainment and literacy and for employment.

There is surprisingly little research that seeks to evaluate specific communication interventions with deaf people. In part, this is because of the heterogeneity that exists among deaf people, making group studies extremely challenging. Nevertheless, much can be learned from series of carefully conducted single case studies, as in many other areas of speech and language therapy. Much of current clinical practice with deaf people draws on interventions developed with other client groups in mind. Research that seeks to evaluate specific interventions with deaf people represents a key area for future developments in this field.

References

Ackley, R.S. & Decker, T.N. (2006) Audiological advancement in the acquisition of spoken language in deaf children. In P.E. Spencer & M. Marschark (Eds) *Advances in the Spoken Language Development of Deaf and Hard-of-Hearing Children*, pp.64–84. New York: Oxford University Press.

Akamatsu, C. & Musselman, C. (1998) Development and use of conversational proficiency interview with deaf adolescents. In M. Marschark and M.D. Clark (Eds) *Psychological Perspectives on Deafness*, vol. 2, pp.265–295. Mahwah, NJ: Lawrence Erlbaum.

Alegria, J., Dejean, K., Capouillez, J. & Leybaert, J. (1990) Role played by Cued Speech in the identification of written words encountered for the first time by deaf children. *Cued Speech Journal*, 4, 4–9.

Allen, M.C., Nikolopoulos, T.P., Tait, M. & O'Donoghue, G.M. (1998) Speech intelligibility in children after cochlear implantation. *American Journal of Otology*, 19, 742–746.

Allen, T.E. (1986) Patterns of academic achievement among hearing impaired students: 1974 and 1983. In A.N. Schildroth & M.A. Karchmer (Eds) *Deaf Children in America*, pp.161–206. San Diego, CA: College-Hill Press.

Alton, S. (2008) Use and generalisation of communication skills learnt in Live English (smiLE) speech and language therapy by deaf primary school pupils. Unpublished MSc dissertation, City University London.

Antia, S.D. & Kreimeyer, K.H. (1992) Social competence for young children with hearing impairments. In S.L. Odom, S.R. McConnel & M.A. McEvoy (Eds) *Social Competence of Young Children with Disabilities*, pp.135–164. Baltimore: Paul H. Brookes.

Bain, L., Scott, S. & Steinberg, A. (2004) Socialisation experiences and coping strategies of adults raised using spoken language. *Journal of Deaf Studies and Deaf Education, 9(1)*, 120–128.

Bamford, J., Carr, G., Davis, A., Gascon-Ramos, M., Lea, R., McCracken, W., Pattison, E., Woll, B., Woolfe, T. & Young, A. (2009) *Positive support in the lives of deaf children and their families*. Final Report to the Big Lottery Fund.

Bat-Chava, Y., Martin, D. & Kosciw, J.G. (2005) Longitudinal improvements in communication and socialization of deaf children with cochlear implants and hearing aids: Evidence from parental reports. *Journal of Child Psychology and Psychiatry, 46(12)*, 1287–1296.

Beazley, S. (1992) Social skills group work with deaf people. In M. Fawcus (Ed.) *Group Encounters in Speech and Language Therapy*, pp.63-75. Kibworth: Far Communications Ltd.

Bench, R.J. (1992) *Communication Skills in Hearing Impaired Children*. London: Whurr Publishers Ltd.

Bernhardt, B., Gick, B., Bacsfalvi, P. & Ashdown, J. (2003) Speech habilitation of hard of hearing adolescents using electropalatography and ultrasound as evaluated by trained listeners. *Clinical Linguistics and Phonetics, 17*, 199–216.

Boone, D.R. (1966) Modification of the voices of deaf children. *Volta Review, 68*, 686–692.

Boone, D.A. & McFarlane, S.C. (2000) *The Voice and Voice Therapy*, 6th edition. Boston: Allyn and Bacon.

Bouvet, D. (1990). *The Path to Language: Bilingual Education for Deaf Children*. Clevedon: Multilingual Matters.

Brackett, D. (1983) Group communication strategies for the hearing-impaired. *Volta Review, 85(5)*, 16–28.

Calderon, R. & Greenberg, M.T. (2000) Challenges to parents and professionals in promoting socioemotional development in deaf children. In P.E. Spencer, C.J. Erting & M. Marschark (Eds) *The Deaf Child in the Family and at School*, pp.167–180. Mahwah, N.J.: Lawrence Erlbaum Associates.

Campbell, R. & Wright, H. (1990) Deafness and immediate memory for pictures: Dissociations between 'inner speech' and the 'inner ear'? *Journal of Experimental Child Psychology, 50*, 259–286.

Carney, A.E. & Moeller, M.P. (1998) Treatment efficacy: Hearing loss in children. *Journal of Speech, Language, and Hearing Research, 41*, S61–S84.

Chamberlain, C. & Mayberry, R.I. (2000) Theorizing about the relationship between ASL and reading. In C. Chamberlain, J. Morford & R.I. Mayberry (Eds) *Language Acquisition by Eye*, pp.221–260. Mahwah, NJ: Lawrence Erlbaum and Associates.

Conrad, R. (1979) *The Deaf School Child*. London: Harper Row.

Cornett, R.O. (1967) Cued speech. *American Annals of the Deaf, 112(3)*, 13.

Crocker, S. & Edwards, L. (2004) Deafness and additional difficulties. In S. Austen & S. Crocker (Eds) *Deafness in Mind*, pp.252–269. London: Whurr Publishers Ltd.

Daneman, M., Nemeth, S., Stainton, M. & Huelsmann, K. (1995) Working memory as a predictor of reading achievement in orally educated hearing-impaired children. *Volta Review, 97*, 225–241.

Dammeyer, J. (2010) Psychosocial development in a Danish population of children with cochlear implants and deaf and hard-of-hearing children. *Journal of Deaf Studies and Deaf Education, 15(1)*, 50–58.

Davis, A., Bamford, J., Wilson, I., Ramkalawan, T., Forshaw, M. & Wright, S. (1997) A critical review of the role of neonatal hearing screening in the detection of congenital hearing impairment. *Health Technology Assessment, 1(10)*.

DiFrancesca, S. (1972) Academic achievement test results of a national testing program for hearing impaired students – U.S. Spring (Series D, No 9). Washington, DC: Gallaudet College, Office of Demographic Studies.

Dyer, A., MacSweeney, M., Szczerbinski, M. & Green, L. (2003) Predictors of reading delay in deaf adolescents: The relative contributions of rapid automatized naming speed and phonological awareness and decoding. *Journal of Deaf Studies and Deaf Education, 8*, 215–229.

Erber, N. (1982) *Auditory Training*. Washington DC: AG Bell Association.

Ertmer, D. (2010) Relationships between speech intelligibility and word articulation scores in children with hearing loss. *Journal of Speech, Language, and Hearing Research, 53*, 1075–1086. DOI:10.1044/1092-4388

Fletcher, S.G., Dagenais, P.A. & Critz-Crosby, P. (1991) Teaching consonants to profoundly hearing-impaired speakers using palatometry. *Journal of Speech and Hearing Research, 34*, 929–943.

Fordham, M. (2003) Cued Articulation with hearing-impaired children: Successful working in education. In J. Passy (Ed.) *A Handful of Sounds: Cued Articulation in Practice*. Cirencester: Acer Press.

Gagne, J.P., Stelmacovich, P. & Yovetich, W. (1991) Reactions to requests for clarification used by hearing-impaired individuals. *Volta Review, 93(3)*, 129–143.

Geffner, D. & Rothman Freeman, L. (1980) Speech assessment at the primary level: Interpretation relative to speech training. In J.D. Subtelny (Ed.) *Speech Assessment and Speech Improvement for the Hearing Impaired*, pp.1–17. Washington, DC: AG Bell Association.

Gilbert, H. & Campbell, M. (1980) Speaking fundamental frequency in three groups of hearing-impaired individuals. *Journal of Communication Disorders, 13*, 195–205.

Gold, T. (1980) Speech production in hearing impaired children. *Journal of Communication Disorders, 13*, 397–418.

Gravenstede, L. (2009) Phonological awareness and decoding skills in deaf adolescents. *Deafness and Education International, 11*, 171–190.

Greenberg, P. & Kusche, C. (1998) Preventive intervention for school-age deaf children: The PATHS curriculum. *Journal of Deaf Studies and Deaf Education, 3(1)*, 49–63.

Gregory, J. (1987) An investigation of speechreading with and without Cued Speech. *American Annals of the Deaf, 132(6)*, 393–398.

Gregory, S., Powers, S. & Thoutenhoofd, T. (1998) *Educational Achievements of Deaf Children*. London: DfEE Publications.

Hale, C.M. & Tager-Flusberg, H. (2003) The influence of language on theory of mind: A training study. *Developmental Science, 6(3)*, 346–359.

Harris, M. & Beech, J.R. (1998) Implicit phonological awareness and early reading development in prelingually deaf children. *Journal of Deaf Studies and Deaf Education, 3*, 205–216.

Hazan, V. (2001) Introduction to acoustics and speech perception. In J. Ballantyne (Ed.) *Deafness*, pp.55–71. London: Whurr Publishers. Ltd

Higgins, P.C. (1980) *Outsiders in a Hearing World: A Sociology of Deafness*. Beverley Hills, CA: Sage Publications.

Hindley, P. (2000) Child and adolescent psychiatry. In P. Hindley & N. Kitson (Eds) *Mental Health and Deafness*, pp.42–74. London: Whurr Publishers Ltd.

Hindley, P. (2004) Promoting social and emotional skills in deaf children: Avoiding deficits that lead to problems. *The British Association of Teachers of the Deaf Magazine*. Retrieved on 19 January 2011 from: http://www.batod.org.uk/index.php?id=/articles/mentalhealth/hindley.htm

Hogan, S., Stokes, J., White, C., Tyszkiewicz, E. & Woolgar, A. (2008) An evaluation of auditory verbal therapy using the rate of early language development as an outcome measure. *Deafness and Education International, 10(3)*, 143–167. DOI: 10.1002/dei.242

Horns, M. & Chasin, J. (2009) Attentional patterns in deaf and hearing infants: The roe of auditory cues. *Journal of Child Psychology and Psychiatry, 46*, 1116–1123.

Hudgins, C. & Numbers, F. (1942) An investigation of the intelligibility of the speech of the deaf. *Genetic Psychology Monographs, 25*, 289–392.

Jeanes, R.C., Nienhuys, T. & Rickards, F. (2000) The pragmatic skills of profoundly deaf children. *Journal of Deaf Studies and Deaf Education, 5(3)*, 237–247.

Joint Committee on Infant Hearing (2007) Position statement: Principles and guidelines for early hearing detection and intervention programs. *Pediatrics, 120(4)*, 898–921. DOI: 10.1542/peds.2007-2333

Kerr, P.C. & Cowie, R.I. (1997) Acquired deafness: A multi-dimensional experience. *British Journal of Audiology, 31(3)*, 177–188.

King, C.M. & Quigley, S.P. (1985) *Reading and Deafness*. London: Taylor & Francis.

Kyle, F. & Harris, M. *Predictors of Reading and Spelling Development in Deaf Children: A Three Year Longitudinal Study*. In press.

Ladd, P. (2003) *Understanding Deaf Culture: In Search of Deafhood*. Clevedon: Multilingual Matters.

Lane, H., Hoffmeister, R. & Bahan, B. (1996) *A Journey into the Deaf-World*. San Diego, CA: Dawn Sign Press.

Lawlor, E. (2009) An investigation into the effectiveness of the functional therapy approach 'Live English' in a sign-bilingual secondary school. Unpublished MSc dissertation.

Lederberg, A.R. & Everhart, V.S. (2000) Conversation between deaf children and their hearing mothers: Pragmatic and dialogic characteristics. *Journal of Deaf Studies and Deaf Education, 5(4)*, 303–322.

Lederberg, A.R. (1991) Social interaction among Deaf pre-schoolers. The effects of language ability and age. *American Annals of Deaf, 136(1)*, 53–59.

Lemanek, K., Williamson, D., Gresham, F. & Jensen, B. (1986) Social skills training with hearing-impaired children and adolescents. *Behaviour Modification, 10(1)*, 55–71.

Lewis, S. (1996) The reading achievements of a group of severely and profoundly hearing-impaired school leavers educated within a natural aural approach. *Journal of British Association of Teachers of the Deaf, 20(1)*, 1–7.

Leybaert, J. (2005) Learning to read with a hearing impairment In M.J. Snowling & C. Hulme (Eds) *The Science of Reading: A Handbook*, pp.379–396. Oxford: Blackwell.

Leybaert, J. & Alegria, J. (1993) Is word processing involuntary in deaf children? *British Journal of Developmental Psychology, 11*, 1–29.

Leybaert, J. & Charlier, B. (1996) Visual speech in the head: The effect of Cued Speech on rhyming, remembering, and spelling. *Journal of Deaf Studies and Deaf Education, 1*, 234–248.

Liebal, K., Behne, T., Carpenter, M. & Tomasello, M. (2009) Infants use shared experience to interpret pointing gestures. *Developmental Science, 12*, 264–271.

Marschark, M. (1993) *Psychological Development of Deaf Children*. Oxford: Oxford University Press.

Marschark, M. (2000) Education and development of deaf children – or is it development and education? In P.E. Spencer, C.J. Erting & M. Marschark (Eds) *The Deaf Child in the Family and at School*, pp.275-292. Mahwah, NJ: Lawrence Erlbaum Associates.

Marschark, M., Rhoten, C. & Fabich, M. (2007) Effects of cochlear implants on children's reading and academic achievement. *Journal of Deaf Studies and Deaf Education, 12*, 269–282.

Martin, K., Herman. R., Hirson. A., Thomas, J. & Pring. T. (2007) The efficacy of speech intervention using electropalatography with an 18-year-old Deaf client: A single case study. *Advances in Speech-Language Pathology, 9(1)*, 46–58.

Mason, K., Rowley, K. Marshall, C.R., Atkinson, J. Herman, R. Woll, B. & Morgan, G. (2010) Identifying specific language impairment in Deaf children acquiring British Sign Language: Implications for theory and practice. *British Journal of Developmental Psychology, 28*, 33–49.

Massaro, D.W. & Light, J. (2004) Using visible speech to train perception and production of speech for individuals with hearing loss. *Journal of Speech, Language, and Hearing Research, 47*, 304–320. DOI:10.1044/1092-4388(2004/025

Maybery, R.I. & Squires, B. (2006) Sign language: Acquisition. In E. Kieven (Ed.) *Language Acquisition*, vol. 11, pp.291–296. Encyclopedia of Language and Linguistics, 2nd ed., Keith Brown (Editor in Chief). Oxford: Elsevier.

Mayer, C. (2008) What really matters in the early literacy development of deaf children? *Journal of Deaf Studies and Deaf Education, 12*, 411–416.

McCracken, W. (2010) Deaf children with additional needs. National Deaf Children's Society publication. Retrieved on 19 January 2011 from http://www.ndcs.org.uk/family_support/our_publications_m/additional_needs.rma

Meadow, K.P. (1980) *Deafness and Child Development*. London: Edward Arnold.

Meadow, K.P. (2005) Early manual communication in relation to the deaf child's intellectual, social and communicative functioning. *Journal of Deaf Studies and Deaf Education, 20(4)*, 321–329.

Meristo, M., Hjelmquist, S. & Morgan, G. (in press). How access to language affects cognitive development in deaf children. In L. Surian & M. Siegal (Eds) *The Impact of Language on Children's Cogntive Development*. Oxford: Oxford University Press.

Mitchell, R. & Karchmer, M. (2004) Chasing the mythical ten percent: Parental hearing status of deaf and hard of hearing students in the United States. *Sign Language Studies, 4*, 138–163.

Moeller, M.P., Hoover, B., Putman, C., Arbataitis, K., Bohnenkamp, G., Peterson, B. & Stelmachowicz, P. (2007) Vocalizations of infants with hearing loss compared with infants with normal hearing: Part I. Phonetic development. *Ear Hear, 28*, 605–627.

Moeller, M.P. & Schick, B. (2006) Relations between maternal input and theory of mind understanding in deaf children. *Child Development, 77*, 751–766.

Monsen, R. (1974) Durational aspects of vowel production in the speech of deaf children. *Journal of Speech and Hearing Research, 17*, 386–398.

Monsen, R. (1979) Acoustic qualities of phonation in young hearing-impaired children. *Journal of Speech and Hearing Research, 22*, 270–288.

Morgan, G., Herman, R. & Woll, B. (2002) The development of complex verb construction in BSL. *Journal of Child Language, 29*, 23–36.

Morgan, G. & Woll, B. (2002) *New Directions in Sign Language Acquisition*. Amsterdam: John Benjamins Publishing Co.

Morgan, G. & Kegl, J. (2006) Nicaraguan sign language and Theory of Mind: The issue of critical periods and abilities. *Journal of Child Psychology and Psychiatry, 47*, 811–819.

National Deaf Children's Society (NDCS) (2001) *My School in Scotland: A Review of Deaf Pupils' Experiences of Mainstream Schools*. London: NDCS.

Newport, E.L. & Meier, R.P. (1985) The acquisition of American Sign Language. In D.I. Slobin (Ed.) *The Crosslinguistic Study of Language Acquisition*, vol. 1. Hillsdale, NJ: Lawrence Erlbaum.

NHS Newborn Hearing Screening Programme (2011) Retrieved on 19 January 2011 from http://hearing.screening.nhs.uk/nationalprog

Nicholas, J.G. & Geers, A.E. (2003) Personal, social and family adjustment in school-aged children with a cochlear implant. *Ear and Hearing*, supplement *24(1)*, 692–780.

Nicholas, J.G & Geers, A.E. (2006) The process and early outcomes of cochlear implantation by three years of age. In P.E. Spencer & M. Marschark, *Advances in the Spoken Language Development of Deaf and Hard-of-Hearing Children*, pp.271–297. Oxford: Oxford University Press.

Novelli-Olmstead, T. & Ling, D. (1984) Speech production and speech discrimination by hearing-impaired children. *Volta Review, 86(2)*, 72–80.

Nunes, T., Pretzlik, U. & Olsson, J. (2001) Deaf children's social relationships in mainstream schools. *Deafness and Education International, 3(3)*, 123–136.

Nurmsoo, E. & Bloom, P. (2008) Preschoolers' perspective taking in word learning: Do they blindly follow eye gaze? *Psychological Science, 19*, 211–215.

O'Halpin, R. (2001) Intonation issues in the speech of hearing impaired children: Analysis, transcription and remediation. *Clinical Linguistics and Phonetics, 15*, 529–550.

Padden, C. & Humphries, T. (1988) *Deaf in America: Voices from a Culture.* Cambridge: Harvard University Press.

Padden, C. & Humphries, T. (2005) *Inside Deaf Culture.* Cambridge: Harvard University Press.

Pantelemidou, V., Herman, R. & Thomas, J. (2003) Efficacy of speech intervention using electropalatography with a cochlear implant user. *Journal of Clinical Phonetics and Linguistics, 17*, 1–11.

Parker, A. & Rose, H. (1990) Deaf children's phonological development. In P. Grunwell (Ed.) *Developmental Speech Disorders.* London: Whurr Publishers Ltd.

Parsloe, R. (1998) Use of the speech pattern audiometer and the electropalatograph to explore the speech production/perception relationship in a profoundly deaf child. *International Journal of Language and Communication Disorders, 33*, 109–121.

Passy, J. (1990) *Cued Articulation.* Cirencester: Acer Press.

Peng, S., Spencer, L.J. & Tomblin, J.B. (2004) Speech intelligibility of pediatric cochlear implant recipients with 7 years of device experience. *Journal of Speech, Language and Hearing Research, 47*, 1227–1236.

Peterson, C.C. (2009) Development of social-cognitive and communication skills in children born deaf. *Scandinavian Journal of Psychology, 50*, 475–483.

Powers, S. (2002) From concepts to practice in deaf education: A United Kingdom perspective on inclusion. *Journal of Deaf Studies and Deaf Education, 7(3)*, 230–243.

Remmel, E. & Peters, K. (2009) Theory of mind and language in children with cochlear implants. *Journal of Deaf Studies and Deaf Education, 14*, 218–236.

Roberts, S.B. & Rickards, F.W. (1994) A survey of graduates of an Australian integrated auditory/oral preschool. Part II: Academic achievement, utilisation of support services and friendship patterns. *Volta Review, 96*, 207–236.

Robinson, S. & Adam, R. (2003) Cultures of disability and deafness: Rethinking links between the disability movement and the deaf community. Paper given at the Australian Social Policy Conference, University of New South Wales.

Royal National Institute of the Deaf (2002) Facts and figures on deafness and tinnitus, RNID Information, March 2006. Retrieved on 19 January 2011 from http://www.rnid.org.uk/ VirtualContent/101697/Facts_and_figures_on_deafness_and_tinnitus_March_2006.pdf

Schamroth, K. & Threadgill, L. (2007) Using a 'Live English' curriculum. *Bulletin of the Royal College of Speech and Language Therapists* (Feb), 12–13.

Schick, B., de Villiers, P., de Villiers, J. & Hoffmeister, R. (2007) Language and theory of mind: A study of deaf children. *Child Development*, 78, 376–396.

Silvestre, N., Ramspott, A. & Pareto, I. (2007) Conversational skills in a semistructured interview and self-concept in Deaf students. *Journal of Deaf Studies and Deaf Education*, 12(1), 38–54.

Spencer, P.E., Erting, C.J. & Marschark, M. (2000) *The Deaf Child in the Family and at School: Essays in Honour of Katherine P. Meadow-Orlans*. London: Lawrence Erlbaum Associates.

Spencer, P.E. & Marschark, M. (Eds) (2006) *Advances in the Spoken Language Language Development of Deaf and Hard-of-Hearing Children*. New York: Oxford University Press.

Steinberg, A.G., Sullivan, V.J. & Loew, R.C. (1998) Cultural and linguistic barriers to mental health service access: The Deaf consumer's perspective. *American Journal of Psychiatry*, 155, 982–984.

Stevenson, E.A. (1964) A study of the educational achievement of deaf children of deaf parents. *California News*, 80, 1–3.

Stinson, M.S. & Antia, S.D. (1999) Considerations in educating deaf and hard-of-hearing students in inclusive settings. *Journal of Deaf Studies and Deaf Education*, 4(3), 163–175.

Stinson, M., Liu, Y., Saur, R. & Long, G. (1996) Deaf college students' perceptions of communication in mainstream classes. *Journal of Deaf Studies and Deaf Education*, 1(1), 40–51.

Stuckless, E.R. & Birch, J.W. (1966) The influence of early manual communication on the linguistic development of deaf children. *American Annals of the Deaf*, 111, 452–460, 499–504.

Subtelny, J.D. (1977) Assessment of speech with implication for training. In F. Bess (Ed.) *Childhood Deafness*. New York: Grune and Stratton.

Svirsky, M., Robbins, A., Kirk, K., Pisoni, D.B. & Miyamoto, R.T. (2000) Language development in profoundly deaf children with cochlear implants. *Psychological Science*, 11, 153–158.

Swanwick, R. & Gregory, S. (2007) *Sign Bilingual Education: Policy and Practice*. Coleford: Douglas McLean.

Taumoepeau, M. & Ruffman, T. (2008) Stepping stones to others' minds: Maternal talk relates to child mental state language and emotion understanding at 15, 24 and 33 months. *Child Development*, 79, 284–302.

Trezek, B.J. & Malmgren, K.W. (2005) The efficacy of utilizing a phonics treatment package with middle school deaf and hard-of-hearing students. *Journal of Deaf Studies and Deaf Education, 10*, 256–271.

Trezek, B.J. & Wang, Y. (2006) Implications of utilizing a phonic-based reading curriculum with children who are deaf or hard-of-hearing. *Journal of Deaf Studies and Deaf Education, 11*, 202–213.

Trybus, R.J. & Karchmer, M.A. (1977). School achievement scores of hearing impaired children: National data on achievement status and growth patterns. *American Annals of the Deaf, 122(2)*, 62–69.

Vieu, A., Mondain, M., Blanchard, K., Sillon, M., Reuillard-Artieres, F., Tobey, E., Uziel, A. & Piron, J. (1998) Influence of communication mode on speech intelligibility and syntactic structure of sentences in profoundly hearing impaired French children implanted between 5 and 9 years of age. *International Journal of Otorhinolaryngology, 44*, 15–22.

Waters, G.S. & Doehring, D.G. (1990) Reading acquisition in congenitally deaf children who communicate orally: Insights from an analysis of component reading, language, and memory skills. In T.H. Carr & B.A. Levy (Eds) *Reading and its Development: Component Skills Approaches*, pp.323–373. San Diego, CA: Academic Press.

Wauters, L.N., Agnes, E.J.M., Tellings, A.E.J.M., van Bon, W.H.J. & Mak W.M. (2007) Mode of acquisition as a factor in deaf children's reading comprehension. *Journal of Deaf Studies and Deaf Education*, published online at: www.doi:10.1093/deafed/enm050

White, K.R. (1982) Defining and prioritising the personal and social competencies needed by hearing-impaired students. *Volta Review, 84(6)*, 266–274.

Wirz, S. (2001) Managing voice with deaf and hearing impaired speakers. In M. Freeman & M. Fawcus (Eds) *Voice Disorders and their Management*, 3rd edition. London: Whurr.

Woll, B. (2008) Deafness and hearing impairment. Paper prepared as part of the Foresight Review on Mental Capital and Wellbeing. Retrieved on January 2011 from: http://www.bis.gov.uk/assets/bispartners/foresight/docs/mental-capital/sr-d5_mcw.pdf

Woll, B. & Morgan, G. (2010) Sign linguistics, sign language learning and sign bilingualism. *Contemporary Applied Linguistics*, vol. 2. Linguistics for the Real World. London: Continuum Press.

Wood, D., Wood, H., Griffiths, A. & Howarth, I. (1986) *Teaching and Talking with Deaf Children*. Chichester: John Wiley & Sons Ltd.

Woolfe, T., Want, S.C. & Siegal, M. (2002) Signposts to development: Theory of mind in deaf children. *Child Development, 73*, 768–778.

Yoshinaga-Itano, C. (2009) Beyond newborn hearing screening: Language outcomes to 84 months. National Hearing Screening Progam Conference, London, March 2009.

8 My Speech, Language and Communication 'A real kind of overwhelming kind of challenge sometime'

Victoria Joffe

City University London, UK

Abigail Beverly and Lavinia Scott

> *It takes a thousand voices to tell a single story*
>   Native American saying

Introduction

This is a book about the impact of communication disability across the lifespan. Eminent researchers and practitioners in the field of developmental and acquired speech, language and communication difficulties (SLCD) have come together to share their research and highlight the impact these difficulties have on the lives of other individuals. This is progress in itself, as any focus on the wider impact of communication disability is relatively recent, particularly in the area of developmental communication difficulties. There are emerging studies looking at the impact of developmental SLCD on the *quality of life* and *wellbeing* of children and young people experiencing these difficulties *from their own perspectives* (see for example, Carroll & Dockrell, 2010; Dockrell, Lindsay, Palikara & Cullen, 2007; Markham, van Laar, Gibbard & Dean, 2009; McCormack, McLeod, McAllister & Harrison, 2010; Myers, Davies-Jones, Chiat, Joffe & Botting, in press; Owen, Hayett & Roulstone, 2004; Palikara, Lindsay & Dockrell, 2009). This work is valuable and provides important insights. The nature of many of these studies is the identification of commonalities and shared experiences across participants and the summarizing of key information collected from groups of people and interpreted with reference to the literature.

This chapter is different. It is different to the research on perspectives and outcomes identified above, and it is also different (although similar to Cruice et al., see Chapter 16, this edition) to the other chapters in this book which report on the impact of communication disability on other individuals. In this chapter, two young people with SLCD share their views and thoughts on their abilities, difficulties and their lives in general. The aim of this chapter is to present to the reader the perspectives and views of the *individual* with communication disability. My co-authors (Beverly and Scott) spoke to me (Joffe) individually over two sessions, with each session lasting between approximately one and three hours. The young people were asked to participate in a chapter on their views and perspectives around language and communication, their own SLCD and its impact on their lives. In order to sufficiently prepare the young people, a selection of topics was sent to them prior to the meetings. The topic areas included: how I see myself; different means of expression; the meaning of speech, language and communication; my speech, language and communication abilities and difficulties; and the impact of my SLCD, past and present.

They were asked to add any areas that they felt they would like to share and that had been omitted. On the day of the meetings, these topics were used to start and facilitate the discussion. There was no other structure to the sessions. The young people were familiar with the first author. The conversations were recorded and transcribed by student and graduate speech and language therapists. Each conversation was transcribed twice by different people, and checked for accuracy. The young people were involved in selecting which parts of the conversation were included in this chapter, and gave their final consent to the version you are reading now. We present their stories.

Abigail (Abby) Beverly

My name is Abigail Beverly. I'm 27 years old and I graduated from Central Saint Martins in 2006, with a degree in textile design. I'm an adult with a speech and language difficulty. I live in London with my parents and have a brother and a sister (both older). Since leaving university I have been doing lots of different things, mainly related to my interest in textiles and art. I also give talks about my speech and language difficulties. I volunteer at the Afasic Youth Project[1] and run regular arts and crafts sessions.

Speech, language and communication is important to me

I think language is like part of you. It's what you understand and I think what communication is about expressing yourself and to others so that's what I see language and communication, language is part of you, and communication is about how you express yourself and how you use language to talk to one another. I think it is really important. I think actually we take speech and language for granted because it is such a quick response. And I think we used language all the time but particularly when we are travelling, asking for directions on the tube or when you are using the phone, emails. It's that kind of, particularly nowadays, it's quite demanding of quick responses [clicks fingers].

I knew early on that I was different

I remember I was at primary school when I be talking or something. I got quite a lot of funny looks from people, from my classmates and from teachers and all because I said the wrong words or I said the phrase in the, not in the right context and they look at me a bit differently. Like they often frowned. So that's when I realized that something wasn't quite right.

If I said a word out of context or if the grammar is not correct or anything, my parents help me to support, realize my mistake. They said like, 'Abby it is "written" not "wrote"' or something like that, whereas I remember at school they did it more like, oh, I'm more clever than you, 'No Abby, it's this'. I remember this girl in particular, she loved to correct me and I really hated that, because it's more about yeah I am smarter than you. Whereas my parents are more doing it for so I could learn my mistakes. But I think it is different and I don't like it when people, that's one of my pet hates, people correcting me because I just feel actually that my speech and language difficulty is a part of Abby. I mean OK they might have the best intentions but no, I find it really rude when people correcting me.

---

1   Afasic is a UK charity which supports children and young people with SLCD and their parents and carers. The Afasic Youth Project is a group run in northeast London for young people with communication difficulties between the ages of 11 and 19 years.

My speech and language difficulties are a part of who I am

If I wouldn't have speech and language difficulty, I wouldn't be Abby. I think it has made me the person that I am today – quite confident. I was going to say like I really pushed hard to get what I am now. I knew from an early age that I had speech and language difficulties so I think that helps. That is why I think I have accepted myself. Being proud of what you are and my family wouldn't change me for the world. I am more confident in myself. I am proud of being Abby right now.

As I look back I can see more clearly what helped and supported me with my speech and language difficulties

Visual cues are important

I'm a very visual learner and always remember things that I've seen rather than read. I really respond to rules and patterns, especially when they are presented in pretty colours. I had Michelle (*specialist teacher*) who really got to know me and she was my teaching support for a very long time and she got to know my strengths as well as my weaknesses and it was what really worked. Her notes or my revision notes, her handwriting was really clear and really visually, loved it, it was good to read. And also she was very self-conscious about layout of text onto a paper and making it visual. She knew that I was very visual learner so she used those skills. Because I didn't get on with my science very well so she used like my strongest skills to help with my weakest subject. Something I remember in science when I said I don't understand, and all he [*teacher*] did was just repeat himself but louder, you know. And he did it twice actually, bless him.

Having the confidence to say I don't understand

I think what really helped was I had the confidence to say I don't understand because I got really really frustrated not keeping up with the others. I wanted to be at the same level as everyone else so I said like, I always said put your hand up if you don't understand something. I wasn't embarrassed by that at all because I was more frustrated by that I couldn't keep up with the others. I'd rather put my hands up and say I didn't understand than you know, being left behind.

Planning and organization is important for me

I learned to be organized quite early. I know it takes me such a long time that I know I start things, projects, straight away. I have my diary or my 'Post-It' notes to keep me organized because I do have this difficulty but I have learned ways to overcome it by like help, tools, phones. I have a reminder on it because yeah when someone tells me, 'Abby, could you send out the, you know, the addresses or something like that'. So I put that straight in the phone to remind me so I use what helpful tools to help me.

It's important to get the right support

I think it did help me to have one-to-one support, definitely. When I left school, I went to sixth form college and I had one-to-one support at the learning support department. And she was great because she really put my words down to paper because that is what I struggled with. I find it really hard to express my ideas, particularly in written form. So she was fantastic like she actually took on, she actually listened to me, what I wanted to say and she wrote my ideas down into paper. So I really remember the day when Mum read a passage and she was 'I can read your voice'.

And sometimes you need to fight for it

It wasn't all plain sailing at uni when I had one-to-one support. I knew quite early on what sort of difficulties I do have. So when I did turn up at uni, I did kind of knew what I was to expect. And actually, I got quite stroppy at one point because I was very good. I filled in all the applications for support and I didn't hear from them for three weeks. I was quite dominant and said, 'That's not good enough' and then actually the next day, I had the support. I do think you have to stand up sometimes and make a fuss. Yeah, I do need support but I am not thick. I was just outraged that they said they can't fit you in. It was just like that is just not good enough.

And I can also clearly see what did NOT help and support me

I was going to mention the support teachers who didn't know their role. They felt their role was to, they think they were trying to give the answers and that's not the point of having a support teacher. The point is for me to work out my own answers you know. The whole point of it is for me to understand the language and the topic and also work out the answers all by myself, not you know answers written for me because I have a speech and language difficulty. That's a bit cheating really. I just felt like I didn't earn it. I need to work it for myself.

I don't have many good memories of school

Moving from special school to mainstream primary school

I began at a special school when I was 4. I wanted to go to the same school as my sister, my local school just around the corner from where I lived. As my language improved, I found the lessons at the special school a bit boring and repetitive, and then when I was 7, I slowly went into mainstream. It was OK but I remember like the work, the written work it wasn't by me, it was by a support teacher. She just wrote it for me. It was about the pyramids. My mum looked at it and she was like that is not yours. It wasn't miserable. I was more miserable in secondary than I was in primary.

To secondary school

I am not a big fan of school. I don't have a lot of good memories. I think the only good times at school was with art and making textiles. I didn't have a lot of great friends. And I got bullied in school. I was just named underneath the run really. I meant I was called everything under the sun really. My glasses, my hair, my back brace, hips, my everything you could think of. I just didn't know how to stand up to them, if I did it would be quite like an explosion. So I think if I didn't have speech and language difficulty then maybe I would have been more assertive and would have stood up or know what to say.

I was going to mention about the homework. Because that what I really remember from school. The homework, it just took over my home life – evenings and weekends. And it just didn't make me socialize, like my friends, they socialized. So they can do their homework in their lunchtime but they spent more time socializing when I spent all my time on homework. It just took over. I had to. It was real difficult.

Starting afresh and moving on to sixth form college

Moving to sixth form, one of my happiest memories. I felt more uplifted and I became more me. And not worried and literally the chance to start fresh, a slate clean. And also you are in a room where people want to learn. It was very positive, particularly in the learning support department. I felt really, really supported and it wasn't an issue, and that was what was really great. Whereas once it made an issue about my speech and language difficulties, whereas I think sixth form, it wasn't an issue. It was they accepted me, that was part of me.

My memories of speech and language therapy were of being tested to a point of failure

I remember I only had one speech and language therapist (SLT). She was very proper. I do remember the tests and stuff but there was one point where she kept testing me to beyond failing and to a point of failure. And I was like it was depressing, like disheartening. And I decided to stop it just because I couldn't carry on. I just get annoyed by some SLTs. They kind of, because it's so contradicting, it's about communication. I find that some have really poor communication skills, you know where they are so hung up on theory and yet they don't put it into context.

My family are my strongest support system

My parents and my family, they really supported me, they really taught me to be confident saying, 'Abby, if you don't understand something you say, just put your hands up' because I think they recognize how I get quite anxious when I don't know what is going on. I think definitely the confidence comes from my family from you know we has a nice family life, like dinners together, holidays together, and quite a fun, you know, play together. We my family played loads of games and it actually helped me, turn-taking, conversation.

Jessie, my sister, she is closer to my age. I tend to ask her advice. But also like, particularly at school when we had those meetings with the SENCO with my parents. She was there and acted as my voice. There was sometimes those days when I just didn't understand what they were talking about. And Jessie often, she was almost like my translator and she also made sure I'd get it, I'd get to have my say.

I think my language and communication difficulties has made my family more aware of children with disability but also getting a fair deal in realizing their potential. They wanted Abby to be treated fairly and yeah to see her potential and not to see her disability. I think I am very fortunate to have a very special network. So, some bits were quite tough, horrible, I think it has made us all stronger as a family.

Having a network of friends who understand me is important

My friends accept me for who I am

I used to be quite anxious meeting new people but I am a bit more better I think. I am a lot more confident to be myself. I have a very good network of friends. The friends I have got today, they don't see you as a disability, they don't see you as you know, like a girl with speech and language difficulty. They just see me as Abby. And also my friends are quite open-minded as well and I think that makes a difference. They just accept it as part of Abby and also like the friends I have now, I have the confidence to say 'Sorry, I didn't understand that' or 'What are we doing?' I couldn't do that with the friends I had at school. Whereas the friends I have met now are much more supportive.

Socializing can be difficult

When I go out to house parties I get really nervous because like I don't know anyone there. I find it quite difficult to make new friendships. Sometimes there are barriers. I think I am one of those people, I don't like going to places I don't feel familiar with. For instance, like getting back home it is like quite tricky to try and get home on your own. The girls are quite independent, sort of they can hold themselves, whereas I find it really difficult.

My boyfriend understands me well

He is quite quiet actually but he does open up. Oh, he is a sweet lad. Since dating me, I think he has more of an awareness of speech and language difficulties and he is also a volunteer for Afasic. I think there have been times, when we get the wrong end of the stick or something, quite early in the relationship. There was this one time when we started dating where again I painfully and stakedly constructed a text message and I thought should I send it. And at the time, none of my friends were around and I was going to phone my friend and I thought that is ridiculous. I can't phone a friend – 'Oh what do you think about the message'? I didn't send it because I wasn't quite sure and then in the evening he texted me first and I was 'Oh, after all that!'

My speech and language difficulties continue to present challenges

The difficulties I still have today is like with text messages and emails. It takes me so long and also particularly with someone not aware of my background. I want to get it so right but it takes me such a long time to kind of get what I want to get across. I get lots of emails from a variety of people all demanding a response but I find it really hard work. Also actually on Facebook as well, the social network, there has been a couple of occasions where I had written something like on your status, and like what I thought were my friends, they like took the mickey out of me. Something I wrote yeah, and was quite innocent, but the way it sounded, it sounded quite rude and I was so embarrassed.

I find it really hard work emailing and typing, you know, I want a direct answer, so I prefer the phone. But I am not very good at options. I think sometimes they are hard, cinemas or train tickets where you have to remember all of the things. I also get, I don't like it when people are on mobile phones and it is really noisy and like for instance my friend Mary.[2] She drives while she uses the free-hand set while driving and I find that really distracting. Because it is like I can hear the noise and I am trying to listen.

It is important for me to be busy

I am busy with my quilting. It has given me routine, I think. The last time I saw you I did not have work. I really struggled not having a routine and that is what I love about work, I like having a routine and that is what I am looking for at the moment, is having a routine. But actually at the moment I'm in a good place where I am quite busy right now.

I am looking for a more permanent job

I tend to go for jobs that don't have a lot of written work because I just don't think that is one of my strengths. And so when I do apply for jobs, I do tend to apply for jobs with a good work team. I tend to focus on my strengths as opposed to my weaknesses. I am very creative, a team player. I don't really mention my speech and language difficulty unless I have to. Like there was one time I had to. I went for an interview for an events assistant and she sort of said how it would work. And she said she would tell me on the day like a half an hour before the programme was going to be started. I was like, 'Oh that is not going to work', and I explained about my difficulties. And she was said 'You look normal to me'. Which is quite a common thing people say to me. So I sort of explained my difficulties and what would work. And I said like you know 'Is it possible to have the schedule beforehand as I can understand it more?' and she said, 'Yeah it is not a problem.'

I express myself in other ways besides language

I love textiles so much because it doesn't involve words. Also art I think is really fascinating. I could do it independently. One aspect of my art is

---

2   Pseudonym supplied by Abby.

quilting. It is ideal for me because, although it is quite technical, there is a formula that you have to follow, with each step of the process mapped out, and you have to be very organized. These are some examples of my quilting. I went to a festival and saw this fabric just like literacy and words. I just really liked it a lot.

The print design is called 'Authentic' – by Moda – and the technique I used is called Log Cabin – which is my favourite – a really simple process which starts off small and then grows as you add strips.

My love/hate relationship with words

I have a fascination with words and symbols – even though I see words as being such a barrier! I am quite fascinated by words and yet I get really frustrated with them sometimes. I am quite fascinated by the word shape and how the words look on the page. But yet there are some days where I just find they are real kind of barrier. A real kind of overwhelming kind of challenge sometime.

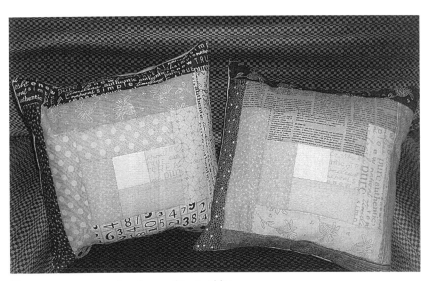

'These are some examples of my quilting' – Abby

▄▄▄▄▄▄▄ Lavinia Scott

My name is Lavinia Scott and I am 19. I live in East London with my mother and younger sister. I am studying for a foundation degree in Creative Industries at the Redbridge College and the University of East London. I like to draw and stay up until 6am talking to people across the world on social networks. I make dolls, keyrings and badges and I represent Afasic as a member of the Council for Disabled Children. I also do volunteer work at Barnardo's.[3]

Words are used as weapons against me

Speech and language, it's kinda like just like a barrier in a way, cos where some people can express themselves easily, I can't. And words are kind of like used as weapons like against me personally. There's some words I can't say compared to other people. Like whatever word is an /n/ before a /m/ like when I say it the /m/ comes first like 'aminal' and 'amination' or 'emeny' and stuff like that. And I can't and 'crips' I can't say it. Like I can say it slow but I can't say it at normal speed and some people they can just like throw words at me and they know I can't say it. So it's just like a weapon and a barrier. When I was in secondary school, people used to say, 'Oh just say this say this or say that' and they used to take the mick out of me cos they knew I couldn't say it.

Memories of being at school

School was my prison

I went to Arcues[4] High School aka prison. I hated that school, and primary school I hated as well. It was a prison cos you've got the big gates and the big scary building and also like the kids are like the prisoners and you've got like gangs in schools like how they would in prison.

---

3   Barnardo's is the UK's largest children's charity.
4   Pseudonym supplied by Lavinia.

Fitting in with the other kids was hard

I was bullied a lot in primary school. I remember in year two we had a new girl in our class and she didn't speak much English and I helped her out with English even though I couldn't really speak myself like properly. And in return of that I got bullied by her. I used to come home with bruises on my back and on arms and legs where she used to punch me and kick me and that.

There were teachers who did not understand my difficulties

When I was in secondary school in GCSEs we read this book called *Things Fall Apart* by Chinua Achebe. And it was loads of African Nigerian terms and obviously no one could really say them and I hate reading out loud and I was picked to read out loud and I was struggling and the teacher snapped and said, 'Can someone else just take over.' I wanted to shoot the teacher.

But there were also teachers who understood and talked to me

The good teachers, outside of lesson they kinda like talk to you more, instead of just inside class, where they just like have the teacher student like 'I'm right you're wrong' type thing. Outside they get to hear your kinda like opinion on different things and if anything was wrong you could go up to them, talk. But they kind of left – the good teachers always left, the bad ones stayed behind.

The support and understanding I did get at school was important to me

In primary school, there was a deputy headteacher who was alright. Who my mum explained to that I have a speech and language impairment and she was really like supportive and understanding. And I had a year three and year four teacher who was understanding, and they knew like that I had speech and language impairment and they knew if I was getting bullied. They all kinda knew how I was creative so they embraced every activity instead of like in a way pushing me to do things like I know I couldn't do. When those teachers left, that's when I kind of like struggled more. Especially in year five and year six when they prepare you for secondary school. It got harder.

College gave me an escape from my school prison

I'm studying a foundation degree in creative industries. I went to college cos I just wanted to escape prison. And with college like you have people who are older and some people who are younger, so it's not always about the same peers and luckily in my class I was like one of the youngest people and the teachers they were more understanding and they helped out more compared to secondary school. When I had interview my mum came with me and she explained to them and they were more understanding. They helped support me. They gave me more time for written work and they gave me like a structure to do and each draft I could hand in they could tell me what to improve on and what not to.

At college I got one-to-one support and with the tutors they kinda had a open-door policy so where if you ever need help you can just go to them and ask for help. This was different to school, where you kind of get scared of going to the staffroom to ask for tutors.

My mum never stopped believing in me

If it wasn't for my mum I wouldn't be kinda like talking right now. Cos my mum never gave up on me when I was younger like when I was younger she kinda saw like yeah there is something wrong but no one seemed to believe her, they kind of said, 'No she will grow out of it there's nothing wrong', and she like took me to so many different youth like nurseries to try and help me socialize with kids. My mum got me to do gymnastics, horse riding to try and like help me.

The anger and frustration I felt became uncontrollable

With English, especially during GCSEs, I used to you know get into tantrums and stuff because what I wanted to write down I couldn't write down so I used to throw my book downstairs and say 'I give up'. And have really bad tantrums like hit my head against the walls, punch walls, rip up paper and stuff like that. It doesn't help being Aries and speech and language.

Hurting others

When I get angry I kinda bottle them up and I either take it out on myself or I take it out on someone who had nothing to do with anything. So my mum was always that kind of person so like if something bad happened at school for a whole week I used to bottle it up and if my mum just like said one thing I used to shout everything at her. But I was always like apologetic afterwards. Saying like 'I'm sorry' and she was like always understanding.

Hurting myself

When I was like around 14 I used to self-harm as well, cos I couldn't say anything. I used to like hide it from school. You kinda like felt numb afterwards. So you don't feel no pain. When my mum found out she was like devasted. All the like anger and like pain and upset I used to take it out on myself. I couldn't express like when I was angry. When I get angry kinda feels like the person who I'm angry at is more dominant so I don't wanna get angry at them but yet I can't express myself I can't find the words or anything, and so just like used to take it out on myself. I was 14 and I stopped when I was 16. I stopped mainly cos I left secondary school and got into college.

Expressing feelings without hurting anyone

And my friend kinda helped me express myself with my drawings a lot more cos he was there to help me with my drawings. And my boyfriend who I got with when I was 16 was like really supportive and like he didn't mind if I got angry or anything. Yeah just like get a pen and just destroyed paper.

Expressing myself creatively through my work

I draw. I started drawing since I was like 7. I was naturally artistic. I started drawing like a certain style of drawings when I first watched *Sailor Moon*. *Sailor Moon*, it's a Japanese cartoon about a girl who has magical powers and turns into a superhero. I like illustrations. I kinda sew and make little dolls, keyrings, badges and like at the moment I'm trying to make my own hoodie cos I want to dress up as Pikachu for Halloween.

Learning a new language makes me feel equal to everyone else

I can learn other languages cos like the paces of everyone else. So you can pick up things at the same pace or even quicker. For me I kinda picked up

Spanish quite quick. I learned Spanish when I was in secondary school. I was quite shocked I was in set one for Spanish. I was like 'What, set one, is that right? No I'm only in set four for things'. [*laughs*] I kinda like languages. And with the speech and language everyone gets to feel like what it feels like expecting to learn something and you can't do it. You're on the same level as everyone else.

Socializing is really hard for me

With social activities I can't really socialize with many young people my age. I can only socialize with like people older than me or younger than me. Cos older people they're like more mature they won't take the mick out of you and they're kind of like more understanding and younger people like they just accept you for who you are. Whereas like people my age they kind of like seem to judge you more.

I have a small circle of friends

I have a few like really small number of friends. Yeah like about five. One friend I met throughout college, she kinda like... didn't care about what I was saying like she just accept me for my wacky like craziness type person and we just like clicked at once. And my other friend, he just sees me for me, he doesn't pick on my imperfections or anything.

The importance of sharing interests and experiences with friends

At college, I am friends with two people. A guy who's kinda like he's quiet at times and that but we have the same interests and a woman who's 36 from Japan and she just like getting to grips with English. Some of my drawings, it's kinda like it was influenced by Japanese culture, so I kinda grew up like wanting to live in Japan and wanted to meet a Japanese person and that was my dream come true. And like with her learning English she kinda gets same struggles as well so it's kinda like yeah I can understand where she's coming from and she can understand where I'm coming from.

Factors that come into play when choosing friends

Well most of my friends are like older than me, like in their late twenties.

Or they're either just male. Girls are bitchy and they find something wrong but guys are like alright they're too lazy to bitch. And I also kinda grew up as a tomboy and I'm not bothered about like what dress suits me or what clothes suit me or like if this make-up is good for me. I just go out as me. Like it or lump it type of thing. Like you don't like me, fine. It hurts as well cos when girls bitch that's what they actually think.

My boyfriend

He's from Ghana, so like English is like a second well third language for him. So he kinda like understands difficulties with different words. I just talk to him. Like we have really private random jokes. And when he heard that I couldn't say certain words he was like, 'OK, that's fine'", he didn't like kind of try and push me to say them.

I have many more friends on social networks

I have Facebook but Facebook bores me. I just log on then forget that it's on. But I go on a site called DeviantART, which is like a social networking site but it is more like for people who are creative. So you upload your art work. And like I've made like few friends on there even though they live across like in America. And also I'm on a pen pal website called InterPals where I have pen pals, 50. I write but if I spell something I always put in brackets 'My spellings suck. I am sorry'.

I'm afraid of people judging me

When I meet new people I'm just like mute, like so quiet. Like on my first week of college, I went in I didn't wanna talk. I didn't wanna say anything. I was like quiet. And when it came to introducing ourselves I was like 'erm erm'. Don't wanna do it in case they kinda judged me for my speech and cos like human beings are just prejudiced.

Feeling lonely

I'm also a young carer as well as a young person with speech and language. So that's why you're like lonely as a young carer and you're lonely as a person with speech and language thing. Squashing that together. Kinda twice as

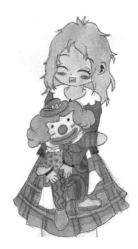

lonely. Yeah like I tend to talk to myself as kinda used to have dolls I tend to talk to myself with the doll and stuff or just like make up random stories and tell the air. I had these clown doll called Sonic which was given to me when I was 3 by my great-aunt Pam. And he was kinda like he's been by my side ever since. Even though I don't really like clowns but this clown was cool. I also got like a knitted doll called Betty. They [*dolls*] don't bitch back at you. And also you can just make them your perfect friend. Someone who just accepts you. The picture I have drawn here is of little me hugging Sonic my toy clown. Sonic was my best friend. He understood everything I said. He didn't judge me, he just loved me. I didn't need friends because of Sonic, he was the only person I needed. Even though he was a toy.

My communication disability still restricts me

It stops me kinda like making phone calls and just going out to different places that I don't know. Stuff like going out in groups like socializing. And like I'd rather stay in than go out to socialize. With social stuff it is cos like especially when my mum sends me round the shops I'm like 'Nah I don't wanna do it', cos like the person might think I'm weird. I don't like making phone calls. Cos you can't see the person. And sometimes when you kinda speak, they kinda make up some they kinda make a assumption about you they've already pictured made a picture about you. Like if you just got a random phone call from someone who speaks slang all the time you kind of imagine that person to be like a hoodie or something.

But it doesn't restrict me so much that I don't have fun

I went Camden last week with a friend. And they had this like truck thing and you know the Nintendo Wii. They have a new dance game for it called Just Dance 2. And they're just advertising it and getting people to try it out. Before I would never go up, I'd just watch it but I managed to drag my friend up. We danced. And I was quite shocked within myself that I managed to do that cos I like the Wii cos I played the Just Dance, the first game and it's really cool and I wanted my friend to do it. And I didn't care like what people thought of me cos like people were just making idiot out of themselves on there already.

Things that I would like to tell people

Don't assume that someone's independent they don't need help in a way. And like, support them, don't bring them down.

Have training cos like I know with teachers it's optional to have training about learning how to deal with students with learning difficulties and that.

But like everyone had that training no matter what field you're going in you'd end up getting either a customer or colleagues with disabilities. Just like no matter what you do, have that training.

Supportive networks and exciting opportunities ahead

Afasic kinda help me cos they got a girls' group and they kinda help you socialize more and help you go out more. Like I remember like on the first trip they were like 'Lavinia, you're going take us from Stratford and take us to the Jubilee line' and I was like 'oh OK' and so it kinda like made me more independent. And also helped me get into more things like I represent Afasic on the council of disabled children. And I do illustrations for the Afasic newsletter. And I'm doing conferences for them and that. They kind of see past the speech and language disability. They're kinda like they're there to support you, not judge you. Yeah, people should see past you. Yeah like live in world peace and have harmony and I feel like a beauty pageant! [*laughs*]

There is only one Lavinia – awesome, man!

It's part of me if you don't like me, if you don't like speech and language then you don't like me, like it or lump it type thing. At times I wish I didn't have them but like that's me. I think I'm kinda like a different person compared to when I was in secondary school. I don't wish to see it as a disability. I think, she's awesome, man. Yeah there's no words to describe her. She has the 80s awesomeness [*laughs*]. She knows music taste, she knows about her stuff. She has a lot of opportunities. There's only one Lavinia who can say it like 'aminal' like, the way she can [*laughs*].

Concluding remarks

At our final meeting, over tea and cakes, the three of us shared our own perspectives and experiences about our involvement in this chapter. Lavinia emphasized how important she felt this chapter was, as 'It's one thing finding out from professionals working with young people about their speech and language difficulties but another thing hearing from the young person themselves. You should hear it first hand, their words themselves.' Abigail remarked what an insight it was: 'They are powerful words and you hope people will take it into account. It's quite positive, it's not all doom and gloom. Our speech and language, it's been a journey.' 'And for me,' interjected Lavinia, 'my speech and language, it's like a rollercoaster.'

My co-authors are clearly committed to sharing their perspectives and educating others around speech, language and communication. This endeavour has given me the opportunity to spend time with two vibrant young people with SLCD and to share their experiences. For me, the overriding memory will be the fun and laughter we shared. And as I read and reread our conversations, what comes through most for me are the insight, honesty, hope and aspirations. Your perceptions, as the reader, will be different and individual. Whatever they may be, I hope these two voices enthuse you to listen to many more such voices, as it probably takes even more than 1000 voices to tell this story.

Acknowledgements

The first author would like to thank her co-authors, Abby and Lavinia, for sharing their stories so generously and for all the fun, laughter and friendship. Thanks also go to the graduate and student speech and language therapists who assisted with the transcriptions so enthusiastically: Hayley Rogers, Michelle Coleman, Saerlaith Murphy and Eleanor Murray.

References

Carroll, C. & Dockrell, J. (2010) Leaving special school: Post-16 outcomes for young adults with specific language impairment. *European Journal of Special Needs Education, 25(2)*, 131–147.

Dockrell, J., Lindsay, G., Palikara, O. & Cullen, M.A. (2007) *Raising the Achievements of Children and Young People with Specific Language and Communication Needs and Other Special Educational Needs Through School, to Work and College.* RR837. Nottingham: Department for Education and Skills.

Markham, C., van Laar, D., Gibbard, D. & Dean, T. (2009) Children with speech, language and communication needs: Their perceptions of their quality of life. *International Journal of Language and Communication Disorders, 44(5)*, 748–768.

McCormack, J., McLeod, S., McAllister, L. & Harrison, L.J. (2010) My speech problem, your listening problem, and my frustration: The experience of living with childhood speech impairment. *Language, Speech, and Hearing Services in Schools, 41*, 379–392.

Myers, L., Davies-Jones, C., Chiat, S., Joffe, V. & Botting, N. (in press) 'A place where I can be me': A role for social and leisure provision to support young people with language impairment. *International Journal of Language and Communication Disorders.*

Owen, R., Hayett, L. & Roulstone, S. (2004) Children's views of speech and language therapy in school: Consulting children with communication difficulties. *Journal of Child, Language, Teaching and Therapy, 20(1)*, 55–73.

Palikara, O., Lindsay, G. & Dockrell, J. (2009) Voices of young people with a history of specific speech and language difficulties in the first year of post-16 education. *International Journal of Language and Communication Disorders, 44(1)*, 56–78.

Section II
The Impact of Communication Disorders in Adulthood

9 Aphasia

Katerina Hilari
City University London, UK

Introduction

Aphasia is a language disability caused by organic damage to the brain, most commonly a stroke. It can affect all language modalities, i.e. speaking and expressing oneself, understanding what other people say, reading and writing. It may also affect non-verbal communication modalities such as gestures. It is estimated that about a third of people who suffer a stroke have aphasia early post-stroke (Engelter, Gostynski, Papa, Frei, Born, et al., 2006), while 15% remain aphasic in the long term (Wade, 1994).

More often than not, aphasia does not occur in isolation. People may have other stroke-related disabilities, such as mobility problems, difficulties with activities of daily living and self-care, and cognitive decline. In a survey of stroke outcomes across western Europe, at one year post-onset, 55% of stroke survivors were still dependent in basic activities of daily living (Wolfe, Tilling, Rudd, Giroud & Inzitari, 2004). The prevalence of cognitive impairment has been estimated at 35% at one year post-stroke (Patel, Coshall, Rudd & Wolfe, 2003). People with aphasia (PWA) may also have other communication problems, such as dyspraxia. Communication may be further compromised by reduced hearing and vision, which typically affect people of older age.

Aphasia has a profound impact on all aspects of people's lives. Chapter 16 of this book illustrates this through the voices of people with aphasia themselves. In this chapter, the research evidence on how aphasia impacts on a person's emotional wellbeing, relationships, social participation and quality of life is presented. The impact on the family is also highlighted. Before considering all this, issues around the assessment of wellbeing and quality of life in PWA are raised. The chapter finishes with drawing clinical implications.

Challenges in assessing the impact of aphasia

Assessing wellbeing and quality of life with PWA is not without challenges. PWA may have difficulty understanding the questions that interviewers ask them or the items on questionnaires. They may also have difficulty finding the words they want to use and expressing their responses. As a result of this, until the late 1990s, stroke studies focusing on psychosocial outcomes either excluded PWA or included only people with mild aphasia. Some studies used proxy data for PWA. This is understandable for people with severe aphasia, but analyzing proxy data together with self-report data can be misleading. There tend to be significant differences in proxy and self-report assessments of functional status and quality of life after stroke (Knapp & Hewison, 1999; Sneeuw, Aaronson, de Haan & Limburg, 1997) and aphasia (Cruice, Worrall, Hickson & Murison, 2005), especially when generic tools for quality of life are used.

In the field of aphasiology, a lot of progress has been made in addressing these issues. From a qualitative paradigm, interviewing techniques, such as semi-structured and structured interviewing, and ethnographic approaches, such as participant or non-participant observation, analysis of artefacts, for example, diaries or published personal accounts, have been used to evaluate the impact of aphasia on people's lives (Cruice, Hill, Worrall & Hickson, 2010; Hinckley, 2006; Parr, Byng & Gilpin, 1997; Parr, 2007).

From a quantitative paradigm, measures specifically for use with people with aphasia have been developed, such as the Visual Analogue Self-Esteem Scales (VASES; Brumfitt & Sheeran, 1999), the Quality of Communication Life Scale (Paul, Holland, Frattali, Thompson, Caperton & Slater, 2004) and the Communication Disability Profile (Swinburn & Byng, 2006). Scales for other groups have also been adapted for use with PWA, such as the Stroke and Aphasia Quality of Life scale (SAQOL-39; Hilari, Byng, Lamping & Smith, 2003; Hilari, Lamping, Smith, Northcott, Lamb & Marshall, 2009) and the Community Integration Questionnaire (Dalemans, de Witte, Beurskens, van den Heuvel & Wade, 2010a).

Ways to facilitate PWA complete self-reported measures have been researched. These include modifying the presentation of scales to make them more aphasia-friendly – key words in bold, large font (minimum 14), few items per page, practice items, lead-in questions and, where appropriate, use of pictures – and administering the scales in an interview format with an interviewer who can facilitate the communication of PWA (Hilari & Byng, 2001; Townend, Brady & McLaughlan, 2007; Worrall, Rose, Howe, Brennan, Egan et al., 2005).

Last but not least, research on proxy and self-report agreement on quality of life scales between PWA and their proxies has shown that agreement is generally poor when generic scales are used (Cruice et al., 2005), whereas it is better when stroke- and aphasia-specific scales, such as the SAQOL-39, are used (Hilari, Owen & Farrelly, 2007).

The approaches identified here may facilitate the assessment of the impact of aphasia on people's lives, yet they have their limitations. Qualitative approaches are hard to implement in clinical practice; and in the case of ethnographic approaches involve value judgements linking an observed behaviour or artefact to what the person with aphasia may feel about it, which is problematic. Using scales and questionnaires, even adapted for PWA, raises questions about whether the most relevant questions are asked for each individual. Each method has its limits but it is important to remember there is no perfect way of assessing wellbeing and quality of life for people with communication disabilities. We need to be aware of the strengths and limitations of each approach and interpret findings accordingly. In the light of this, using the tools and the methods identified above, a substantial body of evidence is emerging on the impact of aphasia on people's lives. This is synthesized below.

Emotional wellbeing

Emotional wellbeing is commonly affected after stroke. A conservative estimate is that 33% of people with stroke suffer depressive symptoms at any time during follow-up (Hackett, Yapa, Parag & Anderson, 2005). Such symptoms affect people's response to rehabilitation and, thus, long-term functional outcomes and quality of life. For PWA, the prevalence of depression is even higher, with 70% being depressed at three months post-stroke and 62% at one year (Kauhanen, Korpelainen, Hiltunen, Maatta, Mononen et al., 2000). In this study, although the overall prevalence of depression decreased from three months to one year, the prevalence of major depression increased from 11% to 33%.

Identifying what factors predict low mood is important in order to detect those at risk for depression and target intervention appropriately. In a recent review, the most consistent variables associated with depressive symptoms after stroke were physical disability, stroke severity and cognitive impairment (Hackett & Anderson, 2005). Fewer studies explored social factors, but when considered together – living alone, place of residence, social support and social isolation – these were also important. However, in most of the studies included in this review (17 out of 20), PWA were excluded.

PWA were included in two recent studies that systematically evaluated predictors of emotional distress after stroke. In the first study, people were assessed one and six months post-stroke. Expressive aphasia and dependence in personal activities of daily living (ADL) predicted distress at one month post-stroke. Stroke severity, expressive aphasia and distress at one month post-stroke predicted distress at six months (Thomas & Lincoln, 2008). In the second study, people were assessed within two weeks of their stroke and then three months and six months later. Stroke severity was the strongest predictor of distress early on, whereas social factors predicted distress at three and six months post-stroke. The baseline factors that predicted distress at six months were levels of distress, loneliness and low satisfaction with one's social network (Hilari, Northcott, Roy, Marshall, Wiggins et al., 2010). In this study, though aphasia was not a predictor of distress at any time point, still, at three months post-stroke, people with aphasia were significantly more likely to suffer from emotional distress (93%) than people without aphasia (50%). These two studies highlight that emotional distress and depression are persistent problems impacting on PWA's lives.

Social wellbeing

Two areas are considered in this section: social participation and social support.

In terms of social participation, i.e. involvement in social life situations, PWA perform fewer social activities than non-aphasic controls and derive less satisfaction from them (Cruice, Worrall & Hickson, 2006). PWA also feel less engaged in their social activities and less integrated (Dalemans, de Witte, Wade & van den Heuvel, 2010c) and are at risk of social isolation and exclusion (Parr, 2007). A recent study looking at factors associated with social participation in PWA found that age, gender, functional activities of daily living (ADL) and aphasia severity were the strongest predictors (Dalemans, De Witte, Beurskens, van den Heuvel & Wade, 2010b). Return to work is also a major issue. For the majority of people, there is no return to work at all after stroke and aphasia; and return to work is often characterized by reduced hours, return to another job or return to the same job with modifications (Dalemans, de Witte, van den Heuvel & Wade, 2008).

Social relationships and social support are also affected. People are at risk of losing their friends after a stroke (Astrom, Asplund & Astrom, 1992) and this is even more the case for those who have aphasia (Davidson, Howe, Worrall, Hickson & Togher, 2008). In a study of 83 people with chronic aphasia,

64% reported that they saw their friends less than before the stroke, and 30% reported having no close friends at all (Hilari & Northcott, 2006).

Maintaining social networks is important after a stroke as friendships can be a protective factor for older people. A meta-analysis of studies on factors affecting wellbeing in later life suggested that contact with friends is associated with higher subjective wellbeing (Pinquart & Sorensen, 2000). Friends-based social networks have also been shown to enhance survival in the elderly (Giles, Glonek, Luszcz & Andrews, 2005).

Using in-depth qualitative interviews, Northcott and Hilari (in press) explored why people lose friends after stroke. The main reasons given were: loss of shared activities; reduced energy levels; physical disability; aphasia; unhelpful responses of others; environmental barriers; and changing social desires. The participants who experienced the most extensive loss of friends were those who described a sense that they were 'closing in' on themselves leading to a withdrawal from social contact. Those with aphasia experienced the most hurtful negative responses from others and found it more difficult to retain their friends unless they had strong supportive friendship patterns prior to the stroke (Northcott and Hilari, in press).

Health-related quality of life

Health-related quality of life (HRQL) reflects the impact of a health state, in this case aphasia, on a person's ability to lead a fulfilling life. It incorporates the individual's perception of and satisfaction with his/her physical, mental/ emotional, family and social functioning (Bullinger, Anderson, Cella & Aaronson, 1993; Berzon, Hays & Shumaker, 1993).

Aphasia has a profound impact on quality of life. A recent population-based study of people living in long-term care facilities in Canada (n=66,193) compared the impact of 60 diseases and 15 conditions on caregiver-assessed preference-based HRQL. After adjusting for age, sex and other diagnoses, aphasia exhibited the largest negative relationship to preference-based HRQL, even over and above cancer and Alzheimer's disease (Lam & Wodchis, 2010). People with aphasia themselves report significantly worse HRQL than non-aphasic stroke controls (Hilari, 2011); and compared to healthy controls they report worse quality of life, particularly in terms of level of independence, social relationships and access to aspects of their environment (Ross & Wertz, 2003).

In terms of the impact of the severity of aphasia, individuals with severe aphasia have significantly lower HRQL compared to their general aphasic peers (Hilari & Byng, 2009). Two studies used both measures of functional communication and language impairment to explore their relative impact. They found that impaired functional communication, and to a lesser degree language impairment, predicted worse HRQL and wellbeing in PWA (Cruice, Worrall, Hickson & Murison, 2003; Hilari, Wiggins, Roy, Byng & Smith, 2003).

A recent systematic review explored the factors associated with or predictive of poor HRQL in PWA post-stroke. This review comprised 14 studies (three qualitative and 11 quantitative reports). The qualitative studies included a total of 98 participants with aphasia and the quantitative studies 742 PWA. Emotional distress/depression, extent of communication disability and aphasic impairment, presence of other medical problems and activity level were the predictors of HRQL emerging from quantitative studies. Social factors also emerged as important. Themes drawn from qualitative studies included looking to the future/having a positive outlook, verbal communication, body functioning, and people and social support, and supported these findings. They also added to them, by identifying adaptation of personal identity and development of a collective identity, and working to remove the barriers that people with aphasia face as ways to reduce aphasic disability and live successfully with aphasia (Hilari, Needle & Harrison, in press).

Impact on the family

A large proportion of disabled stroke survivors live at home and they are primarily supported by informal carers, i.e. their family or, in some cases, friends. A review of studies on the quality of life of informal carers highlighted that they suffer from reduced HRQL and high levels of stress, anxiety and depression (Rombough, Howse, Bagg & Bartfay, 2007). Looking at what happens as time passes (from admission to hospital to three years after stroke), it has been reported that burden decreases but harmony in the relationship and social relations also decrease. Moreover, although carer depression decreases initially post-stroke, it increases in the long term (Visser-Meily, Post, van de Port, Maas, Forstberg-Wärleby & Lindeman, 2009).

Studies on factors affecting carer burden and quality of life identified advancing age and anxiety in patients and carers, high patient dependency and poor family support as main predictors of poor carer outcomes, which could be reduced by carer training (McCullagh, Brigstocke, Donaldson & Karla, 2005). A review of qualitative studies corroborates these findings by identifying lack of information and training and also lack of emotional support to manage distress, feeling undervalued or trapped and lacking freedom as main challenges for carers. It also adds to these findings by highlighting role and relationship changes, such as having to give up paid employment and having to adjust to the new role of being a carer, as main themes identified by the carers (Greenwood, Mackenzie, Cloud & Wilson, 2009).

Studies focusing specifically on the needs of carers of PWA are scarce. One study compared carers of PWA to carers of non-aphasic stroke survivors and found that carers of PWA perceived greater difficulty with tasks and had more negative stroke-related outcomes than carers of non-aphasic survivors. Communication with the person with aphasia was rated as most upsetting and difficult by carers in the aphasic group, followed by managing behaviours (Bakas, Kroenke, Plue, Perkins & Williams, 2006). Two qualitative studies on the challenges that spouses/family members of PWA face raised as main concerns:

1 changes in family/marital life, such as worrying for the person with aphasia and understanding their needs, profoundly changed marital life, dependence on the help of other people and the loss of spare time (Zemva, 1999); and

2 the need for support and respite and the lack of available services (Le Dorze & Signori, 2010).

In summary, carers of people with stroke and aphasia suffer from anxiety, depression and reduced quality of life. Their marital and family relations change, their role in the family changes and their financial circumstances also change. They identify as main challenges the need for training and information and for support and respite.

Clinical implications

Hilari and Cruice (in press) advocate a quality of life approach to intervention for aphasia, which structures assessment and therapy from the client's perspective, having determined their desire for therapy, priorities, standards, and personal aspirations from initial quality of life interviews. Such an approach is not an alternative or addition to, for example, neuropsychological or functional communication approaches. It is more of an overarching philosophy that encompasses different approaches and methods depending on what works best for each client, at different stages of recovery and life after stroke and aphasia (Hilari & Cruice, in press).

To date, few interventions have specifically focused on improving the impact of aphasia on people's lives. There is promising evidence for group therapy for PWA, in terms of psychosocial improvements after therapy (Elman & Bernstein-Ellis, 1999; Ross, Winslow, Marchant & Brumfitt, 2006) and improved social participation and social connection after therapy compared to controls (Vickers, 2010). There is also preliminary evidence that impairment-based therapy for word-finding difficulties, when carefully targeted around an individual's interests, can produce changes not just in the therapy room but also on what people do in real life and on how they feel about it (Best, Greenwood, Grassly & Hickin, 2008).

Yet, other programmes that are generally thought to lead to broader benefits for the lives of PWA do not always have the evidence base to support such assumptions. Simmons-Mackie, Raymer, Armstrong, Holland and Cherney (2010) reviewed the literature on the effects of communication partner training on PWA and their communication partners. They found that communication partner training is effective in improving communication activities and/ or participation of the communication partner and is probably effective in improving communication activities and/or participation of persons with chronic aphasia when they are interacting with trained communication partners. However, there was insufficient evidence to make recommendations related to the impact of partner training on psychosocial adjustment, or quality of life for either the person with aphasia or the communication partner. There is a pressing need for such outcomes to be systematically evaluated in relation to interventions.

In terms of service provision for PWA, some models of community service have been evaluated in terms of psychosocial outcomes for PWA and their families, but lack of appropriate controls limit the validity of their findings. These services include the York-Durham Aphasia Centre in Canada (Hoen, Thelander & Worsley, 1997), the MossRehab Aphasia Centre in the US (Fink & Schwartz, 2000), and in the UK the Volunteer Stroke Service groups (Legg, Stott, Ellis & Sellars, 2007) and Connect, the communication disability network (van der Gaag, Smith, Davis, Moss, Cornelius, et al., 2005).

Interventions for carers also need to be considered. In the UK, a large randomized controlled trial looked at the effectiveness of training carers in reducing the burden of stroke in carers and patients. They compared conventional care mainly involving stroke education, encouragement to attend therapies and help with accessing services (control group), with conventional care plus training in basic nursing and facilitation of personal care (intervention group). In the intervention group, a higher proportion of disabled stroke survivors achieved independence at an earlier stage; both stroke survivors and their carers reported better quality of life and less anxiety and depression; and the cost of stroke care was reduced (Karla, Evans, Perez, Melbourn, Patel et al., 2004). A review of intervention studies for stroke carers concluded that counselling programmes appeared to have the most positive outcomes (Visser-Meily, van Heugten, Post, Schepers & Lindeman, 2005). Such programmes should be made routinely available to stroke survivors and their families in order to reduce the personal, societal and economic burden of stroke.

Conclusion

Aphasia has a profound impact on people's lives. Communication, which is crucial in all domains of people's lives, is affected by aphasia and leads to high levels of emotional distress and depression, reduced HRQL, reduced social participation and the loss of friends. Interventions that aim to improve the impact of aphasia on people's lives by specifically targeting factors that affect HRQL – depression, communication disability, engagement in activities, and diminishing social networks – need to be systematically evaluated.

References

Astrom, M., Asplund, K. & Astrom, T. (1992) Psychosocial function and life satisfaction after stroke. *Stroke, 23,* 527–531.

Bakas, T., Kroenke, K., Plue, L.D., Perkins, S.M. & Williams, L.S. (2006) Outcomes among family caregivers of aphasic versus nonaphasic stroke survivors. *Rehabilitation Nursing, 31(1),* 33–42.

Berzon, R., Hays, R.D. & Shumaker, S.A. (1993) International use, application and performance of health-related quality of life instruments. *Quality of Life Research, 2,* 367–368.

Best, W., Greenwood, A., Grassly, J. & Hickin, J. (2008) Bridging the gap: Can impairment-based therapy for anomia have an impact at the psycho-social level? *International Journal of Language and Communication Disorders, 43(4),* 390–407.

Brumfitt, S. & Sheeran, P. (1999) *Vases: Visual Analogue Self-Esteem Scale.* Bicester: Winslow Press Ltd.

Bullinger, M., Anderson, R., Cella, D., Aaronson, N.K. (1993) Developing and evaluating cross cultural instruments: From minimum requirements to optimal models. *Quality of Life Research, 2,* 451–459.

Cruice, M., Hill, R., Worrall, L. & Hickson, L. (2010) Conceptualising quality of life for older people with aphasia. *Aphasiology, 24(3),* 327–347.

Cruice, M., Worrall, L. & Hickson, L. (2006) Quantifying aphasic people's social lives in the context of non-aphasic peers. *Aphasiology, 20(12),* 1210–1225.

Cruice, M., Worrall, L., Hickson, L. & Murison, R. (2003) Finding a focus for quality of life with aphasia: Social and emotional health, and psychological wellbeing. *Aphasiology, 17(4),* 333–353.

Cruice, M., Worrall, L., Hickson, L. & Murison, R. (2005) Measuring quality of life: Comparing family members' and friends' ratings with those of their aphasic partners. *Aphasiology, 19(2),* 111–129.

Dalemans, R.J.P., de Witte, L., van den Heuvel, W. & Wade, D. (2008) A description of social participation in working age people with aphasia: A review of the literature. *Aphasiology, 22(10),* 1071–1091.

Dalemans, R.J.P., de Witte, L., Beurskens, S., van den Heuvel, W. & Wade, D. (2010a) Psychometric properties of the Community Integration Questionnaire adjusted for people with aphasia. *Archives Physical and Medical Rehabilitation, 91(3),* 395–399.

Dalemans, R.J., de Witte, L.P., Beurskens, A.J., van den Heuvel, W.J. & Wade, D.T. (2010b) An investigation into the social participation of stroke survivors with aphasia. *Disability and Rehabilitation, 32(20),* 1678–1685.

Dalemans, R.J.P., de Witte, L., Wade, D. & van den Heuvel, W. (2010c) Social participation through the eyes of people with aphasia. *International Journal of Language and Communication Disorders, 45(5),* 537–550.

Davidson, B., Howe, T., Worrall, L., Hickson, L. & Togher, L. (2008) Social participation for older people with aphasia: The impact of communication disability on friendships. *Topics in Stroke Rehabilitation, 15(4),* 325–340.

Elman, R.J. & Bernstein-Ellis, E. (1999) Psychosocial aspects of group communication treatment: Preliminary findings. *Seminars in Speech and Language, 20(1),* 65–72.

Engelter, S.T., Gostynski, M., Papa, S., Frei, M., Born, C., Ajdacic-Gross, V. et al. (2006) Epidemiology of aphasia attributable to first ischemic stroke: Incidence, severity, fluency, etiology, and thrombolysis. *Stroke, 37(6),*1379–1384.

Fink, R.B. & Schwartz, M.F. (2000) MossRehab aphasia center: A collaborative model for long-term rehabilitation. *Topics in Stroke Rehabilitation, 7(2),* 32–43.

Giles, L.C., Glonek, G.F.V., Luszcz, M.A. & Andrews, G.R. (2005) Effect of social networks on 10 year survival in very old Australians: The Australian longitudinal study of aging. *Journal of Epidemiology and Community Health, 59,* 574–579.

Greenwood, N., Mackenzie, A., Cloud, G.C. & Wilson, N. (2009) Informal primary carers of stroke survivors living at home – challenges, satisfactions and coping: A systematic review of qualitative studies. *Disability and Rehabilitation, 31(5)*, 337–351.

Hackett, M.L. & Anderson, C.S. (2005) Predictors of depression after stroke. A systematic review of observational studies. *Stroke, 36*, 2296–2301.

Hackett, M.L., Yapa, C., Parag, V. & Anderson, C.S. (2005) Frequency of depression after stroke. A systematic review of observational studies. *Stroke, 36*, 1330–1340.

Hilari, K. (2011) The impact of stroke: Are people with aphasia different to those without? *Disability and Rehabilitation, 33(3)*, 211–218.

Hilari, K. & Byng, S. (2001) Measuring quality of life in people with aphasia: The Stroke Specific Quality of Life Scale. *International Journal of Language and Communication Disorders, 36* (suppl), 86–91.

Hilari K. & Byng S. (2009) Health-related quality of life in people with severe aphasia. *International Journal of Language and Communication Disorders, 44(2)*, 193–205.

Hilari, K., Byng, S., Lamping, D.L. & Smith, S.C. (2003) Stroke and aphasia quality of life scale-39 (SAQOL-39): Evaluation of acceptability, reliability and validity. *Stroke, 34(8)*, 1944–1950.

Hilari, K. & Cruice, M. (in press) Quality of life approach in aphasia. In I. Papathanasiou, P. Coppens & C. Potagas (Eds) *Aphasia and Related Neurogenic Communication Disorders*. Boston: Jones and Bartlett Publishers, LLC.

Hilari, K., Lamping, D.L., Smith, S.C., Northcott, S., Lamb, A. & Marshall, J. (2009) Psychometric properties of the Stroke and Aphasia Quality of Life scale (SAQOL-39) in a generic stroke population. *Clinical Rehabilitation, 23(6)*, 544–557.

Hilari, K., Needle, J. & Harrison, K. (in press) What are the important factors in health-related quality of life for people with aphasia? A systematic review. *Archives of Physical Medicine and Rehabilitation*.

Hilari, K. & Northcott, S. (2006). Social support in people with chronic aphasia. *Aphasiology, 20(1)*, 17–36.

Hilari, K., Northcott, S., Roy, P., Marshall, J., Wiggins, R.D., Chataway, J. & Ames, D. (2010) Psychological distress after stroke and aphasia: The first six months. *Clinical Rehabilitation, 24(2)*, 181–90.

Hilari, K., Owen, S. & Farrelly, S.J. (2007) Proxy and self-report agreement on the Stroke and Aphasia Quality of Life scale (SAQOL-39). *Journal of Neurology, Neurosurgery and Psychiatry, 78*, 1072–1075.

Hilari, K., Wiggins, R.D., Roy, P., Byng, S. & Smith, S.C. (2003) Predictors of health-related quality of life (HRQL) in people with chronic aphasia. *Aphasiology, 17(4)*, 365–382.

Hinckley, J.J. (2006) Finding messages in bottles: Living successfully with stroke and aphasia. *Topics in Stroke Rehabilitation, 13(1)*, 25–36.

Hoen, B., Thelander, M. & Worsley, J. (1997) Improvement in psychological wellbeing of people with aphasia and their families: Evaluation of a community-based programme. *Aphasiology*, *11(7)*, 681–691.

Karla, L., Evans, A., Perez, I., Melbourn, A., Patel, A., Knapp, M. & Donaldson, N. (2004) Training carers of stroke patients: Randomised controlled trial. *British Medical Journal*, *328*, 1099–1103.

Kauhanen, M.L., Korpelainen, J.T., Hiltunen, P., Maatta, R., Mononen, H., Brusin, E., Sotaniemi, K.A. & Myllyla, V.V. (2000) Aphasia, depression, and non-verbal cognitive impairment ischaemic stroke. *Cerebrovascular Disease*, *10*, 455–461.

Knapp, P. & Hewison, J. (1999) Disagreement in patient and carer assessment of functional abilities after stroke. *Stroke*, *30*, 938.

Lam, J.M. & Wodchis, W.P. (2010) The relationship of 60 disease diagnoses and 15 conditions to preference-based health-related quality of life in Ontario hospital-based long-term care residents. *Medical Care*, *48(4)*, 380–387.

Le Dorze, G. & Signori, F.H. (2010) Needs, barriers and facilitators experienced by spouses of people with aphasia. *Disability and Rehabilitation*, *32(13)*, 1073–1087.

Legg, L., Stott, D., Ellis, G. & Sellars, C. (2007) Volunteer stroke service (VSS) groups for patients with communication difficulties after stroke: A qualitative analysis of the value of groups to their users. *Clinical Rehabilitation*, *21(9)*, 794–804.

McCullagh, E., Brigstocke, G., Donaldson, N. & Karla, L. (2005) Determinants of caregiving burden and quality of life in caregivers of stroke patients. *Stroke*, *36*, 2181–2186.

Northcott, S. & Hilari, K. (in press) Why do people lose their friends after a stroke? *International Journal of Language and Communication Disorders*, *46*.

Parr, S. (2007) Living with severe aphasia: Tracking social exclusion. *Aphasiology*, *21(1)*, 98–123.

Parr, S., Byng, S. & Gilpin, S. (1997). *Talking about Aphasia*. Philadelphia: Open University Press.

Patel, M., Coshall, C., Rudd, A.G. & Wolfe, C.D. (2003) Natural history of cognitive impairment after stroke and factors associated with its recovery. *Clinical Rehabilitation*, *17(2)*, 158–166.

Paul, D., Holland, A., Frattali, C., Thompson, C., Caperton, C. & Slater, S. (2004). *Quality of Communication Life Scale (ASHA QCL)*. Rockville, MD: American Speech-Language-Hearing Association.

Pinquart, M. & Sorensen, S. (2000). Influences of socioeconomic status, social network, and competence on subjective wellbeing in later life: A meta-analysis. *Psychology of Aging*, *15(2)*, 187–224.

Rombough, R.E., Howse, E.L., Bagg, S.D. & Bartfay, W.J. (2007) A comparison of studies on the quality of life of primary caregivers of stroke survivors: A systematic review of the literature. *Topics in Stroke Rehabilitation*, *14(3)*, 69–79.

Ross, A., Winslow, I., Marchant, P. & Brumfitt, S. (2006) Evaluation of communication, life participation and psychological wellbeing in chronic aphasia: The influence of group intervention. *Aphasiology*, *20(5)*, 427–448.

Ross, K.B. & Wertz, R.T. (2003) Quality of life with and without aphasia. *Aphasiology*, *17(4)*, 355–364.

Simmons-Mackie, N., Raymer, A., Armstrong, E., Holland, A. & Cherney, L.R. (2010) Communication partner training in aphasia: A systematic review. *Archives in Physical Medicine and Rehabilitation*, *91*, 1814–1837.

Sneeuw, K.C.A., Aaronson, N.K., de Haan, R.J. & Limburg, M. (1997) Assessing quality of life after stroke. The value and limitations of proxy ratings. *Stroke*, *28*, 1541–1249.

Swinburn, K. & Byng, S. (2006) *The Communication Disability Profile*. London: Connect.

Thomas, S.A. & Lincoln, N.B. (2008) Predictors of emotional distress after stroke. *Stroke*, *39(4)*, 1240–1245.

Townend, E., Brady, M. & McLaughlan, K. (2007) A systematic evaluation of the adaptation of depression diagnostic methods for stroke survivors who have aphasia. *Stroke*, *38*, 3076–3083.

van der Gaag, A., Smith, L., Davis, S., Moss, B., Cornelius, V., Laing, S. et al. (2005) Therapy and support services for people with long-term stroke and aphasia and their relatives: A six-month follow-up study. *Clinical Rehabilitation*, *19(4)*, 372–380.

Vickers, C.P. (2010) Social networks after the onset of aphasia: The impact of aphasia group attendance. *Aphasiology*, *24(6–8)*, 902–913.

Visser-Meily, A., Post, M., van de Port, I., Maas, C., Forstberg-Wärleby, G. & Lindeman, E. (2009) Psychosocial functioning of spouses of patients with stroke from initial inpatient rehabilitation to 3 years poststroke: Course and relations with coping strategies. *Stroke*, *40*, 1399–1404.

Visser-Meily, A., van Heugten, C., Post, M., Schepers, V. & Lindeman, E. (2005) Intervention studies for caregivers of stroke survivors: A critical review. *Patient Education and Counselling*, *56*, 257–267.

Wade, D.T. (1994) Stroke (acute cerebrovascular disease). In A. Stevens & J. Raftery (Eds) *Health Care Needs Assessment*. Oxford: Radcliffe Medical Press.

Wolfe, C.D.A., Tilling, K., Rudd, A., Giroud, M. & Inzitari, D. (2004) Variations in care and outcome in the first year after stroke: A Western and Central European perspective. *Journal of Neurology, Neurosurgery and Psychiatry*, *75*, 1702–1706.

Worrall, L., Rose, T., Howe, T., Brennan, A., Egan, J., Oxenham, D. et al. (2005) Access to written information for people with aphasia. *Aphasiology*, *19*, 923–929.

Zemva, N. (1999) Aphasic patients and their families: Wishes and limits. *Aphasiology*, *13(3)*, 219–224.

10 Dementia

Kathryn Bayles
University of Arizona, USA

Nidhi Mahendra
California State University, USA

Tammy Hopper
University of Alberta, Canada

Introduction

The focus of this chapter is Alzheimer's dementia (AD) and its impact on victims, their families and society in general. After defining the dementia syndrome and characterizing the effects of AD by disease stage, the impact of the disease on the quality of life (QoL) of both victims and caregivers will be discussed, followed by suggestions for clinical management.

Dementia defined

Dementia is a syndrome associated with multiple cognitive deficits that are sufficient to interfere with social, occupational and communicative functioning. Although some causes of dementia are reversible (e.g. infection, drug side effects), most are not and include age-related diseases. Because dementia is a manifestation of many diseases, there are disease-specific criteria that can be found in the fourth edition of the *Diagnostic and Statistical Manual of Mental Disorders* (DSM-IV-TR; American Psychiatric Association, 2000).

Table 10.1 lists the most common causes of dementia. As can be seen, most are age-related neurodegenerative diseases. First on the list is Alzheimer's disease, accounting for approximately two-thirds of all dementia cases (Nussbaum & Ellis, 2003). Second is Lewy Body disease, a degenerative process that may account for more cases of dementia than vascular disease (Jellinger, 1996). Although dementia is always present in individuals with Alzheimer's and Lewy Body disease, it is not always present in Parkinson's disease (PD). When dementia occurs, it is typically late in the disease course (Tröster & Woods, 1987). In a longitudinal study, Janvin and colleagues (2005) determined the prevalence of dementia in PD at baseline and after four and eight years, and found an increase with disease duration. At baseline, 26% of the sample had dementia symptoms; at four years, the percentage rose to 52%, and by eight years, the percentage had risen to 78%.

Table 10.1 Most common causes of irreversible dementia

Alzheimer's disease
Vascular disease
Parkinson's disease
Frontotemporal dementia
Huntington's disease
Creutzfeldt-Jakob disease

Many victims of dementia have more than one dementing condition. For example, vascular disease and Alzheimer's commonly co-occur (Nolan, Lino, Seligman & Blass, 1998), as do AD and Lewy Body disease. At autopsy, Lewy bodies are routinely present in the brains of individuals with AD (Gearing, Schneider, Rebeck, Hyman & Mirra, 1995). Then, too, many of the proteins that contribute to Parkinson's disease also play a role in AD and vice versa. Additionally, depression is common in AD, PD, and other dementias (Schrag, Jahanshahi & Quinn, 2001; Lyketsos et al., 2002) and can diminish cognitive function.

Persons diagnosed with irreversible dementing diseases progressively lose the ability to care for themselves, a fact that results in significant burden on families and society in general. Because AD is the most common dementing disease and best studied, it is the focus of this chapter (readers interested in cognitive and communication disorders associated with other dementing diseases are referred to Bayles and Tomoeda, 2007).

Rising prevalence of dementia

The prevalence of dementia worldwide is estimated at 30 million and rising. Each year there are approximately 4.6 million new cases, a rate that amounts to one new case every 7 seconds (Ferri et al., 2005). At this alarming rate, the number of people with Alzheimer's dementia will double every 20 years to more than 81 million by the year 2040 and swell to 100 million by 2050 (Alzheimer's Disease International, 2008).

The prevalence of AD among individuals 65 to 69 years is 1% but rises with age. For every five years after age 65, prevalence doubles (Alzheimer's Disease International, 2008). By age 95, the prevalence approximates 50% (Hy & Keller, 2000). Although most cases are sporadic, approximately 5% are familial, and tend to develop in the fifth decade (Selkoe, 2000). Nonetheless, an individual's risk of developing AD is four times higher if a first-order family member has had the disease.

The rate of increase in the number of dementia cases is expected to be three to four times higher in developing regions of the world than in developed areas (Ferri et al., 2005). Currently 60% of individuals with dementia reside in developing countries but this number is expected to rise to 71% by 2040. The increase in India, China, and their Asian neighbours will exceed 300% (Ferri et al., 2005).

Dementia is costly

In 2010 more than five million Americans carried a diagnosis of Alzheimer's disease and the annual cost of their care approximated $172 billion (Alzheimer's Association, 2010). Incredibly, that figure greatly underrepresents the true cost, because the value of the care provided by unpaid individuals approximates $144 billion. In addition to the monetary cost of the disease, which increases with disease progression (Ernst, Hay, Fenn, Tinklenberg & Yesavage, 1997; Souetre, Thwaites & Yeardley, 1999), there is tremendous cost to quality of life for both victims and caregivers.

Impact of Alzheimer's dementia on affected individuals

Cognition and communication

By definition, individuals with Alzheimer's dementia have multiple cognitive deficits that profoundly affect their lives. These develop insidiously and progressively worsen until intellect is devastated. Early in the disease course episodic memory, or the ability to make a chronologic record of recent events, is compromised because of pathology in the basal forebrain and hippocampal complex. As pathology proliferates throughout the frontal lobes and posterior association cortices, working and semantic memory systems also are affected. Relatively spared until late in the disease are the motor strip and basal ganglia and, as a result, speech remains fluent and procedural memory intact. Unsurprisingly, the communication disorder of individuals with AD reflects this progressive deterioration of episodic, working and semantic memory systems and is best described by stage of disease. Few caregivers are aware of the neurobehavioural sequelae of the disease and how they will affect patients and other family members. Periodic counselling by clinicians can prepare caregivers for the challenges of the disease stages and inform them of evidence-based strategies for maximizing function and QoL.

Early stage

The duration of this stage is two to four years. Typical clinical manifestations include rapid forgetting of recent events, difficulty concentrating and disorientation for time (though not place or person). Information encoding, knowledge retrieval and idea generation are less efficient, though not sufficiently impaired to prevent patients from performing basic activities of daily living. However, they are sufficient to cause problems managing finances and doing complex tasks.

Clinicians should be alert to symptoms of depression because evidence is accumulating that depression may be harbinger of cognitive decline. Kohler and colleagues (2010) studied the temporal association between depressive symptoms and cognitive functioning in a large sample of cognitively intact elders, and reassessed them after three and six years. They observed that depression was present in a significant number of subjects who were later diagnosed with AD. Alterations in personality also are common. Some individuals become unusually talkative, others withdraw, and many become anxious in new situations (Finkel, 2000).

Collectively, these changes in cognition, mood and personality affect the AD patient's ability to communicate; that is, their ability to intentionally share information by means of a linguistic symbol system. Although people with AD retain their knowledge of the symbol system of language, their rapid forgetting of information makes following and sustaining a conversation problematic. Family members commonly report being told the same information repeatedly and answering the same questions. A lack of understanding of why this occurs can produce frustration and even anger toward the individual with dementia.

The early changes in the ability to encode information and generate ideas are apparent in the descriptive discourse of patients in the early stage of AD. In several studies of the descriptive discourse of individuals with early AD, investigators observed significantly less cohesion (number of relevant ideas divided by total number of words), more sentence fragments and greater tangentiality than in healthy elders (Bayles, Tomoeda & Boone, 1985; Bayles, Tomoeda, Kaszniak, Stern & Eagans, 1985; Tomoeda & Bayles, 1993). Similarly, the ability to generate examples of items in a category, also known as verbal fluency, is significantly impaired relative to healthy age mates (Clark et al., 2009; Sailor, Antoine, Diaz, Kuslansky & Kluger, 2004).

Although difficulty retrieving names is common with normal ageing, it becomes more pronounced in early AD (Bayles & Tomoeda, 1983). Bayles and Tomoeda analyzed the naming responses of individuals with early AD and found greater dysnomia (Bayles & Tomoeda, 1983) than in healthy elders. However, at this stage most misnamings still bore a semantic relation to the target word (e.g. 'shoe' for 'sock') or were physically similar (e.g. 'ball' for 'orange'). In those instances when the individual could not recall the name of the stimulus item, they were able to recognize it if given a choice of names.

In sum, the communication skills of individuals with early AD may appear unaffected if the encounter is casual and the demand on episodic memory low. However, formal testing reveals that vocabulary is shrinking, descriptive discourse is less cohesive, dysnomia has increased, reading comprehension has diminished, and information processing has slowed, as has the ability to generate ideas. Most persons in the early stage of dementia are aware of and concerned about their memory problems. Many individuals retreat from activities that could reveal their deficits. Those who are employed fear losing their jobs and the consequences of unemployment. Often early-stage patients and their caregivers want advice about possible pharmacologic interventions to slow the disease course.

Middle stage

The middle stage of AD lasts for two to six years and is characterized by dramatic changes in cognitive and communicative function and the ability to care for self. In addition to disorientation for time, victims become disoriented for place. More cognitive functions are affected because the disease has spread, making it harder for affected individuals to compensate. In essence, cognitive deterioration appears to 'snowball' because of the concurrent decline in myriad abilities. In addition to prominent deficits in episodic memory, mid-stage patients have shorter memory span for both visual and verbal information and marked difficulty focusing attention and processing information (Hopper, Bayles & Kim, 2001; Perry, Watson & Hodges, 2000). Judgement and reasoning are compromised and they need supervision to ensure their safety.

The communication ability of mid-stage individuals clearly reflects problems with the mnemonic, conceptual and inferential systems of the brain, the systems where ideas are born and experience is stored. But speech typically remains fluent. It is the content of language that reflects the disease, both in diminished language output and the amount of meaningful information (Bayles, Tomoeda & Trosset, 1992). Mid-stage patients produce fewer exemplars in generative naming (Bayles & Tomoeda, 1983; Bayles et al., 1989), make more confrontation naming errors, and their written language is peppered with misspellings and grammatical missteps. Although they retain the ability to read aloud and silently, they do not retain the information they read.

Although most persons in mid-stage AD have limited insight about their condition, their dependence on others has dramatically changed their lives. Changes in routine cause anxiety and new environments produce confusion. Travelling and other out-of-the-home activities, that previously gave them pleasure, can become frightening even when they are accompanied by a family member. By mid-stage, the patient's world has shrunk and often the same is true for the caregiver. Having said that, individuals who are cared for at home by caregivers educated in maximizing patient function and dignity have a better quality of life than the individual who is trying to manage alone or is cared for by someone ignorant of the nature of the disease.

Late stage

The duration of the late stage is typically one to three years. Affected individuals have become disorientated for time, place and person. They may not recognize close family members or themselves in a mirror. It is during this stage that incontinence becomes an issue, first for bladder and then bowel. Ultimately, some late-stage patients become non-ambulatory.

Speech typically remains fluent but slower and sometimes halting. Language output is dramatically reduced and often seemingly nonsensical. However, when utterances are analyzed in relation to the environment, the content may in fact be logical. Some individuals become mute or exhibit palilalia, whereas others are able to contribute to a conversation, state their name and read single words aloud (Appell, Kertesz & Fisman, 1982; Bayles & Tomoeda, 1994).

Incontinence is a marker of dementia severity and those who are incontinent only for bladder have more communication skills than those who are incontinent for both bladder and bowel (Bayles, Tomoeda, Cruz & Mahendra, 2000; Kim & Bayles, 2007). In a study supported by the National Institute of Mental Health, Bayles et al. (2000) evaluated the communication skills of 49 late-stage AD patients using the Functional Linguistic Communication Inventory (FLCI) (Bayles and Tomoeda, 1994), a standardized test for evaluating the functional communication skills of advanced dementia patients. Those who were only incontinent for bladder appropriately acknowledged a greeting, compliment and farewell comment. They completed a one-step command, recognized the written form of their name, provided their spouse's name and were able to recognize a common object when presented with a line drawing. In contrast, none of the individuals incontinent for bladder and bowel were able to contribute to a conversation, state their spouse's name or provide relevant information about a common object. The least language and fewest skills were observed in those late-stage patients who were non-ambulatory as well as incontinent for bladder and bowel. This study is important because it calls into question a prevalent view that the language of all incontinent late-stage AD patients is extremely limited and virtually nonexistent, a view influenced by the way language was represented in late-stage patients in the Global Deterioration Scale (Reisberg, Ferris, de Leon & Crook, 1982) a widely used instrument for staging dementia severity.

Impact of AD on quality of life

By definition, dementia comprises multiple cognitive deficits of sufficient severity to interfere with occupational and social functioning. If QoL comprises one's ability to work and maintain social relationships, then QoL is profoundly affected over the disease course. However, in addition to the obviously negative effects of cognitive deterioration, interest is growing as to how AD patients themselves view their QoL. Thus, an evaluation of QoL is now recommended as integral to a patient's evaluation (Rabins & Black, 2007;

Mack & Whitehouse, 2001). However, measuring QoL is challenging because of inter-patient variability in memory deficit profiles, insight to self, ability to communicate and the presence of myriad psychological and behavioural problems (Silberfeld, 2002; Ettema et al., 2005). Nonetheless, some measures have gained credibility for use with individuals with dementia (Smith et al., 2005), particularly the DEMQOL (Smith et al., 2007). The DEMQOL comprises 28 questions, administered by an interviewer, to which the AD patient responds. The items query the individual about whether they are feeling or have recently felt various emotions, whether they are worried about various memory and cognitive problems, and their perception about whether various needs are met. The DEMQOL was developed through rigorous two-stage field testing and subsequently validated on a large sample of dementia patients in the UK along with a caregiver version (DEMQOL-Proxy) that was standardized on caregivers. The patient version was found acceptable for use with mild and moderate dementia patients though not for those with severe dementia. The DEMQOL-Proxy, however, showed promise for use with severe patients as well as individuals with mild and moderate dementia.

Although the literature on the use of QoL measures with AD patients is mixed, some findings have gained credence. First, the neuropsychiatric symptoms of depression and apathy are associated with lower perceived QoL by both mild and moderate AD patients and their caregivers (Sands, Ferreira, Stewart, Bond & Yaffe, 2004; Cheon, Cho & Oh, 2005; Selwood, Thorgrimsen & Orrell, 2005; Snow et al., 2005; Vogel et al., 2006; Hoe, Hancock, Livingston & Orrell, 2006; Fuh & Wang, 2006). Second, insight to self is associated with better perceived QoL in individuals with moderate dementia than in those with mild dementia. Unsurprisingly, being aware of one's deficits and the implications of an AD diagnosis can adversely affect perception of QoL in the early stage of the disease, whereas the reduced self insight of moderate dementia enables patients to view their QoL more positively (Hurt et al., 2010). The third finding with consensus is that the ability to care for self is associated with greater perceived QoL. Fourth, results of several research studies show that the behavioural and psychological problems of persons with AD significantly impact QoL in caregivers, particularly those associated with increased motor activity (Banerjee et al., 2009; Conde-Sala, Garre-Olmo, Turro-Garriga, Lopez-Pousa & Vilalta-Franch, 2009). In the Banerjee et al. study, hallucinations were highly correlated with self-report and caregiver reports. Finally, men generally report better QoL than women (Regier et al., 1993; Copeland et al., 1999) and caregivers perceive better QoL in men.

Conde-Sala and colleagues observed higher levels of depression and anxiety in female AD patients, which reflect what is typical of the general population (Regier et al., 1993; Copeland et al., 1999).

Impact of dementia on the family

Dementia is appropriately characterized as a family affair and clinicians should consider treating the patient and caregiver as a dynamic unit. The lives of the patient and caregiver are interdependent. Indeed, the QoL of a patient will be largely a function of the knowledge, emotional make-up and resources of the caregiver; and the QoL of a caregiver will be largely a function of the behaviour of the patient and severity of their dementia.

Victims of the disease become increasingly dependent on family, who need education and support to cope with ever-increasing responsibilities (Garre-Olmo et al., 2000). Most dementia patients are cared for at home by a family member, typically a spouse or middle-aged daughter. Whereas early in the disease the affected individual may not need round-the-clock supervision, ultimately they do. Thus, caregivers eventually find themselves responsible for bathing, clothing, feeding, providing medications and taking the patient to the bathroom with less and less time for their own pursuits. When unfamiliar environments and travel become disturbing to the patient, caregivers may find themselves homebound and socially isolated. Diminished time for participation in pleasurable activities and social isolation contributes to caregiver depression (Mausbach, Patterson & Grant, 2008).

Over time the financial, social, emotional and physical stresses of caring for someone with a degenerative disease profoundly affect the caregiver's psychological and physical health. They are 3 to 38 times more likely to experience depression (Cuijpers, 2005) and a host of physical problems. Their risk of developing hypertension increases (Shaw et al., 1999; Grant et al., 2002), as does their risk for cardiovascular disease (Lee, Colditz, Berkman & Kawachi, 2003; Mausbach, Patterson, Rabinowitz, Grant & Schulz, 2007). Caregiving can weaken the immune system, causing more frequent illness (Kiecolt-Glaser, Marucha, Malarkey, Mercado & Glaser, 1995; Kiecolt-Glaser, Glaser, Gravenstein, Malarkey & Sheridan, 1996; Shaw et al., 1999). Mausbach et al. (2007) reported that caregiving stress increases the plasma level of tissue-type plasminogen activator antigen that increases the risk of future cardiac events. The fact is that caregivers are at an increased risk of mortality (Schulz & Beach, 1999).

Clinical implications

Counselling caregivers

Ideally, caregivers should be interviewed soon after the diagnosis of dementia and offered education and support. Of relevance to providing support is an understanding of their knowledge of the disease, cultural orientation, health and resources. A brief self-report measure, the 13-item Perceived Change Index (PCI) has been developed to evaluate caregiver appraisals of improvement or deterioration in areas of wellbeing related to the dementia caregiving experience (Gitlin, Winter, Dennis & Hauck, 2006). This measure compares caregiver perceptions at two time periods one month apart. The PCI was evaluated with 255 primary caregivers who provided at least four hours of care each day for at least six months and was reported to be valid with good internal consistency. The items reflect dimensions that can vary in response to caregiving demands, for example, 'energy level', 'feeling upset', 'ability to sleep'. The PCI appears to have potential as a tool for clinicians and researchers but will be strengthened by studies that compare caregiver report with ratings by skilled observers.

Table 10.2 Signs of depression

Somatic symptoms

Poor appetite
Loss of weight
Fatigue
Sleep problems
Agitation
Monotonous voice
Low speaking volume
Slow speaking rate
Apathy
Disregard for personal appearance
Distractible
Cries easily
Indecisive
Makes self-deprecatory comments

Because of the high prevalence of depression in caregivers, clinicians should be alert to its signs (Table 10.2). Some clinicians feel comfortable administering a screening measure for depression and several reliable measures exist: Hamilton Rating Scale for Depression (Hamilton, 1967, 1970); Zung Self-Rating Depression Scales (Zung, 1965); the Beck Depression Inventory (Beck, Ward, Mendelson, Mock & Erbaugh, 1961) and the Geriatric Depression Scale (Yesavage et al., 1983). When depression is suspected, the caregiver should be referred to a mental health professional. It has been shown through randomized controlled trials that psychosocial interventions which are tailored to the caregiver reduce symptoms of depression in family caregivers of AD patients (Brodaty & Gresham, 1989; Brodaty, Gresham & Luscombe, 1997; Mittelman et al., 1995; Mittelman, Roth, Coon & Haley, 2004; Brodaty, Green & Koschera, 2003). Also helpful in reducing caregiver depression is increased exposure to pleasurable activities (Coon, Thompson, Steffen, Sorocco & Gallagher-Thompson, 2003; Gallagher-Thompson et al., 2000).

A large proportion of individuals with dementia cannot be cared for at home and need institutionalization. Miller and Weissert (2000) synthesized results of 78 longitudinal studies of factors contributing to institutionalization and reported that the patient characteristics most associated with nursing home placement were: advanced age, living alone, not owning a home and being white. Other predictors were poor health, low physical functioning, poor cognitive functioning, number of illnesses and low scores on measures of activities of daily living. Cohen-Mansfield and Wirtz (2009) reported that the primary reasons given by American caregivers for nursing home placement were confusion of the patient, an inability to care for self and behaviour problems. Results of a study conducted in the UK by Hope, Keene, Gedling, Fairburn and Jacoby (1998) revealed that the best predictors of institutionalization were: excessive night-time activity; immobility or difficulty walking; incontinence; being away from a caregiver for more than 16 hours a week; and being cared for by a female.

Making the decision to institutionalize a family member is painful and often associated with guilt. Not only do caregivers benefit from guidance in choosing a nursing home, they benefit from counselling during the transition. Gaugler, Roth, Haley and Mittelman (2008) conducted a randomized controlled trial of an enhanced counselling and support programme for spouse caregivers of AD patients compared to usual care. Structured interviews were conducted at baseline and every four months during year one and every six months thereafter for up to 16 years. Their enhanced counselling and support consisted of six sessions of individual and family counselling, support group participation and continuous availability of ad hoc telephone counselling. Using the modified Zarit Burden Interview (Zarit, Reever & Bach-Peterson, 1980) and the Geriatric Depression Scale (Yesavage et al., 1983), they found that burden and depressive symptoms were significantly lower for caregivers in the treatment group compared to controls both at the time of and after institutionalization. Previous work by this New York University group has shown that counselling and support produces a clinically significant and long-lasting effect on the depressive symptoms of caregivers (Mittelman et al., 2004). Clearly, caregiving responsibilities do not end with institutionalization because nursing home admission can produce new forms of stress – for example, having to adapt to staff, having to relinquish control over the patient's care and redefinition of the caregiving role.

In spite of the findings of reduced burden and fewer depressive symptoms in caregiver participants in the New York University programme, the literature is mixed as to whether caregivers benefit from education and support programmes. Thompson and colleagues (2007) identified 44 randomized controlled trials in which technological, group and individualized interventions were provided to dementia caregivers and reviewed them for quality of evidence as to caregiver benefit. They concluded that no evidence exists that interventions are uniformly beneficial, but of the various training formats, group interventions appeared to positively impact caregiver depression. Also, qualitative results suggested possible benefit. It is worth saying that measuring benefit is extremely difficult because there are innumerable hard-to-control variables that can influence caregiver affect. Similarly, it is extremely difficult to measure the benefit to the patient of caregiver education. However, it has been the experience of the authors that education, support group participation and personal counselling are highly valued by most caregivers.

Providing caregiver education to maximize communication

Because communication is vital to caregiving, education to facilitate the expression and comprehension of language is recommended. Professional as well as personal caregivers will benefit and training can be provided individually or to a group. The following modifications that caregivers can make to facilitate language comprehension are subcategorized according to their effect on the form, content and use of language.

Modifications related to the form of language

Avoid complex syntax. Complex syntax, such as sentences with embedded clauses, increases the demand on memory because the subject and verb are separated. To derive sentence meaning the memory-impaired patient has to remember the subject while also processing the embedded clause before the verb is heard. Simple active declarative sentences are those most easily understood by English speakers.

Use common, high-frequency words. More frequently used words have stronger memory engrams and are more readily understood. Consider the following sentences that have the same meaning. Whereas many speakers may be unfamiliar with some words in sentence one, everyone is likely to know the words in sentence two.

1 The philatelist was a centenarian.

2 The stamp collector was a hundred years old.

Replace pronouns with proper nouns. All pronouns have an antecedent that must be remembered for the sentence to be fully comprehended. Remembering the antecedent may be impossible for the individual with dementia.

Use multiple choice or yes/no questions. Questions that require memory-impaired individuals to remember recent events set them up for failure. Examples of such sentences are, 'What did you do yesterday?' and 'What did you have for dinner?' Then, too, questions like, 'What do you want to do?' are challenging even though they do not require chronologic memory. Instead, they require the individual to generate ideas of possible activities, and idea generation is impaired. Easier questions provide a choice for the individual: 'Would you like to take a walk or watch television?' 'Would you like chicken or fish for dinner?' The easiest questions require a simple yes or no: 'Are you hungry?' 'Are you feeling OK?'

Modifications related to the content of language

Simplify content by talking about the here and now, things the patient can see, hear and touch. Or, talk about the individual. Provide an activity to stimulate conversation, such as looking at a photo album, sharing a meal or taking a walk.

Reduce the number of propositions in sentences. Rochon, Waters and Caplan (2000) tested the comprehension of individuals with AD using sentences that varied in number of propositions. When the stimulus sentences contained one proposition, the performance of individuals with AD did not differ from that of normal elders. For two proposition sentences, comprehension was significantly poorer than for healthy elders.

Modifications related to the use of language

Researchers have found that professional caregivers talk less to individuals with dementia (Bohling, 1991). When caregivers communicate with persons who have dementia, the focus is on 'task talk' (Santopietro & Ostuni, 1997, p.132) that mostly consists of instructions given by caregivers to facilitate task completion. Then, too, because individuals with AD have reduced capacity to generate ideas and poor episodic memory, they are handicapped in initiating conversation. As a result, many patients are deprived of the pleasure and attention that comes from having a conversation.

Caregivers should be encouraged to converse with dementia patients and taught that providing a context can produce surprisingly good exchanges. The tone of voice, its loudness and pitch are suprasegmental aspects that convey a message even when the words are no longer understood. Thus, caregivers should be advised to use a pleasant, cheerful tone when talking that is not too loud or high in pitch (Small, Huxtable & Walsh, 2009). Avoid sarcasm and be aware that teasing may confuse late-stage patients who are likely to interpret it literally. Individuals with dementia often make statements that are not true. For example, they may accuse someone of stealing an item they cannot find. Or, they may say that their child is coming home from school and they have to go. Disputing them and arguing is non-productive and usually produces defensiveness and anger. It is far better to verbally validate their feelings and redirect their attention.

Supporting production of language

Many of the strategies that advantage language comprehension also support language production; for example, providing a context for conversation, not asking questions that require episodic memory, and priming. Other supportive techniques include: summarizing what patients have been saying when they lose their train of thought; providing opportunities to read aloud; providing food to stimulate social conversation; and supplying a list of news items and materials when the patient wants to write a letter.

Verbal agitation aka disruptive vocalization

Verbally agitated behaviour is common in individuals with dementia. Prevalence among community dwellers has been reported to be between 19% and 51% (Shahar, Snow, Souchek, Ashton & Kunik, 2004) and between 10% and 52% of those in institutions (Cohen-Mansfield & Werner, 1994; Lai, 1999). Not only is verbal agitation common, it is among the most distressing of behaviours to caregivers (Draper et al., 2000).

A wide range of factors is associated with verbal agitation, but the most common cause is physical or psychological discomfort, or both. Pelletier and Landreville (2007) reported that discomfort explained a significant proportion of the variance in the verbal agitation of 49 individuals with dementia after controlling for dementia severity, gender and disability in activities of daily living. Sloane and colleagues (1999) determined that pain was associated with disruptive vocalization in 60% of their study participants but also that the majority of patients with dementia exhibit verbal agitation when they are alone. Cohen-Mansfield and Marx (1990) reported a relation between disruptive vocalization and sleep problems such as night awakening and fewer hours of sleep.

Identifying the cause(s) of verbal agitation is challenging and requires a careful physical examination to identify possible sources of pain. Similarly, careful consideration should be given to whether the patient is depressed. Finally, careful observation and recording of the antecedent and consequent events associated with episodes of verbal agitation often reveal ways to reduce their frequency. Many interventions have been reported to reduce verbal agitation: pain medication, sensory and cognitive stimulation, companionship, validation therapy, reinforcement of appropriate behaviour, more environmental cues to support way finding and ADLs, elimination of physical restraints, decreased frequency of bathing, nurturing better sleep habits and maintaining a routine (Asp et al., 2006; Cohen-Mansfield, 2001; Kovach et al., 2006; Logsdon, McCurry & Teri, 2007; Rockwood, Fay, Jarrett & Asp, 2007).

Clinical management of patients

The goal of clinicians is to support the highest QoL for persons with dementia. Toward that end, early clinical evaluation is important. It is the means for obtaining a baseline of cognitive and communicative abilities and self-insight against which the benefit of drug and behavioural interventions can be evaluated. Additionally, it provides critical information for professional and personal caregivers about retained abilities that can be used to compensate for deficits. Also, a thorough early evaluation gives clinicians the requisite information for developing a cognitive stimulation programme that can help sustain function. Whereas direct therapy to improve orientation requires patients to confront their problems and, as such, may be counterproductive to improving QoL, cognitive stimulation therapies that aim to capture interest and support function can improve QoL (Hurt et al., 2010).

Historically, it was widely believed that little could be done to improve the cognitive and communicative functioning of individuals with AD. Increasingly this belief was challenged. In addition to the many environmental and linguistic modifications that benefit information processing and comprehension, cognitive stimulation through therapy, reminiscence and activity planning has been shown to improve cognitive function (Arkin, 1992; Arkin, Rose & Hopper, 2000; Bird, 2001; Clare, Wilson, Breen & Hodges, 1999; Clare, Wilson, Carter, Gosses, Breen & Hodges, 2000; Clare, Wilson, Carter & Hodges, 2003; Clare, Wilson, Carter, Hodges & Adams, 2001; Clare et al., 2010; Josephsson et al., 1993; Mahendra & Arkin, 2003; Zanetti et al., 1997, 2001).

Further, we now know that humans have several learning/memory systems with unique architecture that are not equally vulnerable to the degenerative processes of AD (Eichenbaum & Cohen, 2001; Schacter, Wagner & Buckner, 2000; Squire, Stark & Clark, 2004; Braak, Braak & Bohl, 1993; Van Hoesen, 1997; Farkas et al., 1982; Haxby et al., 1986, 1990). Whereas the episodic memory component of declarative, or fact, memory is particularly vulnerable, the procedural memory system is relatively spared, giving clinicians an avenue for teaching new behaviours (Hirono et al. 1997). Thus, although the AD patient may not remember the cognitive stimulation episode, their behaviour reveals that learning occurred.

In conclusion

Alzheimer's disease profoundly changes cognition and communicative function and, indeed, all aspects of the affected individual's life. Similarly, it poses enormous challenges to families because of its length and unremitting course. As understanding of the impact of the disease has grown, so also has the realization that the expertise of many professionals is needed to provide QoL for victims and their caregivers. Speech-language pathologists have a key role throughout the disease course because of the importance of cognition and communication to all of the patient's endeavours and those of the caregiver.

References

Alzheimer's Association (2010) Alzheimer's Disease facts and figures. *Alzheimer's and Dementia: The Journal of the Alzheimer's Association, 6(2),* 158–194.

Alzheimer's Disease International (December 2008) *The Prevalence of Dementia Worldwide.* London: Alzheimer's Disease International.

American Psychiatric Association (2000) *Diagnostic and Statistical Manual of Mental Disorders,* 4th edition. Washington, DC: Author.

Appell, J., Kertesz, A. & Fisman, M. (1982) A study of language functioning in Alzheimer's patients. *Brain and Language, 17,* 73–91.

Arkin, S.M. (1992) Audio-assisted memory training with early Alzheimer patients: Two single subject experiments. *Clinical Gerontologist, 12,* 77–96.

Arkin, S.M., Rose, C. & Hopper, T.L. (2000) Implicit and explicit learning gains in Alzheimer's patients: Effects of naming and information retrieval training. *Aphasiology, 14(7),* 723–742.

Asp, E., Cloutier, F., Fay, S., Cook, C., Robertson, M.L., Fisk, J. et al. (2006) Verbal repetition in patients with Alzheimer's disease who receive donezepil. *International Journal of Geriatric Psychiatry, 21(5),* 426–431.

Banerjee, S., Samsi, K., Petrie, C.D., Alvir, J., Treglia, M., Schwam, E.M. & del Valle, M. (2009) What do we know about quality of life in dementia? A review of the emerging evidence on the predictive and explanatory value of disease specific measures of health related quality of life in people with dementia. *International Journal of Geriatric Psychiatry, 24,* 15–24.

Bayles, K.A., Salmon, D.P., Tomoeda, C.K., Caffrey, J.T., Kaszniak, A.W. & Tröster, A. (1989) Semantic and letter category naming in Alzheimer's patients: A predictable difference. *Developmental Neuropsychology, 5,* 335–347.

Bayles, K.A. & Tomoeda, C.K. (1983) Confrontation and generative naming abilities of dementia patients. In R. Brookshire (Ed.) *Clinical Aphasiology Conference Proceedings,* pp.304–315. Minneapolis, MN: BRK Publications.

Bayles, K.A. & Tomoeda, C.K. (1994) *Functional Linguistic Communication Inventory.* Austin, TX: Pro-Ed.

Bayles, K.A. & Tomoeda, C.K. (2007) *Cognitive–Communication Disorders of Dementia.* San Diego, CA: Plural Publishing.

Bayles, K.A., Tomoeda, C.K. & Boone, D.R. (1985) A view of age-related changes in language function. *Developmental Neuropsychology, 1,* 231–264.

Bayles, K.A., Tomoeda, C.K., Cruz, R.F. & Mahendra, N. (2000) Communication abilities of individuals with late-stage Alzheimer disease. *Alzheimer's Disease and Associated Disorders*, *14(3)*, 176–181.

Bayles, K.A., Tomoeda, C.K., Kaszniak, A.W., Stern, L.Z. & Eagans, K.K. (1985) Verbal perseveration of dementia patients. *Brain and Language*, *25*, 102–116.

Bayles, K.A., Tomoeda, C.K. & Trosset, M.W. (1992) Relation of linguistic communication abilities of Alzheimer's patients to stage of disease. *Brain and Language*, *42(4)*, 450–472.

Beck, A.T., Ward, C.H., Mendelson, M., Mock, J. & Erbaugh, J. (1961) An inventory for measuring depression. *Archives of General Psychiatry*, *4*, 561–571.

Bird, M. (2001) Behavioral difficulties and cued recall of adaptive behaviour in dementia: Experimental and clinical evidence. *Neuropsychological Rehabilitation*, *11(3/4)*, 357–375.

Bohling, H.R. (1991) Communication with Alzheimer's patients: An analysis of caregiver listening patterns. *International Journal of Aging and Human Development*, *33(4)*, 249–267.

Braak, H., Braak, E. & Bohl, J. (1993) Staging of Alzheimer-related cortical destruction. *European Neurology*, *33*, 403–408.

Brodaty, H., Green, A. & Koschera, A. (2003) A meta-analysis of psychosocial interventions for caregivers of people with dementia. *Journal of the American Geriatrics Society*, *51*, 657–664.

Brodaty, H. & Gresham, M. (1989) Effect of a training programme to reduce stress in carers of patients with dementia. *British Medical Journal*, *299*, 1375–1379.

Brodaty, H., Gresham, M. & Luscombe, G. (1997) The Prince Henry Hospital dementia caregivers' training program. *International Journal of Geriatric Psychiatry*, *12*, 183–192.

Cheon, J.S., Cho., W. & Oh, B.H. (2005) Predictors of quality of life in patients with dementia of the Alzheimer's type. *Korean Geriatric Psychiatry*, *9*, 63–69.

Clare, L., Linden, D.E., Woods, R.T., Whitaker, R., Evans, S.J., Parkinson, C.H. et al. (2010) Goal-oriented cognitive rehabilitation for people with early-stage Alzheimer disease: A single-blind randomized controlled trial of clinical efficacy. *American Journal of Geriatric Psychiatry*, *18(10)*, 928–939.

Clare, L., Wilson, B.A., Breen, K. & Hodges, J.R. (1999) Errorless learning of face-name associations in early Alzheimer's disease. *Neurocase*, *5*, 37–46.

Clare, L., Wilson, B.A., Carter, G., Gosses, A., Breen, K. & Hodges, J.R. (2000) Intervening with everyday memory problems in early Alzheimer's disease: An errorless learning approach. *Journal of Clinical and Experimental Neuropsychology*, *22*, 132–146.

Clare, L., Wilson, B.A., Carter, G. & Hodges, J.R. (2003) Cognitive rehabilitation as a component of early intervention in dementia: A single case study. *Aging and Mental Health*, *7*, 15–21.

Clare, L., Wilson, B.A., Carter, G., Hodges, J.R. & Adams, M. (2001) Long-term maintenance of treatment gains following a cognitive rehabilitation intervention in early dementia of Alzheimer type: A single case study. *Neuropsychological Rehabilitation*, *11*, 477–494.

Clark, L.J., Gatz, M., Zheng, L., Chen, Y-L., McCleary, C. & Mack, W.J. (2009) Longitudinal verbal fluency in normal aging, preclinical, and prevalent Alzheimer's disease. *American Journal of Alzheimer's Disease and Other Dementias, 24(6),* 461–468.

Cohen-Mansfield J. (2001) Nonpharmacologic interventions for inappropriate behaviors in dementia: A review, summary, and critique. *American Journal of Geriatric Psychiatry, 9(4),* 361–381.

Cohen-Mansfield, J. & Marx, M.S. (1990) The relationship between sleep disturbances and agitation in a nursing home. *Journal of Aging and Health, 2(1),* 42–57.

Cohen-Mansfield, J. & Werner, P. (1994) Verbally disruptive behaviors in elderly persons: A review. In B.J. Vellas, L. Albarede & P.J. Garry (Eds) *Facts and Research in Gerontology: Dementia and Cognitive Impairments,* pp.73–89. New York, NY: Springer.

Cohen-Mansfield, J. & Wirtz, P. (2009) The reasons for nursing home entry in an adult day care population: Caregiver reports versus regression results. *Journal of Geriatric Psychiatry and Neurology, 22(4),* 274–281.

Conde-Sala, J.L., Garre-Olmo, J., Turro-Garriga, O., Lopez-Pousa, S. & Vilalta-Franch, J. (2009) Factors related to perceived quality of life in patients with Alzheimer's disease: The patient's perception compared with that of caregivers. *International Journal of Geriatric Psychiatry, 24,* 585–594.

Coon, D.W., Thompson, L., Steffen, A., Sorocco, K. & Gallagher-Thompson, D. (2003) Anger and depression management: Psychoeducational skill training interventions for women caregivers of a relative with dementia. *Gerontologist, 43(5),* 678–689.

Copeland, J.R., Beekman, A.T., Dewey, M.E., Hooijer, C., Jordan, A., Lawlor, B.A. et al. (1999) Depression in Europe. Geographical distribution among older people. *British Journal of Psychiatry, 174,* 312–321.

Cuijpers P. (2005) Depressive disorders in caregivers of dementia patients: A systematic review. *Aging and Mental Health, 9(4),* 325–330.

Draper, B., Snowden, J., Meares, S., Turner, J., Gonski, P., McMinn, B. et al. (2000) Case controlled study of nursing home residents referred for treatment of vocally disruptive behavior. *International Psychogeriatrics, 12(3),* 333–344.

Eichenbaum, H. & Cohen, N.J. (2001) *From Conditioning to Conscious Recollection: Memory Systems of the Brain.* New York: Oxford University Press.

Ernst, R.L., Hay, J.W., Fenn, C., Tinklenberg, J. & Yesavage, J.A. (1997) Cognitive function and the costs of Alzheimer disease. An exploratory study. *Archives of Neurology, 54(6),* 687–693.

Ettema, T.P., Droes, R.-M., de Lange, J., Mellenbergh, G.J. & Ribbe. M.W. (2005) A review of quality of life instruments used in dementia. *Quality of Life Research 14(3),* 675–686.

Farkas, T., Ferris, S.H., Wolf, A.P., de Leon, M.J., Christman, D.R., Reisberg, B. et al. (1982) 18F-2-deoxy-2-fluoro-D-glucose as a tracer in positron emission tomographic study of senile dementia. *American Journal of Psychiatry, 139(3),* 352–353.

Ferri, C.P., Prince, M., Brayne, C., Brodaty, H., Fratiglioni, L., Ganguli, M. et al. (2005) Global prevalence of dementia: A Delphi consensus study. *Lancet, 366(9503)*, 2112–2117.

Finkel, S. (2000) Introduction to behavioural and psychological symptoms of dementia (BPSD). *International Journal of Geriatric Psychiatry, 15*(suppl), S2–S4.

Fuh, J.L. & Wang, S.J. (2006) Assessing quality of life in Taiwanese patients with Alzheimer's disease. *International Journal of Geriatric Psychiatry, 21*, 103–107.

Gallagher-Thompson, D., Lovett, S., Rose, J., McKibbin, C., Coon, D., Futterman, A. & Thompson, L.W. (2000) Impact of psychoeducational interventions on distressed family caregivers. *Journal of Clinical Geropsychology, 6(2)*, 91–110.

Garre-Olmo, J., Hernández-Ferrándiz, M., Lozano-Gallego, M., Vilalta-Franch, J., Turón-Estrada, A., Cruz-Reina, M.M. et al. (2000) Burden and quality of life in carers of patients with Alzheimer type dementia. *Revue Neurologique, 31*, 522–527.

Gaugler, J.E., Roth D.L., Haley, W.E. & Mittelman, M.S. (2008) Can counseling and support reduce Alzheimer's caregivers' burden and depressive symptoms during the transition to institutionalization? Results from the NYU caregiver intervention study. *Journal of the American Geriatrics Society, 56(3)*, 421–428.

Gearing, M., Schneider, J.A., Rebeck, G.W., Hyman, B.T. & Mirra, S.S. (1995) Alzheimer's disease with and without coexisting Parkinson's disease changes: Apolipoprotein E genotype and neuropathologic correlates. *Neurology, 45*, 1985–1990.

Gitlin, L.N., Winter, L., Dennis, M.P. & Hauck, W.W. (2006) Assessing perceived change in the well-being of family caregivers: Psychometric properties of the Perceived Change Index and response patterns. *American Journal of Alzheimer's Disease and Other Dementias, 21(5)*, 304–311.

Grant, I., Adler, K.A., Patterson, T.L., Dimsdale, J.E., Ziegler, M.G. & Irwin, M.R. (2002) Health consequences of Alzheimer's caregiving transitions: Effects of placement and bereavement. *Psychosomatic Medicine, 64*, 477–486.

Hamilton, M. (1967) A rating scale for depression. *Journal of Neurology, Neurosurgery, and Psychiatry, 23*, 56–62.

Hamilton, M. (1970) Development of a rating scale for primary depressive illness. *British Journal of Social and Clinical Psychology, 6*, 278–296.

Haxby, J., Grady, C., Duara, R., Schlageter, N., Berg, G. & Rapoport, S.I. (1986) Neocortical metabolic abnormalities precede non memory cognitive defects in early Alzheimer-type dementia. *Archives of Neurology, 43*, 882–885.

Haxby, J.V., Grady, C.L., Koss, E., Holtz, B., Heston, L., Shapiro, M. et al. (1990) Longitudinal study of cerebral metabolic asymmetries and associated neuropsychological patterns in early dementia of the Alzheimer type. *Archives of Neurology, 47*, 753–760.

Hirono, N., Mori, E., Ikejiri, Y., Imamura, T., Shimomura, T. & Ikeda, M. (1997) Procedural memory in patients with mild Alzheimer's disease. *Dementia and Geriatric Cognitive Disorders, 8*, 210–216.

Hoe, J., Hancock, G., Livingston, G. & Orrell, M. (2006) Quality of life of people with dementia in residential care homes. *British Journal of Psychiatry*, *188*, 460–464.

Hope T., Keene, J., Gedling, K., Fairburn, G. & Jacoby, R. (1998) Predictors of institutionalization for people with dementia living at home with a carer. *International Journal of Geriatric Psychiatry*, *13*, 682–690.

Hopper, T., Bayles, K.A. & Kim, E. (2001) Retained neuropsychological abilities of individuals with Alzheimer's disease. *Seminars in Speech and Language*, *22(4)*, 261–273.

Hurt, C.S., Banerjee, S., Tunnard, C., Whitehead, D.L., Tsolake, M. & Mecocci, P. (2010) Insight, cognition, and quality of life in Alzheimer's disease. *Journal of Neurology, Neurosurgery and Psychiatry*, *81*, 331–333.

Hy, L.X. & Keller, D.M. (2000) Prevalence of Alzheimer's disease among whites: A summary by levels of severity. *Neurology*, *55*, 198–204.

Janvin, C.C., Aarsland, D. & Larsen, J.P. (2005) Cognitive predictors of dementia in Parkinson's disease: A community-based, 4 year longitudinal study. *Journal of Geriatric Psychiatry and Neurology*, *18*, 149–154.

Jellinger, K.A. (1996) Structural basis of dementia in neurodegenerative disorders. *Journal of Neural Transmission Supplement*, *47*, 1–29.

Josephsson, S., Backman, L., Borell, L., Bernspang, B., Nygard, L. & Ronnberg, L. (1993) Supporting everyday activities in dementia: An intervention study. *International Journal of Geriatric Psychiatry*, *8*, 395–400.

Kiecolt-Glaser, J.K., Glaser, R., Gravenstein, S., Malarkey, W.B. & Sheridan, J. (1996) Chronic stress alters the immune response to influenza virus in older adults. *Proceedings of the National Academy of Sciences of the USA*, *94*, 3043–3047.

Kiecolt-Glaser, J.K., Marucha, P.T., Malarkey, W.B., Mercado, A.M. & Glaser, R. (1995) Slowing of wound healing by psychological stress. *Lancet*, *346*, 1194–1196.

Kim, E.S. & Bayles, K.A. (2007) Communication in late-stage Alzheimer's disease: Relation to functional markers of disease severity. *Alzheimer's Care Quarterly*, *8*, 43–52.

Kohler S., van Boxtel, M., van Os, J., Thomas, A.J., O'Brien, J.T. & Jolles, J. (2010) Depressive symptoms and cognitive decline in community-dwelling older adults. *Journal of the American Geriatrics Society*, *58*, 873–879.

Kovach, C.R., Logan, B.R., Noonan, P.E., Schlidt, A.M., Smerz, J., Simpson, M. & Wells, T. (2006) Effects of the Serial Trial Intervention on discomfort and behavior of nursing home residents with dementia. *American Journal of Alzheimer's Disease and Other Dementias*, *21(3)*, 147–155.

Lai, C.K.Y. (1999) Vocally disruptive behaviors in people with cognitive impairment: current knowledge and future research directions. *American Journal of Alzheimer's Disease and Other Dementias*, *14(3)*, 172–180.

Lee, A., Colditz, G.A., Berkman, L.F. & Kawachi, I. (2003) Caregiving and risk of coronary heart disease in US women: A prospective study. *American Journal of Preventative Medicine*, *24*, 113–119.

Logsdon, R.G., McCurry, S. & Teri, L. (2007) Evidence-based psychological treatments in disruptive behaviors in individuals with dementia. *Psychology and Aging, 22(1)*, 28–36.

Lyketsos, C.G., Lopez, O., Jones B., Fitzpatrick, A.L., Breitner, J. & DeKosky, S. (2002) Prevalence of neuropsychiatric symptoms in dementia and mild cognitive impairment. *Journal of the American Medical Association, 202(288)*, 1475–1483.

Mack, J.L. & Whitehouse, P.J. (2001) Quality of life in dementia: State-of-the-art report of the International Working Group for Harmonization of Dementia Drug Guidelines and the Alzheimer's Society satellite meeting. *Alzheimer Disease and Associated Disorders, 15*, 69–71.

Mahendra, N. & Arkin, S.M. (2003) Effects of four years of exercise, language, and social interventions on Alzheimer discourse. *Journal of Communication Disorders, 36(5)*, 395–422.

Mausbach, B.T., Patterson, T.L. & Grant, I. (2008) Is depression in Alzheimer's caregivers really due to activity restriction? A preliminary mediational test of the Activity Restriction Model. *Journal of Behavior Therapy and Experimental Psychiatry, 39(4)*, 459–466.

Mausbach, B.T., Patterson, T.O., Rabinowitz, Y., Grant, I. & Schulz, R. (2007) Depression and distress predict time to cardiovascular disease in dementia caregivers. *Health Psychology, 26(5)*, 539–544.

Miller, E.A. & Weissert, W.G. (2000) Predicting elderly people's risk for nursing home placement, hospitalization, functional impairment, and mortality: A synthesis. *Medical Care Research and Review, 57(3)*, 259–297.

Mittelman, M.S., Ferris, S.H., Shulman, E., Steinberg, Ambinder, A., Mackell, J.A. & Cohen, J. (1995) A comprehensive support program: Effect on depression in spouse care-givers of AD patients. *Gerontologist, 35*, 792–802.

Mittelman, M.S., Roth, D.L., Coon, D.W. & Haley, W.E. (2004) Sustained benefit of supportive intervention for depressive symptoms in Alzheimer's caregivers. *American Journal of Psychiatry, 161*, 850–856.

Nolan, K.A., Lino, M.M., Seligman, A.W. & Blass, J.P. (1998) Absence of vascular dementia in an autopsy series from a dementia clinic. *Journal of the American Geriatric Society, 46*, 597–604.

Nussbaum, R.L. & Ellis, C.E. (2003) Alzheimer's disease and Parkinson's disease. *New England Journal of Medicine, 348*, 1356–1364.

Pelletier, I.C. & Landreville, L. (2007) Discomfort and agitation in older adults with dementia. *Biomed Central Geriatrics, 7(27)*, 1–24.

Perry, R.J., Watson, P. & Hodges, J.R. (2000) The nature and staging of attention dysfunction in early Alzheimer's disease: Relationship to episodic and semantic memory impairment. *Neuropsychologia, 38*, 252–271.

Rabins, P.V. & Black, B. (2007) Measuring quality of life in dementia: Purposes, goals, challenges and progress. *International Psychogeriatrics, 19(3)*, 401–407.

Regier, D.A., Farmer, M.E, Rae, D.S, Myers, J.K., Kramer, M. & Robins, L.N. (1993) One-month prevalence of mental disorders in the United States and sociodemographic characteristics: the Epidemiologic Catchment Area study. *Acta Psychiatrica Scandinavica, 88*, 35–47.

Reisberg, B., Ferris, S.H., de Leon, M.J. & Crook, T. (1982) The global deterioration scale (GDS): An instrument for the assessment of primary degenerative dementia (PDD). *American Journal of Psychiatry, 139*, 1136–1139.

Rochon, E., Waters, G.S. & Caplan, D. (2000) The relationship between measures of working memory and sentence comprehension in patients with Alzheimer's disease. *Journal of Speech, Language, and Hearing Research*, 43, 395–413.

Rockwood, K., Fay, S., Jarrett, P. & Asp, E. (2007) Effect of galantamine on verbal repetition in AD: A secondary analysis of the VISTA trial. *Neurology, 68(14)*, 1116–1121.

Sailor, K., Antoine, M., Diaz, M., Kuslansky, G. & Kluger, A. (2004) The effects of Alzheimer's disease on item output in verbal fluency tasks. *Neuropsychology, 18(2)*, 306–314.

Sands, L.P., Ferreira, P., Stewart, A.L., Brod, M. & Yaffe, K. (2004) What explains differences between dementia patients' and their caregivers' ratings of patients' quality of life? *American Journal of Geriatric Psychiatry, 12*, 272–280.

Santopietro, M.J. & Ostuni, E. (1997) *Successful Communication with Alzheimer's Disease Patients: An In-Service Manual.* Boston, MA: Butterworth-Heinemann.

Schacter, D.L., Wagner, A.D. & Buckner, R.L. (2000) Memory systems of 1999. In E. Tulving & F.I.M. Craik (Eds) *Oxford Handbook of Memory*, pp.627–643. New York: Oxford University Press.

Schrag, A., Jahanshahi, M. & Quinn, N.P. (2001) What contributes to depression in Parkinson's disease? *Psychological Medicine, 31*, 65–73.

Schulz, R. & Beach, S. (1999) Caregiving as a risk factor for mortality: The caregiver health effects study. *Journal of the American Medical Association, 282*, 2215–2219.

Selkoe, D.J. (2000) The genetics and molecular pathology of Alzheimer's disease: Roles of amyloid and the presenilins. *Neurologic Clinics, 18*, 903–922.

Selwood, A., Thorgrimsen, L. & Orrell, M. (2005) Quality of life in dementia – a one-year follow-up study. *International Journal of Geriatric Psychiatry, 20*, 232–237.

Shahar, K., Snow A.L., Souchek, J., Ashton, A.M. & Kunik, M.E. (2004) Cutpoint definition of agitation. *Clinical Gerontologist, 27*, 15–23.

Shaw, W.S., Patterson, T.L., Ziegler, M.G., Dimsdale, J.E., Semple, S.J. & Grant, I. (1999) Accelerated risk of hypertensive blood pressure recordings among Alzheimer caregivers. *Journal of Psychosomatic Research, 46*, 215–227.

Silberfeld M. (2002) Content validity for dementia of three generic preference based health related quality of life instruments. *Quality of Life Research, 11*, 71–79.

Sloane, P.D., Davidson, S., Knight, N., Tangen, C. & Mitchell, C.M. (1999) Severe disruptive vocalizers. *Journal of the American Geriatric Society*, *47(4)*, 439–445.

Small, J.A., Huxtable, A. & Walsh, M. (2009) The role of caregiver prosody in conversations with persons who have Alzheimer's disease. *American Journal of Alzheimer's Disease and Other Dementias*, *24*, 469–475.

Smith, S.C. Lamping, D.L., Banerjee, S., Harwood, R.H., Foley, B. et al. (2005) Measurement of health-related quality of life for people with dementia: Development of a new instrument (DEMQOL) and an evaluation of current methodology. *Health Technology Assessment*, *9(10)*, 1–93.

Smith, S.C., Lamping D.L., Banerjee S., Harwood, R.H., Foley, B., Smith, P. et al. (2007) Development of a new measure of health related quality of life for people with dementia: DEMQOL. *Psychologic Medicine*, *37*, 737–746.

Snow, A.L., Dani, R., Souchek, J., Sullivan, G., Ashton, C.M. & Kunik, M.E. (2005) Comorbid psychosocial symptoms and quality of life in patients with dementia. *American Journal of Geriatric Psychiatry*, *13*, 393–401.

Souetre, E., Thwaites, R.M. & Yeardley, H.L. (1999) Economic impact of Alzheimer's disease in the United Kingdom. Cost of care and disease severity for non-institutionalized patients with Alzheimer's disease. *British Journal of Psychiatry*, *174*, 51–55.

Squire, L.R., Stark, C.E.L. & Clark, R.E. (2004) The medial temporal lobe. *Annual Review of Neuroscience*, *27*, 279–306.

Thompson, C.A., Spilsbury, K., Hall, J., Birks, Y., Barnes, C. & Adamson, J. (2007) Systematic review of information and support interventions for caregivers of people with dementia. *Biomed Central Geriatrics*, *7(18)*, 1–12.

Tomoeda, C.K. & Bayles, K.A. (1993) Longitudinal effects of Alzheimer's disease on discourse production. *Alzheimer Disease and Associated Disorders*, *7*, 223–236.

Tröster, A.I. & Woods, S.P. (1987) Neuropsychological aspects of Parkinson's disease and parkinsonian syndromes. In R. Pahwa, K.E. Lyons & W.C. Koller (Eds) *Handbook of Parkinson's Disease*, 3rd edition, pp.127–157. New York: Marcel Dekker.

Van Hoesen, G. (1997) Ventromedial temporal lobe anatomy, with comments on Alzheimer's disease and temporal injury. *Journal of Neuropsychiatry and Clinical Neurosciences*, *9*, 331–341.

Vogel, A., Mortensen E.L., Hasselbalch S.G., Andersen, B.B. & Waldemar, B. (2006) Patient versus informant reported quality of life in the earliest phases of Alzheimer's disease. *Internal Journal of Geriatric Psychiatry*, *21*, 1132–1138.

Yesavage, J.A., Brink, T.L., Rose, T.L., Lum, O., Huang, V., Adey, M.B. & Leirer. V.O. (1983) Development and validation of a geriatric depression screening scale: A preliminary report. *Journal of Psychiatric Research*, *17*, 37–49.

Zanetti, O., Binetti, G., Magni, E., Rozzini, L., Bianchetti, A. & Trabucchi, M. (1997) Procedural memory stimulation in Alzheimer's disease: Impact of a training program. *Acta Neurologica Scandinavia*, *95*, 152–157.

Zanetti, O., Zanieri, G., Di Giovanni, G., De Vreese, L.P., Pezzini, A., Metitieri, T. & Trabucchi, M. (2001) Effectiveness of procedural memory stimulation in mild Alzheimer's disease patients. A controlled study. *Neuropsychological Rehabilitation, 11,* 263–272.

Zarit, S.H., Reever, K.E. & Bach-Peterson, J. (1980) Relatives of the impaired elderly: Correlates of feelings of burden. *Gerontologist, 20,* 649–655.

Zung, W.W.K. (1965) A self-rating depression scale. *Archives of General Psychiatry, 1,* 63–70.

11 Acquired Motor Speech Disorders

Nick Miller
University of Newcastle, UK

Lena Hartelius
University of Gothenburg, Sweden

Introduction

This chapter examines the nature of the impact of acquired motor speech disorders on individuals. It considers issues about how one might assess impact clinically and points to some implications for intervention.

The label 'acquired motor speech disorders' (MSDs) encompasses essentially apraxia of speech and the dysarthrias. Neurogenic voice disorders (e.g. vocal cord palsies) are also commonly included. The label 'MSDs' is a standard term, but the presentation and trajectory of the disorder from individual to individual is far from uniform and standard. To appreciate the impact of MSDs, it is worth bearing in mind some key variables in how they present.

MSDs may be acquired at any age, though for the majority onset in later life is probably the case. They may be confined to aetiologies that affect a single articulator (e.g. tongue, soft palate) through to being the result of systemic changes that alter all speech–voice production components. At one extreme they may entail no perceptible changes in the ear of the listener – only speakers themselves are aware of the added effort and concentration they have in sustaining speech, or they perceive subtle changes compared to previously that only they are aware of. At the opposite end, speech may be entirely incomprehensible even to familiar partners. Onset may be sudden or gradual, over weeks, months or years. Prognosis varies between the extremes of improvement to pre-morbid levels versus inevitable decline to complete unintelligibility or muteness, again over months or decades. Across different underlying disorders speech may or may not be influenced by medical and surgical therapies.

MSDs can appear as the sole sequel of an illness. Typically MSDs co-occur with a host of other cognitive, physical and affective changes that impact on or interact with the MSDs. There may be accompanying aphasia and/or wider cognitive difficulties. Attention, motivation, orientation for time, person and place may be altered. Memory and learning can be affected. Physical impairment, including dysphagia, may be present. Pain, fatigue and changes to vision or hearing are familiar concerns. Neurobehavioural consequences may complicate the picture for the person with MSD and their family. End-of-life issues sometimes feature. Worries around employment and financial status may enter the impact equation.

It is clear from accounts by people with MSDs that all these factors do interact with speech, and extricating the impact of MSDs from other impinging factors can prove a major undertaking. As is also clear, the relationship between elements is neither static nor predictable. At different times in the course of recovery or decline, for a host of individual reasons, different physical, cognitive, emotional, psychological and social variables may assume greater or lesser prominence for shorter or longer periods. Apparently similar formal clinical assessment profiles therefore may be associated with quite disparate impact profiles. This should not be surprising given the varied nature of individuals' own family, work and social circumstances, differing attitudes to wellbeing, reactions to illness and divergent patterns of adjustment or coping. This heterogeneity must be borne in mind when attempting to characterize the nature of the impact of MSDs.

A recent survey of nearly 500 individuals with multiple sclerosis (MS) illustrates this (Baylor, Yorkston, Bamer, Britton & Amtmann, 2010). It concluded that self-reported restrictions in communicative participation were statistically significantly associated with multiple variables. Some of these were more general MS-related worries. Fatigue, slurred speech, depression, problems in thinking, employment status and social support were significantly associated with communicative participation, accounting for around 48% of the variance.

In addition, we know that communicative disability can also affect a number of other life areas besides communication, particularly learning and applying knowledge, interpersonal interactions and relationships, social and civic life, domestic life and perhaps even mobility and self-care.

The impact of MSDs

The *International Classification of Functioning, Disability and Health* (ICF, World Health Organization, 2001) provides a biopsychosocial framework for describing health conditions. The associated model is a complex and dynamic conceptual tool outlining how impairments, activity limitations and participation restrictions caused by a disease or disorder interact with each other to shape a person's perception of their disability. These three aspects also interact with contextual factors such as environmental or personal factors.

The complexity and completeness of the model make an important contribution to our thinking about MSDs and it has indeed been applied to this particular population (e.g. Hartelius & Miller, 2010; Yorkston , Beukelman, Strand & Hakel, 2010). Using the ICF terminology, the defining characteristic of MSDs as structural/functional impairments is loss or abnormality of physiological or anatomical structure or function which results in slow, weak, imprecise and/or uncoordinated movements of the speech musculature (dysarthria) or inability to plan speech movements (apraxia of speech). The resulting activity limitation is a negative effect on speech intelligibility, naturalness, prosody, speaking rate and articulatory adequacy. These limitations in turn restrict communicative participation in different life situations. Several contextual factors, both barriers and facilitators in the environment, as well as personal factors, influence the effects of the person's motor speech disorder, as briefly outlined in the list of factors above that impinge on or interact with communication.

Structure/function, activity and participation constitute independent perspectives on the disorder, in as far as there is generally no straightforward mapping between aspects. There is not necessarily any one-to-one correspondence between the underlying motor or neuropathological status (the impairment) and the life changes perceived by the individuals in terms of activity limitations and participation restriction (Hartelius, Elmberg, Holm, Lovberg & Nikolaidis, 2008; Klasner & Yorkston, 2005; Miller, Allcock, Jones, Noble, Hildreth & Burn, 2007; Walshe, Peach & Miller, 2009).

A person with a severe motor speech impairment profile on clinical assessments might not perceive themselves as impaired at all and their family might not see any significant changes as regards communication. Equally frequently, one finds individuals who are completely acquitted from any signs of dysarthria, but still perceive themselves as being restricted in their communicative participation (Hartelius, Jonsson, Rickeberg & Laakso, 2010; Miller, Noble, Jones, Allcock & Burn, 2008; Yorkston, Baylor, Klasner, Deitz, Dudgeon et al., 2007).

The range of impacts

The emphasis of this chapter is on a portrayal of participation and psychosocial impact changes typically associated with MSDs. In as far as all factors and effects that contribute to or stem from this are inextricably entwined with each other, any division into possible constituent parts might seem artificial. For the purposes of description, the following presents reports from or of people with MSDs on: (1) impacts on communication interaction in conversation; (2) impacts on communication participation in a more general sense; (3) the role of environmental factors as barriers or facilitators; and (4) the effects on personal factors and identity. Lastly, (5) the impact of the communication disability associated with MSDs as perceived by the communication partner will be mentioned.

1 Participating in conversation

As regards the effects of MSDs on conversations, aside from the more obvious possible voice and speech changes, there are several alterations that can impact on communication interaction. People with MSDs may adopt an economizing strategy in conversation, characterized by, for example, adding pauses and shortening phrases, with its consequent restriction on what and how things are expressed; changing words to less taxing ones and similar (Walshe & Miller, 2011; Wilkinson, Yorkston, Strand & Rogers, 1995). Other modifications of verbal and non-verbal behaviour have been described by people with MSDs; for example, individuals with stroke have mentioned shouting over the phone to make themselves understood (Dickson, Barbour, Brady, Clark & Paton, 2008) and individuals with multiple sclerosis report reducing speech rate, keeping a good eye contact and requesting feedback, etc. (Bringfelt, Hartelius & Runmarker, 2006). Overall, individuals may take fewer and shorter turns than unaffected speakers (Comrie, Mackenzie & McCall, 2001), and the less intelligible speakers are, the fewer contributions they make.

2 Impact on communication participation

From the perspective of more general effects on communication participation, individuals with MSDs experience communication difficulties across a range of settings, irrespective of their severity of dysarthria (Dickson et al., 2008; Miller, Noble, Jones & Burn, 2006; Walshe & Miller, 2011). In fact, the changes in voice, speech and intelligibility that people with MSDs experience and which may affect conversation in unpredictable ways can be a leading concern. For instance, nearly 40% of a group of 140 individuals with Parkinson's disease placed speech changes amongst their prime concerns (Miller et al., 2006), alongside all the other challenges of the condition. Dysarthria is viewed as part of a larger picture, where physical disability may be more central compared to speech, or may alternate in prominence (Bringfelt et al., 2006; Walshe & Miller, 2011).

Other factors such as cognitive and linguistic processes influence conversation and have a general impact on participation. For example, individuals with hypokinetic dysarthria caused by Parkinson's disease perform differently, closer to the lower end of their production range, in conversation compared to sentence repetition (Rosen, Kent, Delaney & Duffy, 2006). Talking takes a lot of energy and the experience of having speech difficulties makes you question your own ability as a communication partner, which in turn may lead to avoidance of instigating new conversations or withdrawal. This has been described by several groups of people with MSDs, including Parkinson's disease (Miller et al., 2008), Huntington's disease (Hartelius et al., 2010) and stroke (Brady, Clark, Dickson, Paton & Barbour, 2011).

The presence of dysarthria can cause one to avoid certain communication situations, such as asking for items in shops, telephoning, getting involved in conversations with strangers, talking in a group situation, making financial transactions that involve speech, making speeches, meeting neighbours, going for interviews, making enquiries/asking questions (Walshe & Miller, 2011). In general, the speech problems influence quality of life, affect family and friends, and cause loneliness, social isolation and emotional stress. Persons with stroke have described amongst other things that 'I won't talk to someone for days', 'You feel as if you are left out' (Brady et al., 2011). Reports from individuals with MS (Klugman & Ross, 2002) include, for example, 'People think I'm intoxicated and treat me as such' and 'If you're on your own it doesn't bother you but it does affect a normal lifestyle. It draws you away from the people you need the most.'

The perceived effects on conversation partners and significant others are that they restrict their interaction by limiting the topic of conversation, failing to challenge or avoiding discussion altogether. Persons with dysarthria frequently feel explicitly excluded from social interaction and experience that significant others are frequently turned to initially, and invited to be 'interpreters' (Brady et al., 2011). Listeners seem to talk over you, for you, ignore you and do not wait for an answer (Miller et al., 2006; Dickson et al., 2008), often perceived as a major factor in loss of dignity.

3 Impact on personal factors and identity

The disorder underlying the MSDs may make people feel fundamentally different, but the changes in voice and speech specifically can alter self-image. Family roles and other social roles are described as altered. Many individuals experience that their spouse may now speak on their behalf. This can lead to a sense of loss of independence or identity, or for others is a strategy in conserving energy or last resort to be understood (Miller et al., 2006). Persons with dysarthria due to stroke describe that 'I know I have a speech impediment. All I have to do is go to the answering machine on the phone or tape myself and I would know and that's embarrassing', 'I worry about the way I come across, that type of thing', and 'I hate myself because I can't speak right... People can obviously understand what I'm saying but as I said to you already, it really infuriates me that I can't speak in the same power and fire it out' (Dickson et al., 2008; Walshe & Miller, 2011).

'Your self image and identity is sensitive to other people's labels and comments. You become "Bill that's had a stroke" and not "Bill from the bowling club"' (Brady et al., 2011). Many quotes bear evidence of embarrassment and sensitivity, lack of confidence and feelings of inadequacy as emotions resulting from dysarthria. People feel helpless, scared and stigmatized (Dickson et al., 2008; Miller et al., 2008; Walshe & Miller, 2011).

Over time the negative changes perceived of self as a communicator (competence, adequacy, control and ease in communication) and the self-view can evolve independently of intelligibility and other clinical measures, a picture reported for individuals with Parkinson's disease (Miller, Andrew, Noble & Walshe, 2011). This indicates a heterogeneity and variability of impact on personal factors and identity and points to a possible sensitivity to different contextual factors. However, a negative self-image due to communication difficulties might be altered by conversation partners and more favourable environmental factors.

4 The role of contextual factors

Contextual factors include the attitudes and behaviour of the conversation partners as well as physical environmental factors. Conversation partners seem to be most influential, with several reports describing their impact. Yorkston, Bombardier and Hammen (1994) found that individuals with severe dysarthria perceived conversation partners as more influential and helpful, compared to individuals with mild or moderate dysarthria. Several speakers with different neurological conditions found that receiving time and opportunities to talk affected communication in a positive way and that stress and conversation partners who speak too fast had negative consequences for communication (Hartelius et al., 2010; Walshe & Miller, 2011). Also, impatience on the part of the listeners, poor lighting, background noise and competing attentional factors are perceived as communication barriers. The perceived attitudes and reactions of conversation partners adds to dysarthric speakers' fear of being misunderstood or perceived as unintelligent and can cause the speaker to avoid conversation out of consideration for listener discomfort (Walshe & Miller, 2011).

Persons with dysarthria identify a number of barriers to communication in work situations. These include: physical appearance; giving the impression of being incoherent; fatigue; loss of inflection in one's voice making it difficult to convince others; being afraid to speak; the demands of having to speak efficiently and accurately; noisy environments (Adams, Moon, Dykstra, Abrams, Jenkins & Jog, 2006); speaking on the phone and using voicemail; interacting at a large meeting; listening or speaking at the same time as doing something else (Bunton & Keintz, 2008; Garcia, Laroche & Barrette, 2002); awareness of the pragmatic aspects of communication (breakdown on the part of both listeners and speaker may hinder participation) (McNamara & Durso, 2003; Comrie et al., 2001).

5 The communication partner

There are fewer studies focusing on the attitudes and actions of communication partners involved with speakers with MSDs, but they all describe difficulties and frustration. The communication partners generally become a more active conversation partner and are frequently the main initiator of self-repairs for the dysarthric speaker (Bloch & Wilkinson, 2009). Communication partners are less confident regarding the competence of a speaker with dysarthria compared to controls without a communication problem, at least in a medical situation (Fox & Pring, 2005), and may be inclined to form more negative views of people with dysarthria (Lyons, Tickle-Degnen & DeGroat, 2005; Pentland, Pitcairn, Gray & Riddle, 1987). They may also limit their participation because they feel a sense of failure for not understanding (Lubinski, 1991). Listeners find it more demanding to understand and accept speakers with decreased intelligibility (Dagenais, Watts, Turnage & Kennedy, 1999; Whitehill & Wong, 2006), sometimes not even worthwhile communicating in depth at all (individuals with HD; Hartelius et al., 2010).

Severity of dysarthria is an influencing factor; individuals with moderate dysarthria are given poorer listener comfort ratings than individuals with mild dysarthria. However, in a professional situation, listeners do not seem to let the exchange of information be affected, as shown in a study of service enquiries by individuals with mild and moderate dysarthria caused by traumatic brain injury over the telephone (Guo & Togher, 2008).

Assessment of impact

The above underlines that the impact of MSDs is complex, describable in diverse dimensions. Issues around speech–voice are inextricably bound up with other physical, emotional, cognitive and social variables. Thus, to single out communication for assessment from the total matrix will always lead to an incomplete story. Neither is impact a finite, stable entity. What counts as successful or satisfactory communication or as a detrimental impact on communication varies from one individual to the next and for one individual according to an array of factors – including real and perceived demands of the situation; whom they are speaking to, what about and how they are communicating; what the purpose and goal of the exchange is; the environmental, social and collaborative supports available to achieve goals. Consequently, communication disability is relative, subjective and variable.

This web of factors poses considerable challenges to assessing impact and charting differences over time or across situations, topics and interlocutors. The task is how to balance an instrument that both reflects the overall complexity, and is sensitive and faithful to individual variation and views. Reconciling these two poles, certainly within a single assessment, is scarcely possible. The following paragraphs take a brief look at some of the clinical solutions applied to examine impact in MSDs.

Case-history interviews have always been a method to elicit self-reports on impact, priorities in rehabilitation and perceptions of change. They presuppose, though, that the clinician is a skilled history taker, has the time to conduct in-depth interviews and an individual is able to discuss their situation in detail (no aphasia, clear insights into their circumstances and so forth). Further, in evaluating progress after intervention they should not be coloured by biases in response and recall. To lend some structure to interviews, some more systematic techniques have been employed.

Goal attainment scaling (Malec, 1999; Schlosser, 2004) represents one method to tailor clinical aims and objectives to variables that are valuable to the individual. One progresses through collaborative identification of participatory areas and impact that represent priorities for an individual – for instance, using the telephone. Descriptors that characterize these variables are identified – e.g. apprehension at prospect of using phone; unable to make self understood. Parties then agree on what would count as evidence and markers of successful outcomes, in the example maybe reduced apprehension, more successful transmission of information. Change in therapy is gauged by progression towards these individualized goals. Skill is required to agree goals that are simultaneously meaningful, attainable within the constraints posed by the overall socio-medical context and measureable.

Repertory grid technique (Fransella, 2004; Kelly, 1955) and the closely related semantic differential technique (Ellis-Hill, 2000; Miller et al., 2008; Osgood, Suci & Tannenbaum, 1957) have been used to pinpoint dimensions along which individuals interpret their world, to find continua along which they view variation in behaviours and therefore represent dimensions along which rehabilitation might try to effect change. How we understand our environment and the place and roles of ourselves and others within it arises from our implicit theory of the world. This grows out of our personal experiences. Repertory grid techniques are ways to explore an individual's implicit theory, how they personally construe their world.

The process might start with a topic – e.g. me as a communicator – and elicit elements – e.g. situations, people, feelings – which are instances of or associated with the topic as perceived by the person. Subsequently, 'personal constructs' are established – i.e. terms/contrasts the person uses to make sense of elements – e.g. confident–tentative; confident–frightened; quiet–sociable; quiet–arrogant. Finally individuals, and possibly significant others, rate themselves on scales between the extremes of their constructs. In this fashion one hopes to arrive at a quantification of the meaning of individual constructs to that person. Rehabilitation might then focus on one or more core constructs to gradually modify. Outcomes can be gauged against rating results of 'me now' versus 'how I want to be after therapy'.

Using interviews to identify goals and measure change is not always possible or desirable. To circumvent inherent difficulties such as level of insight, shifting subjectivity and time available to the clinician, a range of questionnaires and checklists has been developed. Some of these are more general purpose (health- related) quality-of-life instruments, or condition-specific tools that may contain items related to communication, such as the Burden of Stroke Scale (BOSS) (Doyle, McNeil, Mikolic, Prieto, Hula et al., 2004) and the Parkinson's Disease Questionnaire (PDQ-39) (Jenkinson, Fitzpatrick, Peto, Greenhall & Hyman, 1997). Others have been devised with speech disorders especially in mind (for examples, see Donovan, Kendall, Young & Rosenbek, 2008; Hartelius et al., 2008; Long, Hesketh, Paszek, Booth & Bowen, 2008; Ma & Yiu, 2001; Walshe et al., 2009).

The format is typically that an individual rates themselves on items on a rating scale, e.g. 'I have difficulty making myself understood in a noisy room', or for presence or absence of an element. Lists may relate to perceived impact of voice or articulation on communication; a list of roles or situations people might be engaged in and how well they manage them; or to psychosocial reactions individuals experience.

Their advantage is speed and ease of application, provided there are no accompanying language or cognitive barriers. They can deliver a broad overview of impact for that individual. However, validity, sensitivity to change and clinical usefulness rest on various assumptions.

They assume items are relevant to individual respondents and adequately capture perceptions of impact as they envisage it. Ideally, tools will have passed through a development phase where items are elicited and honed to be maximally relevant to users, growing out of their views and experiences, not solely from the preconceived ideas of the deviser (Brown, 2009, 2010; Yorkston, Johnson & Klasner, 2005). Nevertheless, it can remain problematic constructing item-sets that simultaneously cover all issues pertinent to all potential repliers without being impossibly long, without containing items irrelevant to many speakers, or, if reduced to a set of items with apparent applicability to all, not missing detail important to a particular person.

Furthermore, rating scales should ideally acknowledge in their scoring/

interpretation that individuals demonstrate varying communicative behaviour before onset of any changes. For instance, a person may be asked to rate agreement with 'I let my spouse do the talking in formal situations', or their position on a continuum between 'talkative–withdrawn', 'confident–not confident in entering situation X'. One needs to bear in mind that they may always have been happy for the spouse to do the communicating or never felt talkative or confident in situation X.

In evaluating or devising own instruments it is important that they gauge participation or impact. Some instruments evidence a degree of blurring between impairment characteristics, activity limitations and participation and impact aspects – not least because these terms are subject to numerous interpretations (Cruice, Hill, Worrall & Hickson, 2010; Noonan, Kopec, Noreau, Singer & Dvorak, 2009; Salter, Jutai, Teasell, Foley, Bitensky & Bayley, 2005; Whiteneck & Dijkers, 2009). Moreover, inferences about communication are often confounded by effects of other variables. Strong agreement that 'I am no longer able to practise my previous leisure activities' may be a result of communication changes, but equally may stem from physical decline, cognitive barriers, financial concerns or the carer lacking time to bring the person to venues.

The impression of significant others regarding an individual's position on rating scales may be important to elicit. They can act as proxies if the person is unable to complete the assessment themselves. Debate continues about how far proxy ratings are accurate reflections of circumstances. However, the very fact that there may be divergences between raters may afford important insights into interactional aspects of communication, as well as highlight listener and speaker variables to target in intervention.

The field of measurement of psychosocial impact in MSDs represents an important area for development. Few of the rating scales and checklists available for MSDs have undergone rigorous psychometric and clinimetric testing to confirm assumptions are met and to exclude confounding variables. Eadie, Yorkston, Klasner, Dudgeon, Deitz et al. (2006) in their review of self-report tools were unable to recommend any as psychometrically fully sound. No instrument exclusively measured communicative participation. Some instruments evidenced low test–retest reliability, whilst others had low internal consistency or had incomplete evidence of construct or concurrent validity. A similar situation is apparent in allied fields (Branski, Cukier-Blaj, Pusic, Cano, Klassen et al., 2008; Franic & Bothe, 2008; Franic, Bramlett & Bothe, 2005; Salter et al., 2005).

Communicative participation item banks

A method pioneered over the last decades that seeks to reconcile attention to impact complexity with individual circumstances, to balance the full array of possible impact factors with what is relevant for any one person, and still remain psychometrically sound has been the communicative participation item-bank approach to patient-reported outcome measures (Baylor, Yorkston, Eadie, Miller & Amtmann, 2009; Bode, Hahn, DeVellis & Cella, 2009; DeWalt, Rothrock, Yount & Stone, 2007).

Tightly relevant items are generated through a lengthy process of focus groups of target populations, refinement in pilot phases and finally psychometric testing of individual items (as opposed to a fixed set of questions) to assure maximum sensitivity to domains and degrees of perceived change.

In this way one builds up a resource of hundreds of items from which one can select for any one individual just those items germane to their situation and concerns. Because each item brings its own psychometric package it does not matter what quantity or combination of items one selects, so long as they are tailored to that individual's circumstances. This simultaneously reduces assessment burden and directly increases validity for that individual.

This represents a core contrast to fixed-menu questionnaires and checklists. On the latter, scores are derived from aggregates across all items/subsections. There is no metric available for individual items. The aggregate mark therefore conceals any variation there may be in relevance of items between respondents or for one respondent over time. Hence, as noted above, scores from such tools are difficult to interpret for their true meaning for an individual. Simply omitting items an individual feels are irrelevant or adding ad hoc dimensions the parties deem appropriate renders the psychometrics invalid and the interpretation even more problematic.

The item-bank approach is in its infancy in MSDs. However, developments promise a more valid and reliable method of describing and quantifying impact than has hitherto been possible. It also offers a method of establishing clearer targets for intervention.

Treatment studies focusing on impact

To date few studies have focused specifically on MSDs. There are more general investigations covering conditions where motor speech difficulties might be an issue, and several interventions or techniques applied in germane fields are ripe for study in relation to MSDs. A broad indication of these is offered here.

Approaches to intervention in the field have always emphasized attention to environmental and listener-related barriers or facilitators. The need to maximize opportunities to speak, to find strategies to cope with varying demands of different situations, to minimize physical and psychological barriers to access is axiomatic in MSDs as in any instance of altered communication. Supporting speakers and listener to establish constructive strategies for managing adaptations to altered speech output is an established principle (Lubinski, 1991; Vogel & Miller, 1991). Methods from conversation analysis have been applied to recognition and negotiation of repair of breakdowns in dysarthric communication (Bloch & Wilkinson, 2009). Attention to speaker and listener strategies to help people with MSDs overcome pragmatic difficulties in entering, staying in and managing conversations have been called for, with some preliminary insights into this (Comrie et al., 2001; Holtgraves & McNamara, 2009), though treatment studies that reach beyond general, largely anecdotal case descriptions to systematic, controlled studies are still awaited.

Education and counselling of people with MSDs and carers have been viewed as important elements in preventative and therapeutic work. A'Campo, Spliethoff-Kamminga, Macht, Roos & EduPark (2010) describe a successful controlled study of psychosocial intervention with people with Parkinson's and their carers. The experience of Ward et al. (2004) cautions that under certain circumstances education programmes can bring negative effects. Simmons-Mackie, Raymer, Armstrong, Holland & Cherney (2010) point to some evidence that communication partner training in aphasia may improve communication activities and/or participation of partners and of speakers when they communicate with trained partners. The full picture remains unclear in aphasia, but the strength of findings warrants application to the field of MSDs.

Interventions applied in other closely related fields lend themselves to solutions in MSDs to help prevent or to ameliorate impact of changes on self-esteem and mood, counteract tendencies to loss of empowerment and control, withdrawal from or restriction of participation. Cohen, Elackattu, Noordzij, Walsh and Langmore (2009) describe approaches to palliative interventions for improving quality of life in relation to voice and dysarthria in people with late-stage neurological and surgical conditions. The use of cognitive behaviour therapy in voice disorders can also apply to people with MSDs (Daniilidou, Carding, Wilson, Drinnan & Deary, 2007). Repertory grid technique has been used as a framework for effecting change in impact in people who stutter (Fransella, 2004), whilst brief solution-focused therapy has shown some initial evidence of effectiveness in a range of disorders germane to MSDs (Ferraz & Wellman, 2008; Kim, 2008).

Music therapy has inherent potential as an intervention aid in MSDs. The physical aspects of singing or instrument playing and other physical activities can have beneficial effects on breathing, fitness and mood (Archer, Fredriksson & Johansson, 2011; Puhan et al., 2006); the social dimension of music groups acts as a counterbalance to isolation and withdrawal (Pacchetti et al., 2000; Tamplin, 2008). For many, listening to music fosters relaxation and improved quality of life, key ingredients to motivation to maintain communication. A range of other relaxation techniques, including visualization, mindfulness and autogenic training approaches, could potentially influence impact in MSDs either alone or as adjuncts to other methods (Bédard et al., 2003; Murray & Kim, 2004).

A hurdle in the past to studies aimed at impact and participation has been the absence of valid frameworks to pinpoint and analyze the nature of impact for groups or individuals (with MSDs), and correspondingly the lack of valid and reliable instruments to quantify outcomes. As outlined above, this situation is changing and the concepts and tools to support principled studies and model assessment and treatments to individual circumstances and aims are becoming available.

Conclusions

It is clear that MSDs do exercise a significant impact on speakers and their circle and, especially when associated with progressive conditions, the nature of impact and changes to participation evolves over time. It is self-evident that the nature of impact is both intricate and highly individualized, rendering assessment correspondingly complex. One may describe MSDs from numerous perspectives and it is true that no straightforward mapping of changes from one level to the other pertains. However, trying to comprehend impact without considering individuals' reactions to impairment and limitation will always remain incomplete. A focus on impairment in intervention that does not assess and act upon limitations and participation is destined to bring about poor maintenance and generalization of improvements. Whilst a challenge, such complexity is not insuperable. The voices of people with motor speech disorder help to delineate sources and consequences of impact, whether these be personal barriers and facilitators, family or societal factors; whether impact is on conversations, participation in a more general sense or for specific contexts. They help to highlight effects on identity and, with the voices of carers and others close to the person, draw attention to the (re)negotiation of relationships that may take place.

Some of these impacts may be part and parcel of experiencing any chronic (neurological) disorder, shared with people without communication changes. Others may be more specific to living with a communication disability, with dimensions in common with people with aphasia, cleft palate or organic voice disorder. Some undoubtedly will be specific to disorders that bring about speech changes and maybe even unique to individual conditions – spasmodic dysphonia, twelfth cranial nerve palsy, or whatever.

In this chapter we have tried to draw out some of these contrasts and identify strands in the complicated knot of influences. There is still a long way to go in untangling these knots, both conceptually and from the point of view of assessment and intervention. Developments in these fields indicate that the near future will bring great gains for all involved.

References

A'Campo, L.E.I., Spliethoff-Kamminga, N.G.A., Macht, M., Roos, R. & EduPark, C. (2010) Caregiver education in Parkinson's Disease: Formative evaluation of a standardized program in seven European countries. *Quality of Life Research, 19*(1), 55–64.

Adams, S., Moon, B., Dykstra, A., Abrams, K., Jenkins, M. & Jog, M. (2006) Effects of multitalker noise on conversational speech intensity in Parkinson's Disease. *Journal of Medical Speech-Language Pathology, 14(4)*, 221–228.

Archer, T., Fredriksson, A. & Johansson, B. (2011) Exercise alleviates Parkinsonism: Clinical and laboratory evidence. *Acta Neurologica Scandinavica, 123(2)*, 73–84.

Baylor, C., Yorkston, K., Bamer, A., Britton, D. & Amtmann, D. (2010) Variables associated with communicative participation in people with multiple sclerosis: A regression analysis. *American Journal Speech-Language Pathology, 19(2)*, 143–153.

Baylor, C., Yorkston, K., Eadie, T.L., Miller, R. & Amtmann, D. (2009) Developing the communicative participation item bank: Rasch analysis results from a spasmodic dysphonia sample. *Journal of Speech, Language, and Hearing Research, 52(5)*, 1302–1320.

Bédard, M., Felteau, M., Mazmanian, D., Fedyk, K., Klein, R., Richardson, J. et al. (2003) Pilot evaluation of a mindfulness-based intervention to improve quality of life among individuals who sustained traumatic brain injuries. *Disability and Rehabilitation, 25(13)*, 722–731.

Bloch, S. & Wilkinson, R. (2009) Acquired dysarthria in conversation: Identifying sources of understandability problems. *International Journal of Language and Communication Disorders, 44(5),* 769–783.

Bode, R., Hahn, E., DeVellis, R. & Cella, D. (2009) Measuring participation: The patient-reported outcomes measurement information system experience. *Archives of Physical Medicine and Rehabilitation, 91(9),* S60–S65.

Brady, M., Clark, A., Dickson, S., Paton, G. & Barbour, R. (2011) The impact of stroke related dysarthria on social participation and implications for rehabilitation. *Disability and Rehabilitation, 33(3),* 178–186.

Branski, R.C., Cukier-Blaj, S., Pusic, A., Cano, S.J., Klassen, A., Mener, D. et al. (2008) Quality of life in dysphonic patients: A systematic review of content development in patient-reported outcomes measures. *Journal of Voice, 24(2),* 193–198.

Bringfelt, P., Hartelius, L. & Runmarker, B. (2006) Communication problems in multiple sclerosis: A 9 year follow-up. *International Journal of MS Care, 8,* 130–140.

Brown, M. (2009) Perspectives on outcome: What disability insiders and outsiders each bring to the assessment table. *Archives of Physical Medicine and Rehabilitation, 90(11),* S36–S40.

Brown, M. (2010) Participation: The insider's perspective. *Archives of Physical Medicine and Rehabilitation, 91(9),* S34–S37.

Bunton, K. & Keintz, C. (2008) Use of dual task paradigm for assessing speech intelligibility in clients with Parkinson's Disease. *Journal of Medical Speech-Language Pathology, 16(3),* 141–155.

Cohen, S., Elackattu, A., Noordzij, J., Walsh, M. & Langmore, S. (2009) Palliative treatment of dysphonia and dysarthria. *Otolaryngologic Clinics of North America, 42(1),* 107–121.

Comrie, P., Mackenzie, C. & McCall, J. (2001) The influence of acquired dysarthria on conversational turn-taking. *Clinical Linguistics and Phonetics, 15(5),* 383–398.

Cruice, M., Hill, R., Worrall, L. & Hickson, L. (2010) Conceptualising quality of life for older people with aphasia. *Aphasiology, 24(3),* 327–347.

Dagenais, P., Watts, C., Turnage, L. & Kennedy, S. (1999) Intelligibility and acceptability of moderately dysarthric speech by three types of listeners. *Journal of Medical Speech-Language Pathology, 7(2),* 91–95.

Daniilidou, P., Carding, P., Wilson, J., Drinnan, M. & Deary, V. (2007). Cognitive behavioral therapy for functional dysphonia: A pilot study. *Annals of Otology Rhinology and Laryngology, 116(10),* 717–722.

DeWalt, D., Rothrock, N., Yount, S., Stone, A. and on behalf of the PROMIS Cooperative Group (2007) Evaluation of item candidates: The PROMIS qualitative item review. *Medical Care, 45(5),* S12–S21.

Dickson, S., Barbour, R., Brady, M., Clark, A. & Paton, G. (2008) Patients' experiences of disruptions associated with post-stroke dysarthria. *International Journal of Language and Communication Disorders, 43(2),* 135–153.

Donovan, N., Kendall, D., Young, M. & Rosenbek, J. (2008) The Communicative Effectiveness Survey: Preliminary evidence of construct validity. *American Journal of Speech-Language Pathology*, *17*(4), 335–347.

Doyle, P., McNeil, M., Mikolic, J., Prieto, L., Hula, W., Lustig, A. et al. (2004) The burden of stroke scale (BOSS). *Journal of Clinical Epidemiology*, *57(10)*, 997–1007.

Eadie, T., Yorkston, K., Klasner, E., Dudgeon, B.., Deitz, J., Baylor, C. et al. (2006) Measuring communicative participation: A review of self-report instruments in speech-language pathology. *American Journal of Speech-Language Pathology*, *15(4)*, 307–320.

Ellis-Hill, C. (2000) Changes in identity and self-concept: A new theoretical approach to recovery following stroke. *Clinical Rehabilitation*, *14*, 279–287.

Ferraz, H. & Wellman, N. (2008) The integration of solution-focused brief therapy principles in nursing: A literature review. *Journal of Psychiatric and Mental Health Nursing*, *15(1)*, 37–44.

Fox, A. & Pring, T. (2005) The cognitive competence of speakers with acquired dysarthria: Judgements by doctors and speech-language therapists. *Disability and Rehabilitation*, *27(23)*, 1399–1403.

Franic, D. & Bothe, A. (2008) Psychometric evaluation of condition-specific instruments used to assess health-related quality of life, attitudes, and related constructs in stuttering. *American Journal of Speech-Language Pathology*, *17(1)*, 60–80.

Franic, D., Bramlett, R. & Bothe, A. (2005) Psychometric evaluation of disease specific quality of life instruments in voice disorders. *Journal of Voice*, *19(2)*, 300–315.

Fransella, F. (2004) *Manual for Repertory Grid Technique*, 2nd edition. Chichester: John Wiley & Sons Ltd.

Garcia, L., Laroche, C. & Barrette, J. (2002) Work integration issues go beyond the nature of the communication disorder. *Journal of Communication Disorders*, *35(2)*, 187–211.

Guo, Y. & Togher, L. (2008) The impact of dysarthria on everyday communication after traumatic brain injury: A pilot study. *Brain Injury*, *22(1)*, 83–98.

Hartelius, L., Elmberg, M., Holm, R., Lovberg, A. & Nikolaidis, S. (2008. Living with dysarthria: Evaluation of a self-report questionnaire. *Folia Phoniatrica*, *60*, 11–19.

Hartelius, L., Jonsson, M., Rickeberg, A. & Laakso, K. (2010) Communication and Huntington's disease: Qualitative interviews and focus groups with persons with Huntington's disease, family members, and carers. *International Journal of Language and Communication Disorders*, *45*(3), 381–393.

Hartelius, L. & Miller, N. (2010) The ICF Framework and its relevance to the assessment of people with motor speech disorders. In A. Lowit & R. Kent (Eds) *Assessment of Motor Speech Disorders*, pp.1–20. San Diego: Plural.

Holtgraves, T. & McNamara, P. (2009) Pragmatic comprehension deficit in Parkinson's disease. *Journal of Clinical and Experimental Neuropsychology*, *32(4)*, 388–397.

Jenkinson, C., Fitzpatrick, R., Peto, V., Greenhall, R. & Hyman, N. (1997) The Parkinson's

Disease Questionnaire (PDQ-39): Development and validation of a Parkinson's Disease summary index score. *Age Ageing, 26(5)*, 353–357.

Kelly, G. (1955) *The Therory of Personal Constructs*, vols I and II. New York: Norton.

Kim, J.S. (2008) Examining the effectiveness of solution-focused brief therapy: A meta-analysis. *Research on Social Work Practice, 18(2)*, 107–116.

Klasner, E. & Yorkston, K. (2005) Speech intelligibility in ALS and HD dysarthria: The everyday listener's perspective. *Journal of Medical Speech-Language Pathology, 13(2)*, 127–139.

Klugman, T. & Ross, E. (2002) Perceptions of the impact of speech, language, swallowing, and hearing difficulties on quality of life of a group of South African persons with multiple sclerosis. *Folia Phoniatrica, 54(4)*, 201–221.

Long, A., Hesketh, A., Paszek, G., Booth, M. & Bowen, A. (2008) Development of a reliable self-report outcome measure for pragmatic trials of communication therapy following stroke. *Clinical Rehabilitation, 22(12)*, 1083–1094.

Lubinski, R. (1991) Dysarthria: A breakdown in inter-personal communication. In D. Vogel & M. Cannito (Eds) *Treating Disordered Speech-Motor Control*, pp.153–181. Austin, TX: Pro-Ed.

Lyons, K., Tickle-Degnen, L. & DeGroat, E. (2005) Inferring personality traits of clients with Parkinson's Disease from their descriptions of favourite activities. *Clinical Rehabilitation, 19(7)*, 799–809.

Ma, E. & Yiu, E. (2001) Voice activity and participation profile: Assessing the impact of voice disorders on daily activities. *Journal of Speech, Language, and Hearing Research, 44(3)*, 511–524.

Malec, J. (1999) Goal attainment scaling in rehabilitation. *Neuropsychological Rehabilitation, 9(3)*, 253–275.

McNamara, P. & Durso, R. (2003) Pragmatic communication skills in patients with Parkinson's Disease. *Brain and Language, 84(3)*, 414–423.

Miller, N., Allcock, L., Jones, D., Noble, E., Hildreth, A. & Burn, D. (2007) Prevalence and pattern of perceived intelligibility changes in Parkinson's Disease. *Journal of Neurology, Neurosurgery, and Psychiatry, 78(11)*, 1188–1190.

Miller, N., Andrew, S., Noble, E. & Walshe, M. (2011) Changing perceptions of self as a communicator in Parkinson's Disease: A longitudinal follow-up study. *Disability and Rehabilitation, 33*, 204–210.

Miller, N., Noble, E., Jones, D., Allcock, L. & Burn, D. (2008) How do I sound to me? Perceived changes in communication in Parkinson's Disease. *Clinical Rehabilitation, 22(1)*, 14–22.

Miller, N., Noble, E., Jones, D. & Burn, D. (2006) Life with communication changes in Parkinson's Disease. *Age Ageing, 35(3)*, 235–239.

Murray, L.L. & Kim, H.-Y. (2004) A review of select alternative treatment approaches for acquired neurogenic disorders: Relaxation therapy and acupuncture. *Seminars in Speech and Language, 25(2)*, 133–149.

Noonan, V., Kopec, J., Noreau, L., Singer, J. & Dvorak, M. (2009) A review of participation instruments based on the International Classification of Functioning, Disability and Health. *Disability and Rehabilitation, 31(23)*, 1–19.

Osgood, C., Suci, G. & Tannenbaum, P. (1957) *The Measurement of Meaning*. Urbana: University of Illinois Press.

Pacchetti, C., Mancini, F., Aglieri, R., Fundaro, C., Martignoni, E. & Nappi, G. (2000) Active music therapy in Parkinson's disease: An integrative method for motor and emotional rehabilitation. *Psychosomatic Medicine, 62(3)*, 386–393.

Pentland, B., Pitcairn, T., Gray, J. & Riddle, W. (1987) The effects of reduced expression in Parkinson's Disease on impression formation by health professionals. *Clinical Rehabilitation, 1*, 307–313.

Puhan, M.A., Suarez, A., Lo Cascio, C., Zahn, A., Heitz, M. & Braendli, O. (2006) Didgeridoo playing as alternative treatment for obstructive sleep apnoea syndrome: Randomised controlled trial. *British Medical Journal, 332(7536)*, 266–270.

Rosen, K., Kent, R., Delaney, A. & Duffy, J. (2006) Parametric quantitative acoustic analysis of conversation produced by speakers with dysarthria and healthy speakers. *Journal of Speech, Language, and Hearing Research, 49(2)*, 395–411.

Salter, K., Jutai, J., Teasell, R., Foley, N., Bitensky, J. & Bayley, M. (2005) Issues for selection of outcome measures in stroke rehabilitation: ICF participation. *Disability and Rehabilitation, 27(9)*, 507–528.

Schlosser, R.W. (2004) Goal attainment scaling as a clinical measurement technique in communication disorders: A critical review. *Journal of Communication Disorders, 37(3)*, 217–239.

Simmons-Mackie, N., Raymer, A., Armstrong, E., Holland, A. & Cherney, L.R. (2010) Communication partner training in aphasia: A systematic review. *Archives of Physical Medicine and Rehabilitation, 91(12)*, 1814–1837.

Tamplin, J. (2008) A pilot study into the effect of vocal exercises and singing on dysarthric speech. *NeuroRehabilitation, 23(3)*, 207–216.

Vogel, D. & Miller, L. (1991) A top-down approach to treatment of dysarthric speech. In D. Vogel & M. Cannito (Eds) *Treating Disordered Speech Motor Control*, pp.87–109. Austin, TX: Pro-Ed.

Walshe, M. & Miller, N. (2011) Living with acquired dysarthria: The speaker's perspective. *Disability and Rehabilitation, 33*, 95–203.

Walshe, M., Peach, R. & Miller, N. (2009) Dysarthria Impact Profile: Development of a scale to measure the psychosocial impact of acquired dysarthria. *International Journal of Language and Communication Disorders, 44(5)*, 693–715.

Ward, C.D., Turpin, G., Dewey, M.E., Fleming, S., Hurwitz, B., Ratib, S. et al. (2004) Education for people with progressive neurological conditions can have negative effects: Evidence from a randomized controlled trial. *Clinical Rehabilitation, 18(7)*, 717–725.

Whitehill, T. & Wong, C. (2006) Contributing factors to listener effort for dysarthric speech. *Journal of Medical Speech-Language Pathology, 14(4)*, 335–341.

Whiteneck, G. & Dijkers, M. (2009) Difficult to measure constructs: Conceptual and methodological issues concerning participation and environmental factors. *Archives of Physical Medicine and Rehabilitation, 90(11)*, S22–S35.

World Health Organization (WHO) (2001) *International Classification of Functioning, Disability, and Health.* Geneva: World Health Organization.

Wilkinson, C., Yorkston, K., Strand, E. & Rogers, M. (1995) Features of spontaneous language in speakers with amyotrophic lateral sclerosis and dysarthria. *American Journal of Speech-Language Pathology, 4(4)*, 139–142.

Yorkston, K., Baylor, C., Klasner, E., Deitz, J., Dudgeon, B., Eadie, T. et al. (2007) Satisfaction with communicative participation as defined by adults with multiple sclerosis: A qualitative study. *Journal of Communication Disorders, 40*, 433–451.

Yorkston K., Beukelman D., Strand E. & Hakel M. (2010) *Management of Motor Speech Disorders in Children and Adults*, 3rd edition. Austin, TX: Pro-Ed.

Yorkston, K., Bombardier, C. & Hammen, V. (1994) Dysarthria from the viewpoint of individuals with dysarthria. In J. Till, K. Yorkston & D. Beukelman (Eds) *Motor Speech Disorders*, pp.19–25. Baltimore: Brookes.

Yorkston, K., Johnson, K. & Klasner, E. (2005) Taking part in life: Enhancing participation in multiple sclerosis. *Physical Medicine and Rehabilitation Clinics of North America, 16(2)*, 583–594.

12 Adults with Learning Disabilities

Karen Bunning and Susan Buell

University of East Anglia, UK

Introduction

Learning disability (LD) is not a fixed condition with a uniform presentation; rather it is a relative construct affected by factors both within and around the individual. There is a significant intellectual impairment with deficits in social functioning (usually measured through basic everyday skills – communication, socialization and functional living skills) that are manifested during the developmental period (Emerson, Hatton, Felce & Murphy, 2001). Adults with learning disabilities (LDs) form a heterogeneous population, ranging from those with more mild or moderate cognitive difficulties requiring variable support, to those who are functioning at the earliest stages of development and reliant on significant others for most aspects of daily living (Coupe O'Kane & Goldbart, 1998). Whilst 'LD' does not necessarily equate with 'communication problem', it is not uncommon for the two conditions to co-occur (Rondal & Edwards, 1997). The strong likelihood of additional motor and sensory impairments is a further consideration, with at least 40% of adults with LDs having some form of hearing impairment (Yeates, 1995).

Estimates on prevalence of communication difficulties vary according to survey methodologies used, ranging from 50% (Enderby & Davies, 1989) to 78% (Parker & Liddle, 1987). An earlier survey by Blackwell et al. (1989) found that 62% of the learning disabled population had identifiable communication problems, with 33% demonstrating some verbal communication difficulty (25% demonstrating marked problems) and 29% who were non-verbal. Law and Lester (1991) reported slightly higher levels of need, with 81% recognized as needing help with communication. Despite variance in reported prevalence figures, it is clear that there is an increased risk of communication difficulties in people with LDs compared with the general population (Kerr, Fraser & Felce, 1996; McLean, Brady & McLean, 1996).

Impact on people's lives

The impact of communication difficulties on adults with LDs is inseparable from the underlying cognitive deficit and therefore both are considered in the context of people's lives.

Everyday communication

Adults with LDs are reliant, to lesser or greater extents, on the support of trained staff or family members for carrying out everyday activities. However, erroneous estimation of an individual's communicative capacity is a frequently encountered problem amongst services for adults with LDs (Bartlett & Bunning, 1997; McConkey, Purcell & Morris,1999; Purcell, McConkey & Morris, 2000). Studies of support staff communication have revealed tendencies to overestimate comprehension levels (Bartlett & Bunning, 1997; Money, 1997), to underestimate problems with hearing, to ignore non-verbal behaviours when there is no accompanying speech (Couchman, 1995), and to take the initiative, direct conversation and repeat what service users say (McConkey et al., 1999; Money, 1997). Conversely, spontaneous contributions to social interaction by people with LDs seem to increase when staff adopt a more facilitative style, avoiding closed questions and directives, and increasing non-verbal feedback (Money, 1997). Staff use of augmentative and alternative communication techniques in the natural environment supports more effective usage by children and adults with LDs (Powell, 2001). Purcell et al. (2000) also reported an increase in service user communication as staff learned to be more responsive to them.

The accounts of the main carers are used frequently, not only in communication assessment procedures (van der Gaag, 1989; Purcell et al., 2000; Iacono, Bloomberg & West, 2005), but also in health consultations (Iacono & Sutherland, 2006; Law, Bunning, Byng, Heyman & Bryars, 2005); psychiatric and challenging behaviour assessments (Moss et al., 1998); and quality of life evaluations (Miller & Chan, 2008; Skea, 2008). However, poor levels of agreement between staff accounts and researcher observations on the developmental stage of communication in adults with severe and multiple disabilities have been reported by a number of researchers (see Iacono, West, Bloomberg & Johnson, 2009). Purcell et al. (2000) found that staff experienced some difficulty in identifying and determining the non-verbal signals emanating from the individuals they supported. The challenge of deciphering the meaning behind observable behaviours is particularly relevant to those individuals with more severe to profound and multiple LDs who lack conventional verbal skills and express themselves through eye gaze, body movement, vocalization and facial expression (see Grove, Bunning, Porter & Olsson, 1999). There is a strong reliance on their communication partners to work out what these non-verbal signals might mean and the chances of inaccurate reporting are high (Grove et al., 1999), all of which may have implications for health, social support, daily activity and self-determination.

Social engagement and inclusion

Having a large network of socially supportive staff, family and friends has been determined as one of the most significant correlates to objectively measured quality of life amongst people with LDs (Campo, Sharpton, Thompson & Sexton, 1997). However, it is generally the case that such individuals tend to have impoverished social networks (Lippold & Burns, 2009). The evidence suggests that people with LDs engage in fewer friendship activities, and tend to gravitate to people with similar disabilities (Emerson & McVilly, 2004; Forrester-Jones et al., 2006; Skea, 2008).

The extent to which social networking difficulties are attributable to communication problems as opposed to LD, or indeed to social stigma, has not been established. Lippold and Burns (2009) found significant differences between the social networks of adults with LDs and a comparator group of people with physical disabilities. Whilst those cast in the role of 'carer', e.g. family members and residential staff, made up the majority of the networks identified by adults with LDs, friends occupied the major part of the social networks for the group with physical disabilities. The authors suggest that disability alone does not account for network restrictions, but type of disability. As all the participants had 'simple conversational skills', communication as a possible factor cannot be ignored. Difficulties in forging friendships have been attributed to problems in cognition, language, communication and social development (Parker, Rubin, Price & Derosier, 1995), but also indirectly to the negative perceptions of others regarding social competence and status of the person with LDs. Friendship development is dependent on the availability of appropriate social opportunities and participatory activities, which research suggests is more restricted for the learning disabled population compared to their typically developing peers (Cowart, Saylor, Dingle & Mainor, 2004). Forrester-Jones et al. (2006) cite a limited ability to reciprocate that affects relationship development brought about by the culture of 'being cared for' and reliance on significant other support in everyday events. Relationship formation is not unidirectional and facilitation of friendships for people with LDs calls for greater responsibility in society at large (Milner & Kelly, 2009). Support staff have a role in establishing the social inclusion of the people they support; however, care tasks appear to be given higher priority (McConkey & Collins, 2010).

Problem and challenging behaviour

Problem or challenging behaviour occurs in 5–15% of people with LDs (Emerson et al., 2001a). It often develops early and then persists throughout the life course (Totsika, Toogood, Hastings & Lewis, 2008). The social constructive nature of challenging behaviour, i.e. that it is related to both individual and environmental characteristics, is widely accepted. This underlines the relevance of interactions between the individual with LDs and the people providing support to the development and maintenance of challenging behaviour (Hastings, 2005). Challenging behaviour sometimes serves as a means of communicating and controlling the environment around the individual. Not surprisingly, multiple forms of problem behaviour are more likely amongst individuals with more severe LDs and those who are non-verbal or experience particular difficulty with reception and expression of language (Borthwick-Duffy, 1994; Emerson et al., 2001b).

A correlation between communication difficulties and behavioural problems has been suggested by a number of researchers (e.g. Bott, Farmer & Rohde, 1997; Chamberlain, Chung & Jenner, 1993). Bott et al. (1997) conducted a large-scale investigation of communication skills using a population-based information system. Registration data completed by the carers revealed a decline in all types of behaviour problems, except acts of delinquency and withdrawal, as expressive skills increased. Conversely, those with more limited communication skills were more likely to have behaviour problems. In a follow-up study of people who had moved into small-scale accommodation, Chung, Jenner, Chamberlain and Corbett (1995) found that those with better communication skills were more likely to show improvements in both communication and behaviour after one year. It would appear that having the ability to verbalize feelings and articulate internal judgements in a common code of reference with significant others has a positive effect on behaviour.

Self-injurious behaviour (SIB) includes, for example, striking self, skin picking/piercing, self-biting and bringing body into forceful contact with inanimate objects to cause varying degrees of tissue damage. Whilst it has been associated with particular genetic syndromes such as Lesch Nyhan, Cornelia de Lange and Prader-Willi, it has also been found to be more common in people with lower ability levels generally (Emerson et al., 2001c). However, there is some variance in the published research regarding associated factors. Lower levels of ability, visual impairment, attention deficit hyperactivity disorder and not having Down syndrome were some of the factors independently related to SIB and aggressive behaviour in two studies carried out by Cooper et al. (2009a, b). Neither study identified communication impairment as a factor. This is supported by Totsika and colleagues (2008), who found no linkage between challenging behaviour and either sensory impairment or communication skills level in their study of the persistence of challenging behaviours over an 11-year period. The fact that lower levels of ability were positively identified amongst the sample displaying SIB calls into question the operational definition of communication impairment used. In contrast, an earlier study by Borthwick-Duffy (1994), noted that 17% of those who were described by carers as non-verbal also exhibited SIB. Other researchers have reported positive associations between SIB emission levels and presence of communication impairment (Deb, Thomas & Bright, 2001), and hearing impairment and autistic-like symptoms (Collacott, Cooper, Branford & McGrother, 1998).

Whilst the studies cited here provide a variable view on the relevance of communicative competence and hearing capacity to the emission of challenging behaviour, it must be noted that many of them relied on carer or support staff narratives. There is a possible resonance with the questionable validity and accuracy of significant other accounts regarding communication skills mentioned earlier in this chapter (see Iacono et al., 2009; Purcell et al., 2000). For example, only 27% of Cooper et al.'s (2009a, b) sample were reported as having a hearing impairment, which is below reported prevalence (see Yeates, 1995). Whilst the evidence falls short of absolute conclusions regarding associations between communication difficulties and challenging behaviour, it is also the case that sensory status and communicative ability cannot be discarded as potentially relevant factors. Just as growing up with a communication difficulty and/or associated hearing impairment may have deleterious effects on social behaviour, people who exhibit such problem behaviour may also be vulnerable to the negative effects of isolation and reduced opportunities for learning and functioning (Emerson, 1995). For example, frontline support staff may avoid or seek restricted contact with the person displaying undesirable behaviour (Hastings & Remington, 1994). Negative consequences include difficulties accessing resources and integrating with local community, problems establishing and maintaining social networks, breakdown of support packages and even exclusion from services (Cooper et al., 2009a). The relationship between communication and challenging behaviour should be viewed as a reciprocal one: abnormal behaviour patterns may challenge and hinder the communication process and failure to communicate effectively may be a catalyst in the establishment and maintenance of problem behaviour.

Access to and maintenance of health

Adults with LDs have a thinner margin of health (Dejong, 1997) and experience difficulties in accessing adequate and timely healthcare (Scheepers et al., 2005). High incidence of premature death (Hollins et al., 1998) has led to a number of policy initiatives in the UK (e.g. DoH, 2001, 2009). The contribution that communication makes to this situation is not clear. The complex nature of presenting symptomatologies combined with communication difficulty may lead to the type of 'secondary complexities' described by Heyman, Swain and Gillman (2004). For example, Law et al. (2005) describe the case of a man with LDs whose broken shin bone was left untreated for five days due to a failed negotiation between practitioner and service user regarding the site of the problem. Chauhan, Kontopantelis, Campbell, Jarrett and Lester (2010) found that recorded health information was significantly higher for individuals undergoing routine health checks compared to those who were not. It might be that the health check procedure circumvented the need for symptom negotiation between practitioner and patient, which is so reliant on communication skills.

Communication difficulties and consent issues have been identified as particular issues in the care and treatment of adults with LDs in general hospitals (National Patient Safety Agency, 2004). Failure to understand the implications of treatment options and other medical procedures impacts directly on human rights (see Law et al., 2005). Poor verbal communication was identified as a particular factor in agitation levels of learning disabled patients as a result of long waits or when hospital staff displayed impatience or anger to them (Gibbs, Brown & Muir, 2008). In their study of experiences of general hospital stays, Iacono and Davis (2003) found that many people with LDs did not have their personal needs met, particularly in relation to accessing the toilet and making a choice from the hospital menu – the latter being exacerbated by limited literacy skills (Emerson et al., 2001a). Such inequalities in the healthcare system also featured in Mencap's 2004 report *Treat Me Right*. Among the recommendations articulated by Backer, Chapman and Mitchell (2009) in their review of secondary healthcare for people with LDs were improving communication and information through the use of a range of tools.

Self-determination

Self-determination encompasses a number of domains such as 'behavioural autonomy, psychological empowerment, self-regulation and self-realisation' (Miller & Chan, 2008, p.1040). Greater self-determination has been found to correlate with improved scores on the Quality of Life Questionnaire (Wehmeyer & Schwartz, 1998). Living with a communication difficulty means that there are frequent problems with influencing what happens in your immediate environment (Bradshaw, 2000; Bartlett & Bunning, 1997). Everyday functioning is certainly affected by a range of factors, which includes the receptive and expressive abilities of the individual, but also the culture of support that is available (Lippold & Burns, 2009). Antaki, Finlay, Walton and Pate (2008) demonstrated how the communication partner is integral to interactive success. Staff practice in this study, far from leading to unequivocal choice-making by the residents, resulted in unclear expression of preferences. Smyth and Bell (2006) concluded that even the most apparently straightforward of choices may have far-reaching ramifications for the individual's health and wellbeing.

Strategically gauged linguistic input by staff has been found to affect the interaction positively (see Money, 1997; Purcell et al., 2000). Nota, Ferrari, Soresi and Wehmeyer (2007) emphasized the role of the social environment, reporting that the *opportunity* to make choices far outweighed a person's actual social ability in terms of successful outcomes in self-determination. This is reiterated by Miller and Chan (2008), who found that frequency and quality of interpersonal exchanges were factors in improved levels of life satisfaction amongst people with LDs. The fact that the research sample all possessed sufficient verbal skills to complete the Quality of Life interview begs the question – if daily interactions are closely related to improved quality of life for the more communicatively able in the population, what is the situation for those with deficits in the speech, language and communication areas?

Initiatives in self-advocacy have grown up over the last 30 years with the overarching purpose of enabling people with LDs to stand up and speak for themselves (Goodley, 2000). Positive outcomes associated with membership of a self-advocacy group include the expression of ideas, the experience of being listened to (Goodley, 2000) and changes in self-concept (Beart, Hardy & Buchan, 2004). However, there has been no specific report of individuals with communication difficulties participating in self-advocacy initiatives. Does this mean that only the verbally more able people are active participants in the self-advocacy movement?

Beyond everyday self-determination and even participation in self-advocacy initiatives, taking part in local and national elections is one way that most adults are able to exercise their human rights; however, adults with LDs are underrepresented at the polls (Keeley, Redley, Holland & Clare, 2008). Physical access to polling stations and the challenges of reading and using voting literature have contributed to poor uptake of voting opportunities (Morris, Roddy & Barnet, 2003). Keeley et al. (2008) identified the critical importance of significant others in registering adults in the electoral roll and providing support that they might exercise the right to vote.

Employment and further education

Work and education bring new opportunities for improving quality of life (Kober & Eggleton, 2005) although the specific impact of communication difficulties has yet to be clearly established. Employment has been associated with growth in personal autonomy and a decrease in behavioural difficulties (Martorell, Gutierrez-Recacha, Pereda & Ayuso-Mateos, 2008), whilst students with LDs on a two-year certificated course at university reported feeling more accepted by peers, more socially included and with greater belief in own competence (O'Brien et al., 2009). However, a reasonably high level of communicative competence amongst participants is indicated, because data collection involved them making diary entries and being interviewed. Despite these examples, school leavers with LDs are often launched into a comparative no-man's-land of patchy further educational provision. For some people, the lack of job prospects challenges the value of being educated in the first place (Wright, 2006). Interestingly, the specific impact of a communication difficulty on adults with LDs in the workplace has been shown to be less of a problem than might have been expected. Martorell et al. (2008) place more emphasis on friendship levels at work and the people contributing to interaction than on the communication itself. It is possible that the studies cited did not include any participants with specific communication difficulties, or alternatively that communication was less of an issue for colleagues once support was in place and the job was being done. Conversely, Cramm, Finkenflügel, Kuijsten and van Exel (2009) reported that some adults with LDs view work as 'structure' over and above 'participation', i.e. getting the job done was the primary focus.

Clinical implications

The evidence asserts the relevance of communication in the establishment of social networks, uptake of occupation and further educational opportunities, its role in self-determination, the emission of problem behaviour and in accessing healthcare. Thus communication should not be viewed as an isolated skill set, but as the cornerstone of human functioning in context. Speech and language therapy practice, therefore, needs to take an ecological view of communicative capacities by locating them in the events of daily life that are relevant to the individual.

Community-based multi-disciplinary practice already exists in the UK and mechanisms such as 'person-centred planning' are designed to bring agencies together around the person who is at the centre of all activity. To what extent real and active collaboration is achieved is a question for all teams serving the adult learning disabled community. What are the ways in which baseline assessment and intervention planning are coordinated, such that the mutual contributions of the relevant stakeholders are supported? For example, given the potential relevance of communication in problem behaviour emission, intervention in this area should be seen as a shared enterprise between challenging behaviour workers, clinical psychologists and speech and language therapists. Beyond an agreed service policy, there is the need to resist separate intervention approaches as dictated by professional orientations, but to come together in an integrated approach to assessment, differential diagnosis and progressive planning of intervention (see, Bradshaw, 2002).

The drive to establish the principle that communication is 'everybody's business' has seen the rise of service-wide strategies involving Total Communication (TC) development and training (see, for example, Bradshaw, 2000; Jones, 2000). Whilst there has been very little research on clinical effectiveness published in this area, outcomes cited as a result of local survey initiative have included: positive change in staff attitudes; evidence of TC use within environments; marked improvement in access to TC tools; and the production of accessible formats of many different documents. Areas of concern have included variable compliance rates amongst staff and limited address of individuals who are at the earliest stages of communication development (Jones, 2000). Clearly there is a need to develop ways of measuring the impact of ecologically framed interventions.

Address of an individual's communication needs to be viewed in a partnership milieu, which means assessment of the contributions made by the person with LD *and* the significant other during social interaction. This indicates a place for sampling, recording and transcribing of communication in the natural environment and the application of linguistic methodologies, such as conversation or discourse analysis (see Antaki et al., 2008). Therefore, bringing about change in the communication of both the person with an LD and the people with whom they communicate becomes the focus of interventions. For example, Intensive Interaction (Nind & Hewett, 2005) is an approach where the main objective is to broaden interactions between communication partners (Firth, Elford, Leeming & Crabbe, 2008). The case of Sandra (see opposite) demonstrates how opposing views of the parents and support staff were resolved through a focus on the partnership milieu.

Case Study 1: Sandra

Sandra is 22 years old and has multiple and complex LDs. She sits with support and is a wheelchair user. All her limbs are affected by her condition, although she does have some use of her arms. She might also have some use of eyesight and hearing, but this is uncertain. Sandra is now cared for by staff in a residential home, where she has been for the last three years. During this time her parents became increasingly unhappy and felt that her communication was being limited by her routine in the home. They were always closely involved in her care when she lived at home, and her mother particularly spent a lot of time with her. Sandra began to express frustration through loud groaning vocalizations and wide arm movements, and then started to go through long periods of silence where she withdrew into herself. Her eating habits changed and she no longer seemed to enjoy food. Sandra started communicating her isolation, sadness and frustration through negative behaviours and these were being noticed. Her key worker identified Intensive Interaction as a possible route to re-engaging Sandra with the world around her. However, some of the staff felt that this was not appropriate to the 'adult' Sandra and wanted her to become more independent. Intensive Interaction was finally introduced and progress was slow. According to reports from most staff members, Sandra now appears to understand environmental cues and contexts – e.g. mealtimes, going 'out', bedtime – and she can anticipate using the multi-sensory area in the day centre she attends. She shows recognition and anticipation by smiling and moving her head to the right and down. She maintains a 'looking' posture for longer when faced with another familiar adult who is giving eye contact, and has started to vocalize with a cooing sound when she is 'looking'. The change is particularly noticeable to Sandra's parents, who say they have now got their daughter back. The aims of the Intensive Interaction sessions between Sandra and her key worker focused on process rather than outcome. However, even the more sceptical staff members, through regular and dedicated close contact with Sandra, have recognized her increased communicative independence.

Future research

Heterogeneity of population makes defining the way forward in terms of research and development a challenging proposition.

Culture of inclusion

Over the last decade in the UK, the Government White Papers *Valuing People* and *Valuing People Now* have assumed great significance to adult service provision (DoH, 2001, 2009). These major policy initiatives are based on an 'enabling philosophy' where there is a conscious move towards 'social inclusion and emancipation' (Grant & Ramcharan, 2002; p.27). The first paper (DoH, 2001) was structured around the four major principles of independence, choice, civil rights and social inclusion. The second paper set out the Government's three-year strategy to improve the lives of people with LDs (DoH, 2009). Importantly, a social constructivist view of LD is taken, which acknowledges the role of environment in individual attainment. Communication was not identified specifically as a core principle, although it is generally acknowledged that it is the cornerstone of implementation (Jones, 2000). An editorial in the *Journal of Intellectual Disability Research* stressed the importance of establishing and maintaining the highest ethical standards in research in obtaining consent from such a vulnerable group of people (Holland, 2008). The author goes on to urge the setting up of research initiatives in areas that directly affect the lives of people with LDs, leading 'best practice and to practical and conceptual advances' (Shakespeare, 2006, cited by Holland, 2008, p.1).

Importance of communication

What does this all mean for research and development in the area of communication? If the impact of communication difficulties on the lives of people with LDs is to be fully understood and interventions to be reliably informed, then comprehensive information regarding the scale and nature of communication difficulties is needed. Published estimates vary broadly, provide insufficient detail and too often rely exclusively on significant other perspectives. There is a need to objectify research in this area by employing the technologies developed specifically for the identification and evaluation of speech, language and communication skills, so the accounts of familiar other persons may be supplemented, e.g. using criterion-related assessments and systematic observation procedures. A population-wide survey of communication skills needs to be linked to quality of life domains such as social network and behaviour, self-determination and activity participation, which may inform future policy initiatives.

Interpersonal advocacy

Communication is a dynamic, interpersonal construct, which acknowledges the presence of 'bidirectional influences in communication' (Nind, Kellett & Hopkins, 2001, p.144). Empirical evidence supports this view where the changing input of the adult has been found to affect both the quality and quantity of the individual's output (e.g. Money, 1997; Purcell et al., 2000). It follows, therefore, that an individual's difficulties with communication should not be seen as deriving solely from the primary cognitive deficit, but rather as by-products of the interactional process (Nind et al., 2001). This calls for exploration of interpersonal advocacy as one outcome of the communication taking place between people with LDs and their caregivers.

Summary

The interaction of cognition and communication means that assessing the impact of communication on quality of life for adults with LDs is far from straightforward. Communication appears to be a factor in challenging behaviour, but the evidence is inconclusive. It seems that reduced friendship groups and limited opportunities for employment and further education are part of the lived experience. Access to health is often determined by the supporting role of significant others, and the extent to which they are able to understand and facilitate the individual's communication. Thus there is ample opportunity for something to go wrong with assessment, diagnosis and treatment procedures. Self-determination and uptake of the same rights that are available to others in society are frequently hard-won. In conclusion, adults with LDs who also have communication difficulties are subject to a kind of double jeopardy, which makes them vulnerable to disempowerment in society.

References

Antaki, C., Finlay, W., Walton, C. & Pate, L. (2008) Offering choices to people with intellectual disabilities: An interactional study. *Journal of Intellectual Disability Research*, *52(12)*, 1165–1175.

Backer, C., Chapman, M. & Mitchell, D. (2009) Access to secondary healthcare for people with intellectual disabilities: A review of the literature. *Journal of Applied Research in Intellectual Disabilities*, *22(6)*, 514–525.

Bartlett, C. & Bunning, K. (1997) The importance of communication partnerships: A study to investigate the communicative exchanges between staff and adults with learning disabilities. *British Journal of Learning Disabilities*, *25(4)*,148–153.

Beart, S., Hardy, G. & Buchan, L. (2004) Changing selves: A grounded theory account of belonging to a self-advocacy group for people with intellectual disabilities. *Journal of Applied Research in Intellectual Disabilities*, *17(2)* 91–100.

Blackwell, C.L., Hulbert, C.M., Bell, J., Elston, L., Morgan, W., Robertshaw, B.A. & Thomas, C. (1989) A survey of the communication abilities of people with a mental handicap. *British Journal of Mental Subnormality*, *35(1)*, 63–71.

Borthwick-Duffy, S.A. (1994) Epidemiology and prevalence of psychopathology in people with mental retardation. *Journal of Consulting and Clinical Psychology*, *62(1)*, 17–27.

Bott, C., Farmer, R. & Rohde, J. (1997) Behaviour problems associated with lack of speech in people with disabilities. *Journal of Intellectual Disability Research*, *41(1)*, 3–7.

Bradshaw, J. (2000) A total communication approach: Towards meeting the communication needs of people with learning disabilities. *Tizard Learning Disability Review*, *5(1)*, 27–30.

Bradshaw, J. (2002) The management of challenging behaviour within a communication framework. In S. Aburdarham & A. Hurd (Eds) *Management of Communication Needs in People with a Learning Disability,* pp.246–275. London: Whurr Publishers Ltd.

Campo, S.F., Sharpton, W.R., Thompson, B. & Sexton, D. (1997) Correlates of the quality of life of adults with severe or profound mental retardation. *Mental Retardation, 35(5),* 329–337.

Chamberlain, L., Chung, M.C. & Jenner, L. (1993) Preliminary findings on communication and challenging behaviour in learning difficulty. *British Journal of Developmental Disabilities, 39(2),* 118–125.

Chauhan, L., Kontopantelis, E., Campbell, S., Jarrett, H. & Lester, H. (2010) Health checks in primary care for adults with intellectual disabilities: How extensive should they be? *Journal of Intellectual Disability Research, 54(6),* 479–486.

Chung, M.C., Jenner, L., Chamberlain, L. & Corbett, J. (1995) One year follow up pilot study on communication skills and challenging behaviour. *European Journal of Psychiatry, 9(2),* 83–95.

Collacott, R.A., Cooper, S.A., Branford, D. & McGrother, C. (1998) Epidemiology of self-injurious behaviour in adults with learning disabilities. *British Journal of Psychiatry, 173(5),* 428–432.

Cooper, S.A., Smiley, E., Allan, L.M., Jackson, A., Finlayson, J., Mantry, D. & Morrison, J. (2009a) Adults with intellectual disabilities: Prevalence, incidence and remission of self-injurious behaviour, and related factors. *Journal of Intellectual Disability Research, 53(3),* 200–216.

Cooper, S.A., Smiley, E., Jackson, A., Finlayson, J., Allan, L.M., Mantry, D. & Morrison, J. (2009b) Adults with intellectual disabilities: Prevalence, incidence and remission of aggressive behaviour and related factors. *Journal of Intellectual Disability Research, 53(3),* 217–232.

Couchman, W. (1995) Using video and conversation analysis to train staff working with people with learning disabilities. *Journal of Advanced Nursing, 22(6),* 1112–1119.

Coupe O'Kane, J. & Goldbart, J. (1998) *Communication Before Speech: Development and Assessment.* London: David Fulton.

Cowart, B.L., Saylor, C.F., Dingle, A. & Mainor, M. (2004) Social skills and recreational preferences of children with and without disabilities. *North American Journal of Psychology, 6(1),* 27–42.

Cramm, J.M, Finkenflügel, H., Kuijsten, R. & van Exel, N.J.A. (2009) How employment support and social integration programmes are viewed by the intellectually disabled. *Journal of Intellectual Disability Research, 53(6),* 512–520.

Deb, S., Thomas, M. & Bright, C. (2001) Mental disorder in adults with intellectual disability. 2: The rate of behaviour disorder among a community-based population aged between 16 and 64 years. *Journal of Intellectual Disability Research, 45(6),* 506–514.

Dejong, G. (1997) Primary care for persons with disabilities. *American Journal of Physical Medicine and Rehabilitation, 76(3),* Suppl.2–8.

Department of Health (DoH) (2001) *Valuing People: A New Strategy for Learning Disability in the 21st Century*. London: Department of Health Publications.

Department of Health (DoH) (2009) *Valuing People Now: A New Three-year Strategy for People with Learning Disabilities*. London: Department of Health Publications.

Emerson, E. (1995) *Challenging Behaviour: Analysis and Intervention in People with Learning Difficulties*. Cambridge: Cambridge University Press.

Emerson, E., Hatton, C., Felce, D. & Murphy, G. (2001a) *Learning Disabilities – The Fundamental Facts*. London: The Foundation for People with Learning Disabilities, London.

Emerson E., Kiernan, C., Alborz, A., Reeves, D., Mason, H., Swarbrick, R., Mason, L. & Hatton, C. (2001b) The prevalence of challenging behaviors: A total population study. *Research in Developmental Disabilities, 22(1)*, 77–93.

Emerson, E., Kiernan, C., Alborz, A., Reeves, D., Mason, H., Swarbrick, R., Mason, L. & Hatton, C. (2001c) Predicting the persistence of severe self-injurious behaviour. *Research in Developmental Disabilities, 22(1)*, 67–75.

Emerson, E. & McVilly, K. (2004) Friendship activities of adults with intellectual disabilities in supported accommodation in Northern England. *Journal of Applied Research in Intellectual Disabilities, 17(3)*, 191–197.

Enderby, P. & Davies, P. (1989) Communication disorders: Planning a service to meet the needs. *British Journal of Disorders of Communication, 24(3)*, 310–331.

Firth, G., Elford, H., Leeming, C. & Crabbe, M. (2008) Intensive Interaction as a novel approach in social care: Care staff's views on the practice change process. *Journal of Applied Research in Intellectual Disabilities, 21(1)*, 58–69.

Forrester-Jones, R., Carpenter, J., Coolen-Schrijner, P., Tate, A., Beecham, J., Hallam, A., Knapp, M. & Wooff, D. (2006) The social networks of people with intellectual disability living in the community 12 years after resettlement from long stay hospitals. *Journal of Applied Research in Intellectual Disabilities, 19(4)*, 285–295.

Gibbs, S.M., Brown M.J. & Muir, W.J. (2008) The experiences of adults with intellectual disabilities and their carers in general hospitals: A focus group study. *Journal of Intellectual Disability Research, 52(12)*, 1061–1077.

Goodley, D. (2000) *Self-advocacy in the Lives of People with Learning Difficulties*. Buckingham: Open University Press.

Grant, G. & Ramcharan, P. (2002) Researching valuing people. *Tizard Learning Disability Review, 7(3)*, 27–33.

Grove, N., Bunning, K., Porter, J. & Olsson, C. (1999) See what I mean: Interpreting the meaning of communication by people with severe and profound intellectual disabilities. *Journal of Applied Research in Intellectual Disabilities, 12(3)*, 190–203.

Hastings, R.P. (2005) Staff in special education settings and behaviour problems: Towards a framework for research and practice. *Educational Psychology, 25(2/3)*, 207–221.

Hastings, R.P. & Remington, B. (1994) Staff behaviour and its implications for people with learning disabilities and challenging behaviours. *British Journal of Clinical Psychology*, *33(4)*, 423–438.

Heyman, B., Swain, J. & Gillman, M. (2004) Organisational simplification and secondary complexity in health services for adults with learning disabilities. *Social Science and Medicine*, *58(2)*, 357–367.

Holland, A. (2008) Determining priorities in intellectual disability research. *Journal of Intellectual Disability Research*, *52(1)*, 1–2.

Hollins, S., Attard, M.T., von Fraunhofer, N., McGuigan, S. & Sedgewick, P. (1998) Mortality in people with learning disability: Risks causes and death certification findings in London. *Developmental Medicine and Child Neurology*, *40(1)*, 50–56.

Iacono, T., Bloomberg, K. & West, D. (2005) A preliminary investigation into the internal consistency and construct validity of the Triple C: Checklist of Communicative Competencies. *Journal of Intellectual and Developmental Disability*, *30(3)*, 139–145.

Iacono, T. & Davis, R. (2003) The experiences of people with developmental disability in emergency departments and hospital wards. *Research in Developmental Disabilities*, *24(4)*, 247–264.

Iacono, T. & Sutherland, G. (2006) Health screening and developmental disability. *Journal of Policy and Practice in Intellectual Disabilities*, *3(3)*, 155–163.

Iacono, T., West, D., Bloomberg, K. & Johnson, H. (2009) Reliability and validity of the revised Triple C: Checklist of Communicative Competence for adults with severe and multiple disabilities. *Journal of Intellectual Disability Research*, *53(1)*, 44–53.

Jones, J. (2000) A total communication approach to meeting the communication needs of people with learning disabilities. *Tizard Learning Disability Review*, *5(1)*, 20–26.

Keeley, H., Redley, M., Holland, A.J. & Clare, I.C.H. (2008) Participation in the 2005 general election by adults with intellectual disabilities. *Journal of Intellectual Disability Research*, *52(3)*, 175–181.

Kerr, M., Fraser, W. & Felce, D. (1996) Primary health care for people with a learning disability. *British Journal of Learning Disabilities*, *24(1)*, 1–8.

Kober, R. & Eggleton, I.R.C. (2005) The effect of different types of employment on quality of life. *Journal of Intellectual Disability Research*, *49(10)*, 756–760.

Law, J., Bunning, K., Byng, S., Heyman, B. & Bryars, R. (2005) Making sense in primary care: Levelling the playing field for people with communication difficulties. *Disability and Society*, *20(2)*, 169–184.

Law, J. & Lester, R. (1991) Speech therapy provision in a social education centre: Is it possible to target intervention? *Mental Handicap*, *19(1)*, 22–28.

Lippold, T. & Burns, J. (2009) Social support and intellectual disabilities: A comparison between social networks of adults with intellectual disability and those with physical disability. *Journal of Intellectual Disability Research*, *53(5)*, 463–473.

Martorell, A., Gutierrez-Recacha, P., Pereda, A. & Ayuso-Mateos, J.L. (2008) Identification of personal factors that determine work outcome for adults with intellectual disability. *Journal of Intellectual Disability Research, 52(12),* 1091–1101.

McConkey, R. & Collins, S. (2010) The role of support staff in promoting the social inclusion of persons with an intellectual disability. *Journal of Intellectual Disability Research, 54(8),* 691–700.

McConkey, R., Purcell, M. & Morris, I. (1999) Staff perceptions of communication with a partner who is intellectually disabled. *Journal of Applied Research in Intellectual Disabilities, 12(3),* 204–210.

McLean, L.K., Brady, N.C. & McLean, J.E. (1996) Reported communication abilities of individuals with severe mental retardation. *American Journal on Mental Retardation, 100(6),* 580–591.

Mencap (2004) *Treat Me Right! Better Healthcare for People with a Learning Disability.* London: Mencap.

Miller, S.M. & Chan, F. (2008) Predictors of life satisfaction in individuals with intellectual disabilities. *Journal of Intellectual Disability Research, 52(12),* 1039–1047.

Milner, P. & Kelly, B. (2009) Community participation and inclusion: People with disabilities defining their place. *Disability and Society, 24(1),* 47–62.

Money, D. (1997) A comparison of three approaches to delivering a speech and language therapy service to people with learning disabilities. *European Journal of Disorders of Communication, 32(4),* 449–466.

Morris, G., Roddy, G. & Barnet, E. (2003) *Disability Access Review.* Swansea: The Pollen Shop.

Moss, S., Prosser, H., Costello, A., Simpson, N., Patel, P., Rowe, S., Turner, S. & Hatton, C. (1998) Reliability and validity of the PAS-ADD checklist for detecting psychiatric disorders in adults with intellectual disability. *Journal of Intellectual Disability Research, 42(2),* 173–183.

National Patient Safety Agency (2004) *Understanding the Patient Safety Issues for People with Learning Disabilities.* London: NPSA.

Nind, M. & Hewett, D. (2005) *Access to Communication: Developing the Basics of Communication with People with Severe Learning Difficulties through Intensive Interaction,* 2nd edition. London: David Fulton.

Nind, M., Kellett, M. & Hopkins, V. (2001) Teachers' talk styles: Communicating with learners with severe and complex learning difficulties. *Child Language Teaching and Therapy, 17(2),* 143–159.

Nota, L., Ferrari, L., Soresi, S. & Wehmeyer, M. (2007) Self-determination, social abilities and the quality of life of people with intellectual disability. *Journal of Intellectual Disability Research, 51(11),* 850–865.

O'Brien, P., Shevlin, M., O'Keefe, M., Fitzgerald, S., Curtis, S. & Kenny, M. (2009) Opening up a whole new world for students with intellectual disabilities within a third level setting. *British Journal of Learning Disabilities, 37(4)*, 285–292.

Parker, J.G., Rubin, K.H., Price, J. & Derosier, M.E. (1995) Peer relationships, child development, and adjustment: A developmental psychopathology perspective. In D. Cicchetti & D.J. Cohen (Eds) *Developmental Psychopathology*, pp.96–161. Chichester: John Wiley & Sons Ltd.

Parker, M. & Liddle, K. (1987) The communication needs of the mentally handicapped population in West Berkshire: A survey. *RCSLT Bulletin, 428*, 1–2.

Powell, G. (2001) Children with severe learning disabilities. In M. Kersner & J.A. Wright (Eds) *Speech and Language Therapy: The Decision-Making Process when Working with Children*, pp.244–255. London: David Fulton.

Purcell, M., McConkey, R. & Morris, I. (2000) Staff communication with people with intellectual disabilities: The impact of a work-based training programme. *International Journal of Language and Communication Disorders, 35(1)*, 147–158.

Rondal, J. & Edwards, S. (1997) *Language in Mental Retardation*. London: Whurr Publishers Ltd.

Scheepers, M., Kerr, M., O'Hara, D., Bainbridge, D., Cooper, S.A., Davis, R., Fujuira, G., Helle, T., Holland, A., Krahn, G., Lennox, N., Meaney, J. & Wehmeyer, M. (2005) Reducing health disparity in people with intellectual disabilities: A report from Health Issues Special Interest Research Group of the International Association for the Scientific Study of Intellectual Disabilities. *Journal of Policy and Practice in Intellectual Disabilities, 2(3/4)*, 249–255.

Skea, D. (2008) Quality of life for adults with learning disabilities in private residential care: Monitoring aspects of life experiences over time. *Mental Health and Learning Disabilities Research and Practice, 5(2)*, 252–265.

Smyth, C.M. & Bell D. (2006) From biscuits to boyfriends: The ramifications of choice for people with learning disabilities. *British Journal of Learning Disabilities, 34(4)*, 227–236.

Totsika, V., Toogood, S., Hastings, R.P. & Lewis, S. (2008) Persistence of challenging behaviours in adults with intellectual disability over a period of 11 years. *Journal of Intellectual Disability Research, 52(5)*, 446–457.

van der Gaag, A. (1989) Joint assessment of communication skills: Formulating the role of the carer. *British Journal of Mental Subnormality, 35*, 22–28.

Wehmeyer, M. & Schwartz, M. (1998) The relationship between self-determination and quality of life for adults with mental retardation. *Education and Training in Mental Retardation and Developmental Disabilities, 33(1)*, 3–12.

Wright, A. (2006) Provision for students with learning difficulties in general colleges of further education – have we been going round in circles? *British Journal of Special Education, 33(1)*, 33–39.

Yeates, S. (1995) The incidence and importance of hearing loss in people with severe learning disability: The evolution of a service. *British Journal of Learning Disability, 23(2)*, 79–84.

13 Traumatic Brain Injury

Skye McDonald
University of New South Wales, Australia

Leanne Togher
University of Sydney, Australia

Introduction

Traumatic Brain Injury (TBI) is the commonest form of brain injury in the Western world, with prevalence rates at approximately 1 in 1000 per annum (Tate, McDonald & Lulham, 1998). In such injuries, typically due to motor vehicle accidents, falls or assault, the brain is subjected to blunt force and rapid acceleration–deceleration resulting in contusions and bleeding, especially in the ventrolateral surfaces of the frontal and temporal lobes, as well as white matter shearing (Bigler, 2001; Gentry, Godersky & Thompson, 1988). Widespread cognitive and physical impairment is common after severe TBI. However, for people who experience such injuries and their families, the most significant changes are in emotion, psychosocial functioning and communication (e.g. Brooks & McKinlay, 1983; Oddy, Humphrey & Uttley, 1978).

Early observational studies (Levin, Grossman, Rose & Teasdale, 1979; Thomsen, 1975) alerted the research community to the unique difficulties that people with TBI experienced when communicating. Aphasic disorders occurred in only the minority of cases (2–30%) (Heilman, Safran & Geschwind, 1971; Sarno & Levita, 1986). Far more prevalent were difficulties with communication including problems of slowness, hesitancy, lack of initiative, reliance on set expressions, tangentiality, inappropriateness and over-talkativeness (Thomsen, 1975). These characteristics were not clearly defined as aphasia, although some were considered to represent a sub-clinical aphasic language disorder (e.g. Sarno & Levita, 1986).

In the ensuing decades, evidence has gradually accrued to suggest that such communication disturbances reflect underlying cognitive impairment arising from fronto-temporal pathology and diffuse axonal injuries rather than disruption to language per se. Slowed information processing, impaired working memory/attention and executive dyscontrol may translate into deficiencies, including inertia, rigidity, poor conceptualization and planning or, alternatively, poor regulation and control (i.e. excesses) of cognition and behaviour (Tate, Fenelon, Manning & Hunter, 1991). Constellations of communication disturbances have been described that reflect the relative influence of these different kinds of cognitive deficits. Thus, adults with severe TBI have been described as over-talkative (Hagan, 1984; Milton & Wertz, 1986) although inefficient (Hartley & Jensen, 1991), tangential (Prigatano, Roueche & Fordyce, 1986), drifting from topic to topic (Snow, Douglas & Ponsford, 1997). Alternatively, they may produce little language at all (Chapman et al., 1992; Hartley & Jensen, 1991), their speech characterized by slow, incomplete responses, numerous pauses and a reliance on set expressions (Thomsen, 1975). People with TBI may also demonstrate confused, inaccurate and confabulatory verbal behaviour (Hartley & Jensen, 1992) with frequent interruptions, disinhibited inappropriate responses, swearing, tangential topic changes or perseveration on topics, or some other combination of these basic features (Hartley & Jensen, 1992). Likewise, in adolescents with TBI, there is reduced conversational fluency and inability to juggle multiple demands of conversation (Douglas, 2010).

Impact on people's lives

While the majority of people with TBI achieve independence in activities of daily living (Tate, Lulham, Broe, Strettles & Pfaff, 1989), they experience poor outcomes in their psychosocial functioning. Almost 50% of people with a severe TBI have no social contacts and few leisure interests one year or more after the injury (Tate et al., 1989), with a greater reliance on family for emotional support which continues long term. In a cohort of 100 consecutive severe TBI patients studied longitudinally, 73% had unmet social participation needs, 66% were affected with regard to their employability and 54% had difficulty with interpersonal relationships. Additionally, one third of the group had no friends 23 years post-injury (Tate, Broe, Cameron, Hodgkinson & Soo, 2005). Depression and anxiety are very common following TBI – depression is reported by approximately 30% of those with severe TBI, both acutely and in the longer term (Gomez-Hernandez, Max, Kosier, Paradiso & Robinson, 1997) and some sort of emotional disorder in up to 60% (Kinsella, Moran, Ford & Ponsford, 1988). Family distress can also be very high when caring for an individual with

TBI. This is related to cognitive changes (Wallace et al., 1998), emotional and behavioural disturbance (Kinsella, Packer & Olver, 1991; Knight, Devereux & Godfrey, 1998) and problems communicating with the affected individual (MAA, 1998). Importantly, impaired ability to communicate has been identified as critical to psychosocial recovery, hampering participation and friendship (Shorland & Douglas, 2010) and employment status (Isake & Turkstra, 2000). In turn, absence of close interpersonal friendships and problems with employment predict depression (Gomez-Hernandez et al., 1997; Kinsella et al., 1988). Thus, impaired interpersonal function and communicative competence are critical to quality of life for both people with TBI and their families.

In order to find sensitive measures of communication disturbances and how these impact upon everyday life, researchers have explored the interaction between language and context and the role of other facets of interpersonal behaviour in communication. For example, we have used both pragmatic and sociolinguistic theory to describe how everyday context influences language use in order to understand how and why people with TBI experience difficulties. We have also used recent advances in social cognition theory to consider what other kinds of judgements are important in social settings, and how these might be affected following TBI.

Disorders in language use

Descriptions of discourse problems following TBI such as lack of initiative, reliance on set expressions, over-talkativeness, tangentiality and inappropriateness indicate that people with TBI have problems adhering to implicit conversational conventions. For example, they fail to follow the maxims of quality (truthfulness), quantity (say what is sufficient), manner (orderliness) and relevance as outlined by Grice (1975). Two measures of everyday conversation based on these maxims are the Pragmatic Protocol (Prutting & Kirchner, 1987) and the Latrobe Communication Questionnaire (LCQ). The LCQ can be answered by self or a significant other and is a reliable and valid measure of communication impairment (Douglas, Bracy & Snow, 2007; Douglas, O'Flaherty & Snow, 2000), sensitive to discourse difficulties in both adults and adolescents with TBI (Douglas, 2010). Difficulties adhering to conversational rules are also evident when performing specific communicative tasks. When asked to explain how to play a game to a naive listener (McDonald & Pearce, 1995), adults with TBI typically fail to mention essential information (maxim of quantity), include irrelevant and therefore misleading information (maxim of relevance), repeat information and fail to sequence important steps in their correct chronological sequence (maxim of manner). Similar problems with the orderly transfer of information have been reported using different procedural tasks (Prince, Haynes & Haak, 2002; Snow, Douglas & Ponsford, 1999). Similarly, conversational topics have been reported as repetitive (Body & Parker, 2005) and narratives insufficient or inaccurate with respect to communicating essential content (Brookshire, Chapman, Song & Levin, 2000).

Adults with TBI also have difficulty using language flexibly and diplomatically to suit the social context (Milton & Wertz, 1986). For example, they may be unable to hint effectively, or address potential obstacles to compliance on the part of the addressee (McDonald & Pearce, 1998; McDonald & Van Sommers, 1993). They can also have great difficulty understanding the implied meaning when others choose to speak indirectly, as when being sarcastic or ironic (Channon, Pellijeff & Rule, 2005; McDonald & Flanagan, 2004; McDonald & Turkstra, 1998). These problems directly correspond to poor social skills. For example, people with TBI who fail to understand sarcasm, white lies and irony are also rated by independent observers as lacking appropriate humour, and being insensitive and egocentric when relating to another (McDonald, Flanagan, Martin & Saunders, 2004).

It is also possible to demonstrate that people with TBI have difficulties in the shared task of communication using a sociolinguistic system of analysis known as systemic functional linguistics (SFL) (Jorgensen & Togher, 2009; Kilov, Togher & Grant, 2009; Togher, Taylor, Aird & Grant, 2006). People with TBI have problems with particular aspects of discourse tasks such as in service encounters, where they have difficulty formulating the service request and ending the encounter (Togher, Hand & Code, 1997). There is also a tendency to confuse the discourse genre with abrupt shifts to casual conversation at inappropriate times (such as in the middle of a service encounter). Another example of a sensitive interactional task is a problem-solving task where two people (the person with TBI and a communication partner) are asked to work together to determine the function and name of an unknown object (Kilov et al., 2009). Using such a task it is possible to examine the capacity to develop hypotheses about the possible identity of the object, arguments to support this thesis, possible solutions to the task, challenges to the other person's suggestions and personal comments. People with TBI have responded well to completing this task with a familiar friend, but in some cases their memory difficulties result in an overreliance on describing the object rather than determining its possible name and function. Another novel approach to discourse elicitation is jointly produced or co-constructed narrative where the person with TBI and a friend retell a story to a third party, such as a friend (Jorgensen & Togher, 2009). This task was facilitatory for people with TBI, as it provided equal opportunity for the person with TBI and their conversational partner to contribute to the retelling.

Clinical implications

Conversational skills in people with TBI are amenable to remediation (Cramon & Cramon, 1992) using both treatment aimed narrowly at narrative production (Cannizzaro & Coelho, 2002; Peach & Wong, 2004) and more broadly at conversation and social skills (Dahlberg et al., 2007; McDonald et al., 2008). Social skills approaches are one of the most effective of all remediation approaches for adults with TBI (Carney et al., 1999). They typically occur in a group setting, using group problem-solving and practice, role plays, homework, feedback and positive reinforcement to shape more socially skilled behaviour. Two recent randomized controlled trials examined the effectiveness of a 12-week social skills programme with people with chronic moderate to severe TBI (Dahlberg et al., 2007; McDonald et al., 2008). The treatment programmes differed but used many of these common elements, and both demonstrated improvements.

As an alternative perspective, sociolinguistic approaches stress that there are always two parties in any conversation and that the behaviour of the conversational partner is critically important – facilitating, or diminishing, opportunities for the individual with brain injury to continue the conversation in a successful manner. Indeed, TBI individuals can be disadvantaged because of the way their communication partners interact with them. For example, in a study of telephone conversations where TBI participants requested information from a range of communication partners, they were asked for and were given less information than matched control participants (Togher et al., 1997). Therapists and mothers never asked people with TBI questions to which they did not already know the answer. Additionally, TBI participants were more frequently questioned regarding the accuracy of their contributions and contributions were followed up less often than matched control participants. Communication partners used patronising comments, flat voice tone and slowed speech production when talking to people with TBI. In contrast, controls were asked for unknown information, encouraged to elaborate, did not have their contributions checked frequently and had their contributions followed up.

This research has a number of clinical implications. Firstly, modifying the communicative environment might be expected to change the discourse behaviour of the person with TBI and we now have evidence for this. For example, when people with TBI were placed in an information-giving role, where they were a guest speaker talking about the experience of having a serious injury, their communication approximated matched control participants (who had a spinal injury) (Togher, 2000). People with TBI also had better levels of participation when placed in an environment with a trained mentor who provided prompts, modelling and structured activities, compared to pre-intervention and post-intervention baseline periods (Bellon & Rees, 2006). Similarly, in interactions between staff members and people with TBI, there was a trend towards increased compliance, attention and participation of the person with TBI when the staff member used more positive communication strategies (Shelton & Shryock, 2007). These results suggest that greater opportunities and increased conversational competence can be created for the person with TBI using a facilitative context.

Secondly, by adopting a broader perspective that regards communication as an interaction between at least two speakers, we can widen our scope of practice to include both the person with TBI *and* their communication partners. We have developed training packages for everyday communication partners (Togher & Grant, 2001) that use a combination of education about the structure of different conversations – e.g. service enquiries and casual conversations, as well as strategies of collaboration and elaboration (Ylvisaker, 1998). This kind of training has proven effective for police officers, enabling them to have more efficient, focused interactions with adults with TBI (Togher, McDonald, Code & Grant, 2004). We have also expanded this programme to provide a 10-week programme, 'TBI Express', of weekly individual and group training to adults with TBI and an everyday communication partner (ECP) to train strategies to maximize communicative effectiveness using behavioural approaches including role plays, conversational practice, cues to assist self-monitoring, positive reinforcement and home practice for the pair (Togher, McDonald, Tate, Power & Rietdijk, 2009). Most ECPs were wives and mothers, who had changed their communication styles following their husband's or son's injury, and which, in some cases, were detrimental to successful everyday interactions (see Case study 1 for an example). Sensitively targeting the behaviours of the ECP, such as their use of test questions and speaking on behalf of the person with TBI, led to a significant change in everyday interactions. The joint training group made significantly more improvement in conversational skills than training of the TBI person alone, or their carer alone (Togher, McDonald, Tate, Power & Rietdijk, 2010b).

Case study 1: Participant in the TBI Express treatment programme

BP is a 21-year-old male medical science student who sustained a severe TBI 18 months previously as the result of a sports accident. At the time of the treatment study he was living at home with his parents and two siblings and was unemployed. He experienced bilateral brain injuries in the accident, which was extremely severe (with a post-traumatic amnesia of 127 days). BP attended training with his mother, who was previously a schoolteacher but had given up work to care for her son. BP's pre-training assessment showed that he had poor communication with others and had become socially isolated, rarely seeing his friends. His mother did not trust him to organize his own activities, so he never went out on his own. He had difficulty reading social and emotional cues in conversation, word-finding difficulties and problems starting and maintaining conversations. His mother spoke for her son in conversation, and tended to ask him teacher-like questions to which she already knew the answer (e.g. 'What did we do today?') and to not give him enough time to have his turn in a conversation.

When asked about what his goals were for the training, he stated that he 'wanted to be normal again' and to share conversation 50:50, especially with his mum. He also wanted to be able to start conversations with his family and friends, to extend his conversations by developing new topics and to use less formal vocabulary and grammar. His mother's goals were to 'communicate with him as an adult child and to enjoy conversations again'. She specifically aimed to slow down, pause more, ask questions one at a time and wait for his response, to avoid correcting him, to preserve his dignity in group situations and support his communication. Other goals included providing information rather than testing questions, using a balance of questions and comments and supporting his organization of conversations by planning tasks together.

Cont. overleaf

Training involved a one-hour individual session and a two-and-a-half-hour group session each week for 10 weeks. At the completion of training, conversations of BP were rated as significantly improved by two independent speech pathologists using the Modified Kagan scales (Togher, McDonald, Tate, Power & Rietdijk, 2010a) and the Bond and Godfrey (1997) scales. The mother's skill in supporting BP's conversation was improved and his skill in communication and sharing the conversation had also improved. The interaction post-training was judged to be more appropriate, interesting and engaged and rewarding, although it was still effortful, and it was clear that the mother was concentrating on her contributions carefully.

Six months later, the interactions had continued to improve and were no longer judged to be effortful, showing habituation to the newly learned conversational behaviours. Improvement was best summed up by BP, who said after the training: 'I found it nothing but beneficial. Nothing negative has come out it. I've now regained myself, level of self-confidence. I've regained my social standing, I used to be scared to get involved in conversations but now I know how to get into conversations, I know how to get into them properly without being rude.'

Some of the general strategies for communication partners from this training included:

(a) Help maintain adult dignity for the person with TBI:
  – Use a natural sounding voice (not patronizing)
  – Choose adult and complex topics involving opinions
  – Acknowledge difficulties and frustrations – 'I know you know'
  – Avoid testing questions

(b) Aim for collaborative, shared conversation:
  – Help understanding by using short simple sentences
  – Use writing or other supports
  – Reduce distractions (e.g. noise, cluttered documents)

- Model good communication behaviours to family and friends
- Keep your sense of humour and make conversations enjoyable

Social perception

Competence in communication and social skills entails the ability to use not only language appropriately in context, but also a range of non-verbal social signals (Trower, 1980). We need to be sensitive to both non-verbal and verbal messages in order to modulate our behaviour to meet social goals and to respond to feedback from others. Non-verbal cues are also critical in order to understand the emotional and cognitive state of others engaged in the interaction. Several kinds of difficulties in social perception have now been empirically established in people with TBI, including problems recognizing emotions in others, problems understanding other people's perspectives (Theory of Mind) and difficulties with empathy.

Emotion

Clinicians working with people with severe TBI have long been aware that many such individuals lack sensitivity to emotions in others and there are now many studies demonstrating that a significant proportion of adults with severe TBI have difficulty identifying emotional expressions in others in static displays of facial expressions, dynamic visual portrayals, emotionally charged voices and audiovisual displays (Dimoska, McDonald, Pell, Tate & James, 2010; Green, Turner & Thompson, 2004; McDonald & Flanagan, 2004; Milders, Fuchs & Crawford, 2003).

Theory of Mind

The ability to make judgements concerning what another person is thinking or feeling is known as Theory of Mind (ToM) (Galski, Tompkins & Johnston, 1998). While ToM deficits were first recognized in respect to autism, such problems have also been identified in many people with TBI (Bibby & McDonald, 2004; Dennis, Purvis, Barnes, Wilkinson & Winner, 2001; Milders et al., 2003). Both emotion perception and ToM are critical in order to accurately understand everyday language, especially situations where language is indirect, such as when speaking sarcastically or diplomatically. For example, people with TBI who experience difficulties understanding second order ToM inferences (i.e. what one person wants another person to believe) are also those most likely to experience problems understanding the meaning of sarcastic exchanges (Channon et al., 2005; McDonald & Flanagan, 2004).

Empathy

Empathy is also critical for successful interpersonal relations as it provides an individual with the ability to understand and respond to the emotional experiences of others (Decety & Jackson, 2004). Individuals who have sustained a severe TBI can be egocentric, self-centred and insensitive to another person's needs (Elsass & Kinsella, 1987; Grattan & Eslinger, 1989). Over 60% of individuals with TBI self-report a loss of empathy (Williams & Wood, 2009). Further, many self-report blunting of emotional experience more generally post-injury (Croker & McDonald, 2005; Hornak, Rolls & Wade, 1996) and show reduced facial mimicry (McDonald et al., 2011) and skin conductance (de Sousa et al., 2010), especially when viewing angry facial expressions. The role of poor empathy in communication skills following TBI has never been examined empirically. However, it is obvious that failure to empathize will render social exchanges more difficult for the person with TBI to negotiate, as they are unable to respond appropriately to another person's emotional state.

Clinical implications

There has been relatively little work conducted to evaluate treatments for difficulties with social perception following TBI. The one area where research has commenced is in the area of emotion perception (Bornhofen & McDonald, 2008b), including randomized controlled trials to evaluate remediation techniques (Bornhofen & McDonald, 2008a, 2008c). These programmes typically spanned 12 weeks of bi-weekly sessions. Techniques included errorless learning (Wilson, Baddley, Evans & Shiel, 1994), i.e. repeated practice of identifying facial patterns where the participant is explicitly told not to guess if unsure. A second technique, self-instructional training (Meichenbaum & Cameron, 1973), involved verbalization of procedural steps by participants when engaged in complex tasks. We also employed: distributed and massed practice to facilitate learning; rehearsal via different modes including mirror practice, role play of facial, body and verbal cues, and games; positive reinforcement for effort and adherence to task structure (e.g. not guessing, in accordance with errorless learning principles); and cumulative review of material both during session and outside of session structured by the use of written outlines and explicitly scheduled for regular times at home. The outcome of both trials indicated that these techniques can be effective, even for people with very severe injuries as illustrated in Case study 2.

Case study 2: Participant in our Emotion Remediation programme

MP, a 22-year-old man with a severe traumatic brain injury, reported experiencing marked difficulty understanding others' feelings and intentions following his injury, which led him to be suspicious and distrusting of others, even members of his family. He said that friends and family regarded his manner as somewhat stiff and wooden compared to before his injury, when, he said, he had enjoyed an active social life with friends and family, often assuming the role of 'life of the party'. He reported diminished confidence in his ability to relate well with others, and in social situations he tended to become irritable and withdrawn.

After completing a 12-week bi-weekly treatment programme (see Clinical implications), MP reported a more positive picture of social functioning. He described greater ease and confidence in communicating with others, especially his family, and far fewer incidences of conflict or confusion due to misinterpretation of people's emotional state. He had begun socializing more frequently and others had noted that he seemed more comfortable, cheerier, and back to his 'old self'.

Conclusions

In conclusion, there is no doubt that communication disturbances are prevalent following severe traumatic brain injury, even though aphasia is relatively infrequent. Such communication disorders pervade every facet of the individual's life post-injury and represent a major obstacle, impeding successful negotiation of life with family, friends, partners, colleagues and the broader community. Using socially oriented theoretical frameworks, it is possible to elucidate problems, not only in the capacity of the individual with TBI to negotiate social interactions in an effective and persuasive manner, but also in terms of the manner in which others interact, which influences communication options available to the person with TBI. These approaches are an important advance because they address the ability to use language in context and all that this entails. In doing so, they reveal subtle but pervasive disorders of communication wherein basic language abilities remain intact but the ability to apply these sensitively and adaptively in everyday life is impaired.

In addition, consideration of language use as inseparable from its social function, makes it clear that cultural differences are critical when conceptualizing normal communication skills. Language use is intertwined with sociolinguistic variables such as level of education, socioeconomic status and cultural background. These facets influence how everyday language proceeds. Certainly, socially oriented theories of communication challenge the assumption that professionally trained therapists can judge the competence of their clients' communication skills solely on the basis of their own interactions in the clinic (Ylvisaker, 1998). Language use varies from one context to the next, from one cultural group to the next, from one age group to another. Finally, many people with TBI experience various deficits in social information processing. New advances in our understanding of social cognition and how this becomes disordered following TBI combined with sophisticated developments in characterising discourse and communication as detailed in this chapter provide us with exciting new directions for characterizing the communication difficulties seen following brain injury and how best these may be remediated.

References

Bellon, M.L. & Rees, R.J. (2006) The effect of context on communication: A study of the language and communication skills of adults with acquired brain injury. *Brain Injury, 20(10)*, 1069–1078.

Bibby, H. & McDonald, S. (2004) Theory of Mind after traumatic brain injury. *Neuropsychologia, 43*, 99–104.

Bigler, E.D. (2001) The lesion(s) in traumatic brain injury: Implications for clinical neuropsychology. *Archives of Clinical Neuropsychology, 16(2)*, 95–131.

Body, R. & Parker, M. (2005) Topic repetitiveness after traumatic brain injury: An emergent, jointly managed behaviour. *Clinical Linguistics and Phonetics, 19(5)*, 379–392.

Bond, F. & Godfrey, H.P.D. (1997) Conversation with traumatically brain-injured individuals: A controlled study of behavioural changes and their impact. *Brain Injury, 11*(5), 319–329.

Bornhofen, C. & McDonald, S. (2008a) Comparing strategies for treating emotion perception deficits in traumatic brain injury. *Journal of Head Trauma Rehabilitation, 23*, 103–115.

Bornhofen, C. & McDonald, S. (2008b) Emotion perception deficits following traumatic brain injury: A review of the evidence and rationale for intervention. *Journal of the International Neuropsychological Society, 15*, 511–525.

Bornhofen, C. & McDonald, S. (2008c) Treating emotion perception deficits following traumatic brain injury. *Neuropsychological Rehabilitation, 18*, 22–24.

Brooks, D.N. & McKinlay, W. (1983) Personality and behavioural change after severe blunt head injury – a relative's view. *Journal of Neurology, Neurosurgery and Psychiatry, 46(4)*, 336–344.

Brookshire, B.L., Chapman, S.B., Song, J. & Levin, H.S. (2000) Cognitive and linguistic correlates of children's discourse after closed head injury: A three-year follow-up. *Journal of the International Neuropsychological Society, 6(7)*, 741–751.

Cannizzaro, M.S. & Coelho, C.A. (2002) Treatment of story grammar following traumatic brain injury: A pilot study. *Brain Injury, 16(12)*, 1065–1073.

Carney, N., Chesnut, R., Maynard, H., Mann, N., Patterson, P. & Helfand, M. (1999) Effect of cognitive rehabilitation on outcomes for persons with traumatic brain injury: A systematic review. *Journal of Head Trauma Rehabilitation, 14(3)*, 277–307.

Channon, S., Pellijeff, A. & Rule, A. (2005) Social cognition after head injury: Sarcasm and theory of mind. *Brain and Language, 93*, 123–134.

Chapman, S.B., Culhane, K.A., Levine, H.S., Harward, H., Mendelsohn, D., Ewing-Cobbs, L. et al. (1992) Narrative discourse after closed head injury in children and adolescents. *Brain and Language, 43*, 42–65.

Cramon, D. & Cramon, G. M.-v. (1992) Reflections on the treatment of brain injured patients suffering from problem solving disorders. *Neuropsychological Rehabilitation, 2*, 207–230.

Croker, V. & McDonald, S. (2005) Recognition of emotion from facial expression following traumatic brain injury. *Brain Injury, 19*, 787–789.

Dahlberg, C.A., Cusick, C.P., Hawley, L.A., Newman, J.K., Morey, C.E., Harrison-Felix, C.L. et al. (2007) Treatment efficacy of social communication skills training after traumatic brain injury: A randomized treatment and deferred treatment controlled trial. *Archives of Physical Medicine and Rehabilitation, 88(12)*, 1561–1573.

de Sousa, A., McDonald, S., Rushby, J., Li, S., Dimoska, A. & James, C. (2010) Why don't you feel how I feel? Insight into the absence of empathy after severe Traumatic Brain Injury. *Neuropsychologia, 48*, 3585–3595.

Decety, J. & Jackson, P.L. (2004) The functional architecture of human empathy. *Behavioral and Cognitive Neuroscience Reviews, 3*, 71–100.

Dennis, M., Purvis, K., Barnes, M.A., Wilkinson, M. & Winner, E. (2001) Understanding of literal truth, ironic criticism, and deceptive praise following childhood head injury. *Brain and Language, 78*, 1–16.

Dimoska, A., McDonald, S., Pell, M.C., Tate, R.L. & James, C.M. (2010) Recognising vocal expressions of emotion following traumatic brain injury: Is the 'what' more important than the 'how'? *Journal of the International Neuropsychological Society, 16*, 369–382.

Douglas, J.M. (2010) Using the La Trobe Communication Questionnaire to measure perceived social communication ability in adolescents with traumatic brain injury. *Brain Impairment, 11(2)*, 171–182.

Douglas, J.M., Bracy, C.A. & Snow, P.C. (2007) Measuring perceived communicative ability after traumatic brain injury: Reliability and validity of the La Trobe Communication Questionnaire. *Journal of Head Trauma Rehabilitation, 22(1)*, 31–38.

Douglas, J.M., O'Flaherty, C.A. & Snow, P.C. (2000) Measuring perception of communicative ability: The development and evaluation of the La Trobe Communication Questionnaire. *Aphasiology, 14(3)*, 251–268.

Elsass, L. & Kinsella, G. (1987) Social interaction following severe closed head injury. *Psychological Medicine, 17(1)*, 67–78.

Galski, T., Tompkins, C. & Johnston, M.V. (1998) Competence in discourse as a measure of social integration and quality of life in persons with traumatic brain injury. *Brain Injury, 12(9)*, 769–782.

Gentry, L.R., Godersky, J.C. & Thompson, B. (1988) MR imaging of head trauma: Review of the distribution and radiopathologic features of traumatic lesions. *American Journal of Roentgenology, 150*, 663–672.

Gomez-Hernandez, R., Max, J.E., Kosier, T., Paradiso, S. & Robinson, R.G. (1997) Social impairment and depression after traumatic brain injury. *Archives of Physical Medicine Rehabilitation, 78*, 1321–1326.

Grattan, L.M. & Eslinger, P.J. (1989) Higher cognition and social behavior: Changes in cognitive flexibility and empathy after cerebral lesions. *Neuropsychology, 3(3)*, 175–185.

Green, R.E.A., Turner, G.R. & Thompson, W.F. (2004) Deficits in facial emotion perception in adults with recent traumatic brain injury. *Neuropsychologia, 42*, 133–141.

Grice, H.P. (1975) Logic and conversation. In P. Cole & J. Morgan (Eds) *Syntax and Semantics: Speech Acts*, vol. 3. New York: Academic Press.

Hagan, C. (1984) Language disorders in head trauma. In A. Holland (Ed.) *Language Disorders in Adults*. San Diego: College Hill Press.

Hartley, L.L. & Jensen, P.J. (1991) Narrative and procedural discourse after closed head injury. *Brain Injury, 5*, 267–285.

Hartley, L.L. & Jensen, P.J. (1992) Three discourse profiles of closed-head-injury speakers: Theoretical and clinical implications. *Brain Injury, 6*, 271–282.

Heilman, K.M., Safran, A. & Geschwind, N. (1971) Closed head trauma and aphasia. *Journal of Neurology, Neurosurgery and Psychiatry, 34*, 265–269.

Hornak, J., Rolls, E. & Wade, D. (1996) Face and voice expression identification in patients with emotional and behavioural changes following ventral frontal lobe damage. *Neuropsychologia, 34(4)*, 247–261.

Isake, E. & Turkstra, L. (2000) Communication abilities and work re-entry following traumatic brain injury. *Brain Injury, 14(5)*, 441–453.

Jorgensen, M. & Togher, L. (2009) Narrative after traumatic brain injury: A comparison of monologic and jointly-produced discourse. *Brain Injury, 23(9)*, 727–740.

Kilov, A.M., Togher, L. & Grant, S. (2009) Problem solving with friends: Discourse participation and performance of individuals with and without traumatic brain injury. *Aphasiology, 23(5)*, 584–605.

Kinsella, G., Moran, C., Ford, B. & Ponsford, J. (1988) Emotional disorder and its assessment within the severe head-injured population. *Psychological Medicine, 18*, 57–63.

Kinsella, G., Packer, S. & Olver, J. (1991) Maternal reporting of behaviour following very severe blunt head injury. *Journal of Neurology, Neurosurgery and Psychiatry, 54(5)*, 422–426.

Knight, R.G., Devereux, R. & Godfrey, H.P. (1998) Caring for a family member with a traumatic brain injury. *Brain Injury, 12(6)*, 467–481.

Levin, H.S., Grossman, R.G., Rose, J.E. & Teasdale, G. (1979) Long term neuropsychological outcome of closed head injury. *Journal of Neurosurgery, 50*, 412–422.

MAA (1998) *Training Needs of Attendant Carers*. Sydney: Motor Accident Authority.

McDonald, S. & Flanagan, S. (2004) Social perception deficits after traumatic brain injury: Interaction between emotion recognition, mentalizing ability, and social communication. *Neuropsychology, 18(3)*, 572–579.

McDonald, S., Flanagan, S., Martin, I. & Saunders, C. (2004) The ecological validity of TASIT: A test of social perception. *Neuropsychological Rehabilitation, 14*, 285–302.

McDonald, S., Li, S., de Sousa, A., Rushby, J., James, C. & Tate, R.L. (2011) Impaired mimicry response to angry faces following severe traumatic brain injury. *Journal of Clinical and Experimental Neuropsychology, 33*, 17–29.

McDonald, S. & Pearce, S. (1995) The 'dice' game: A new test of pragmatic language skills after closed-head injury. *Brain Injury, 9(3)*, 255–271.

McDonald, S. & Pearce, S. (1998) Requests that overcome listener reluctance: Impairment associated with executive dysfunction in brain injury. *Brain and Language, 61*, 88–104.

McDonald, S., Tate, R., Togher, L., Bornhofen, C., Long, E. & Gertler, P. (2008) Social skills treatment for people with severe, chronic acquired brain injuries: A multicenter trial. *Archives of Physical Medicine and Rehabilitation, 89*, 1648–1659.

McDonald, S. & Turkstra, L. (1998) Adolescents with traumatic brain injury: Issues in the assessment of pragmatic language. *Clinical Linguistics and Phonetics, 12*, 237–248.

McDonald, S. & Van Sommers, P. (1993) Pragmatic language skills after closed head injury: Ability to negotiate requests. *Cognitive Neuropsychology, 10(4)*, 297–315.

Meichenbaum, D. & Cameron, R. (1973. Training schizophrenics to talk to themselves: A means of developing attentional controls. *Behavior Therapy, 4(4)*, 515–534.

Milders, M., Fuchs, S. & Crawford, J.R. (2003) Neuropsychological impairments and changes in emotional and social behaviour following severe traumatic brain injury. *Journal of Clinical and Experimental Neuropsychology, 25(2)*, 157–172.

Milton, S.B. & Wertz, R.T. (1986) Management of persisting communication deficits in patients with traumatic brain injury. In B.P. Uzzell & Y. Gross (Eds) *Clinical Neuropsychology of Intervention*. Boston: Martinus Nijhoff Publishing.

Oddy, M., Humphrey, M. & Uttley, D. (1978) Stresses upon the relatives of head-injured patients. *British Journal of Psychiatry, 133*, 507–513.

Peach, R.K. & Wong, P.C. (2004) Integrating the message level into treatment for agrammatism using story retelling. *Aphasiology, 14*, 429–441.

Prigatano, G.P., Roueche, J.R. & Fordyce, D.J. (1986) *Neuropsychological Rehabilitation after Brain Injury*. Baltimore: Johns Hopkins University Press.

Prince, S., Haynes, W.O. & Haak, N.J. (2002) Occurrence of contingent queries and discourse errors in referential communication and conversational tasks: A study of college students with closed head injury. *Journal of Medical Speech Language Pathology, 10(1)*, 19–39.

Prutting, C.A. & Kirchner, D.M. (1987) A clinical appraisal of the pragmatic aspects of language. *Journal of Speech and Hearing Disorders, 52*, 105–119.

Sarno, M.T. & Levita, E. (1986) Characteristics of verbal impairment in closed head injured patients. *Archives of Physical Medicine Rehabilitation, 67*, 400–405.

Shelton, C. & Shryock, M. (2007) Effectiveness of communication/interaction strategies with patients who have neurological injuries in a rehabilitation setting. *Brain Injury, 21(12)*, 1259–1266.

Shorland, J. & Douglas, J.M. (2010) Understanding the role of communication in maintaining and forming friendships following traumatic brain injury. *Brain Injury, 24(4)*, 569–580.

Snow, P.C., Douglas, J.M. & Ponsford, J. (1997) Conversational assessment following traumatic brain injury: A comparison across two control groups. *Brain Injury, 11(6)*, 409–429.

Snow, P.C., Douglas, J.M. & Ponsford, J.L. (1999) Narrative discourse following severe traumatic brain injury: A longitudinal follow-up. *Aphasiology, 13(7)*, 529–551.

Tate, R.L., Broe, G.A., Cameron, I.D., Hodgkinson, A.E. & Soo, C.A. (2005) Pre-injury, injury and early post-injury predictors of long-term functional and psychosocial recovery after severe traumatic brain injury. *Brain Impairment, 6*, 75–89.

Tate, R.L., Fenelon, B., Manning, M. & Hunter, M. (1991) Patterns of neuropsychological impairment after severe blunt head injury. *Journal of Nervous and Mental Disease, 179(3)*, 117–126.

Tate, R.L., Lulham, J., Broe, T., Strettles, B. & Pfaff, A. (1989) Psychosocial outcome for the survivors of severe blunt head injury: The results from a consecutive series of 100 patients. *Journal of Neurology, Neurosurgery and Psychiatry, 52*, 1128–1134.

Tate, R.L., McDonald, S. & Lulham, J.M. (1998) Incidence of hospital-treated traumatic brain injury in an Australian community. *Australian and New Zealand Journal of Public Health, 22(4)*, 419–423.

Thomsen, I.V. (1975) Evaluation and outcome of aphasia in patients with severe closed head trauma. *Journal of Neurology, Neurosurgery and Psychiatry, 38*, 713–718.

Togher, L. (2000) Giving information: The importance of context on communicative opportunity for people with traumatic brain injury. *Aphasiology, 14(4)*, 365–390.

Togher, L. & Grant, S. (2001) *Communication Training Program for Carers*. Sydney: University of Sydney.

Togher, L., Hand, L. & Code, C. (1997) Analysing discourse in the traumatic brain injury population: Telephone interactions with different communication partners. *Brain Injury, 11(3)*, 169–189.

Togher, L., McDonald, S., Code, C. & Grant, S. (2004) Training communication partners of people with traumatic brain injury: A randomised controlled trial. *Aphasiology, 18(4)*, 313–335.

Togher, L., McDonald, S., Tate, R., Power, E. & Rietdijk, R. (2009) Training communication partners of people with traumatic brain injury: Reporting the protocol for a clinical trial. *Brain Impairment, 10(2)*, 188–204.

Togher, L., McDonald, S., Tate, R., Power, E. & Rietdijk, R. (2010a) Measuring the social interactions of people with traumatic brain injury and their communication partners: The adapted Kagan scales. *Aphasiology, 24(6–8)*, 914–927.

Togher, L., McDonald, S., Tate, R., Power, E. & Rietdijk, R. (2010b) Training communication partners of people with traumatic brain injury (TBI) improves casual conversational interactions. *Brain Injury, 24(3)*, 269–270.

Togher, L., Taylor, C., Aird, V. & Grant, S. (2006) The impact of varied speaker role and communication partner on the communicative interactions of a person with traumatic brain injury: A single case study using systemic functional linguistics. *Brain Impairment,* *7(3)*, 190–201.

Trower, P. (1980) Situational analysis of the components and processes of behaviour of socially skilled and unskilled patients. *Journal of Consulting and Clinical Psychology, 3,* 327–339.

Wallace, C.A., Bogner, J., Corrigan, J.D., Clinchot, D., Mysiw, W.J. & Fugante, L. (1998) Primary caregivers of persons with brain injury: Life change 1 year after injury. *Brain Injury, 12,* 483–493.

Williams, C. & Wood, R.L. (2009) Alexithymia and emotional empathy following traumatic brain injury. *Journal of Clinical and Experimental Neuropsychology, 22,* 1–11.

Wilson, B.A., Baddley, A.D., Evans, J.J. & Shiel, A. (1994) Errorless learning in the rehabilitation of memory impaired people. *Neuropsychological Rehabilitation, 4,* 307–326.

Ylvisaker, M. (1998) *Traumatic Brain Injury Rehabilitation: Children and Adolescents.* Boston, MA: Butterworth-Heinemann.

14 Voice Impairment

Jennifer Oates
La Trobe University, Australia

Introduction

The human voice is a powerful communication tool. The voice provides the major source of sound for speech and singing via vibration of the vocal folds in the larynx and the resonant functions of the vocal tract. As well as its critical role as the carrier of speech, the human voice plays other key roles in life (Aronson & Bless, 2009; Colton, Casper & Leonard, 2006; Mathieson, 2001). Variations in the pitch, loudness, quality and resonance of our voices allow us to express emotion, to command attention, to persuade or dissuade, to attract or repel other people, to influence the emotional state of others and to communicate the subtleties of meaning and intention. In addition, a great deal of information about a person is conveyed by the characteristics of their voice: their sex, age, personality, attitudes, and physical and psychological health. Although less well understood, the voice is also thought to function as an important outlet for intense emotions, thus contributing to maintaining emotional equilibrium (Aronson & Bless, 2009; Colton et al., 2006). Further, now that a large proportion of the workforce in western countries are in job roles where their voices are their 'primary tool of trade' (Titze, Lemke & Montequin, 1997, p.254), an effective and reliable voice has become one of the keys to economic and vocational success. It comes as no surprise, then, that impairment of vocal functioning may have a profound impact at both the individual and societal level.

Vocal impairments are associated with a wide range of symptoms and signs (Aronson & Bless, 2009; Colton et al., 2006; Oates, 2004). Symptoms reported by people with vocal impairments include throat discomfort and pain, vocal fatigue, increased vocal effort, and changes in voice quality, pitch, loudness, resonance and/or vocal projection. Similarly, observable signs of vocal impairment include abnormal voice quality, pitch, loudness, resonance and/or impaired control of the aerodynamics of voice production. Signs of vocal impairment are also observable in the acoustic features of the vocal signal, in the structural anatomy of the larynx and supraglottic vocal tract, and in the physiological characteristics of vocal aerodynamics, vocal fold vibration and vocal tract constriction.

The distinction between normal and impaired voice is not straightforward. The most frequently cited definitions of vocal impairment state that a voice is abnormal whenever any of the structures of voice production and/or the auditory-perceptual, physiological and acoustic characteristics of the voice differ from those of people of the same age and sex. However, there is wide inter-individual variation in every one of these aspects of voice and there are no absolute criteria for so-called normality (Aronson & Bless, 2009). Further, a wide range of voice characteristics are accepted in society as within normal limits; cultural, ethnic and social factors are associated with a wide range of accepted vocal variations and vocal impairment does not inevitably result in disability (Aronson & Bless, 2009). For these reasons, most definitions of voice disorder also incorporate considerations of whether the individual's voice meets their social and occupational needs, whether their voice draws attention to itself because it differs from that of others in the individual's cultural and social environments, and whether the individual believes that their voice is disordered.

There is no universally accepted classification system for voice disorders, but most systems are aetiologically based. Aetiologically based systems classify voice disorders broadly as 'functional' or 'organic'. It is acknowledged, however, that the aetiology of some disorders is unknown, equivocal or is multifactorial (Baker, Ben-Tovim, Butcher, Esterman & McLaughlin, 2007). Functional disorders are those whose fundamental cause is behavioural and/ or psychosocial. There may or may not be concomitant mucosal change on the vocal folds. Common examples include muscle tension dysphonia, vocal nodules, psychogenic aphonia and dysphonia, and mutational falsetto. In contrast, organic voice disorders are those whose fundamental cause is an underlying disease process. This category includes disorders of neurological origin such as vocal fold palsy and spasmodic dysphonia, inflammatory conditions such as specific laryngitis, benign neoplasms such as papilloma, trauma-induced disorders such as laryngeal dislocation, and endocrine and auto-immune conditions such as amyloidosis and hyperthyroidism.

The prevalence of voice disorders in the general adult population has been under-researched, but two recent and well-designed epidemiological studies have provided an indication of likely prevalence rates. Roy et al. (2004) determined that, of 1288 non-teachers from Iowa and Utah, 6.2 % reported having a current voice disorder and 28.8% reported experiencing a voice disorder during their lifetime. Russell, Oates and Greenwood (2005) determined that, of 2210 adults from the general population of South Australia, 3.1% reported having a voice disorder on the day of the survey, 4% reported having experienced a voice problem in the last 12 months and 6.8% reported experiencing a voice disorder during their adult life. The results of both studies confirmed that women were more likely to experience voice disorders than were men.

There is also a considerable body of research on the prevalence of voice disorders in occupational groups considered to be at high risk for voice disorders. Most of this research has focused on schoolteachers and all studies have demonstrated that teachers are at greater risk than non-teachers. Roy et al. (2004) and Russell, Oates and Greenwood (1998), for example, examined the rates of self-reported voice disorders among teachers in Iowa and Utah, and South Australia respectively. Roy et al. determined that, of 1243 teachers, 11% reported having a current voice disorder and 57.7% reported experiencing a voice disorder during their lifetime. Russell et al. established that, of 1168 teachers, 16% reported having a voice disorder on the day of the survey, 20% reported having experienced a voice problem in the last 12 months and 19% reported experiencing a voice disorder during their adult life. Again, both studies demonstrated that women were at greater risk than were men.

These prevalence rates for voice disorders in both the general population and among teachers indicate that large numbers of adults experience voice disorders. The following section provides a review of the evidence as to whether these voice problems also have significant negative impacts on individuals and society more generally.

Evidence for the impact of voice impairment in adulthood

Virtually every textbook on voice disorders claims that voice impairments can have significant negative impacts on the person experiencing the impairment as well as on their families, associates and employers (see, for example, Aronson & Bless, 2009; Colton et al., 2006; Mathieson, 2001). Domains of life that may be affected are reported to include employment, leisure activities, interpersonal relationships, activities of daily living and emotional wellbeing. Overall quality of life is also said to be compromised in people with voice impairments. These claims are based on anecdotal clinical evidence, logical extrapolation from our understanding of the role of voice in communication and other aspects of life, and some research evidence. Several authors caution, however, that the impact of voice disorders is not necessarily proportional to the severity of the vocal impairment and that it may vary considerably from person to person (see, for example, Mathieson, 2001). The relationship between the severity of the impairment and its impact is said to be moderated by factors such as the individual's level of dependence on an effective voice for employment or social activities, their age and gender, their level of vocal awareness and on cultural factors. Further, it is not unusual for adults with vocal impairments to list numerous vocal symptoms but at the same time to state unequivocally that they do not have a voice disorder, perhaps implying that their impairment does not have a major impact on their lives. This phenomenon has been demonstrated particularly in studies examining the prevalence of voice problems in occupational voice users (e.g. Russell et al., 1998).

The impact of voice disorders at the societal level is rarely mentioned in the general voice literature. A small number of journal papers and chapters in general speech-language pathology texts suggests that impacts at this level may include economic costs resulting from lost productivity and healthcare interventions, public safety risks due to ineffective communication, loss of qualified and experienced professionals from the workforce, and negative educational effects on students due to the reduced vocal capabilities of their teachers (Oates, 2004; Roy et al., 2004; Titze et al., 1997; Smith, Gray, Dove, Kirchner & Heras, 1997).

Current research evidence

Impact of vocal impairment at the individual level

Prior to the late 1990s, which saw the development of psychometrically evaluated self-report tools for measuring vocal impairment, the impact of impairment on the individual's participation in various life domains and emotional wellbeing, reports of systematic research on the impact of voice disorders were scarce. Most of the earlier studies used questionnaires designed by the researchers (see, for example, Sapir, 1993; Sapir, Mathers-Schmidt & Larson, 1996; Scott, Robinson, Wilson & MacKenzie, 1997; Smith, Taylor, Mendoza, Barkmeier, Lemke & Hoffman, 1998; Smith, Taylor, Mendoza, Lemke & Hoffman, 1998; Smith et al., 1996), or scales not specific to the impact of *voice* impairment, such as standardized scales for evaluation of general or health-related quality of life (see for example, Liu et al., 1998) and/or standardized and non-standardized measures of psychosocial factors such as depression, anxiety, stress, self-esteem and somatic complaints (see, for example, Deary, Scott, Wilson, White, MacKenzie & Wilson, 1997; Goldman, Hargrave, Hillman, Holmberg & Gress, 1996; Liu et al., 1998; Murry, Cannito & Woodson, 1994). None of these early studies used qualitative research methods such as in-depth interviews, although Scott et al. (1997) used an open-ended questionnaire asking participants to list any 'difficulties' they had experienced because of their voice problems. The participant groups in these studies included adults with a range of different voice conditions, specific occupational groups such as singers and students of singing, and adults with specific conditions such as spasmodic dysphonia and vocal nodules.

The findings of these early studies support the contention that adults with voice disorders experience a wide range of activity and participation restrictions as well as reduced psychosocial wellbeing. Frequently reported examples include reduced communicative effectiveness, reduced participation in vocational and social activities requiring voice use, and elevated anxiety, depression, somatisation and stress. In particular, Scott et al. (1997) reported that activity limitations as a result of voice impairment (e.g. inability to project over noise) were more frequently listed by participants than were participation restrictions (e.g. reduced ability to perform job requirements). However, the level and strength of the evidence provided through this body of research is mixed. Although sample sizes in most of these studies were large enough to provide adequate statistical power, and although most studies incorporated control groups, some investigated only people with voice disorders, some used very small sample sizes, most used convenience or ad hoc methods for participant sampling and most used non-standardized study-specific questionnaires. While a small number of studies compared activity and participation restrictions before and after intervention, most studied participants at only one point in time. It is therefore difficult to determine, for example, whether the common pattern of reduced psychosocial wellbeing is a consequence of the voice disorder, a coincidental finding unrelated to vocal impairment, or a pre-existing or even causal factor. Further, the number of studies at that time was very small and there were not enough of them to allow robust conclusions about the impact of specific types of voice disorders or the impacts on specific groups of occupational voice users.

From the late 1990s to the present time, the field of speech-language pathology has seen considerable activity in the development of self-report instruments for measuring communicative impairment and the effects of that impairment on the individual's participation in life roles and on emotional wellbeing. This research activity was no doubt induced, at least in part, by the advent of the World Health Organization's *International Classification of Functioning, Disability and Health* – ICF (WHO, 2001) which has been associated with a paradigm shift in healthcare generally from a focus mainly on impairment to a broader conceptualization of health. This paradigm shift appears to have had a particularly strong effect in the field of voice disorders, where a substantial number of self-report instruments have been developed and evaluated.

The major self-report instruments that have been subject to at least some psychometric evaluation and which claim to measure the impact of voice disorders in adults are, in order of their development, the Voice Handicap Index (VHI; Jacobson et al., 1997), the Voice-Related Quality of Life (V-RQOL; Hogikyan & Sethuraman, 1998), the Voice Activity and Participation Profile (VAPP; Ma & Yiu, 2001); and the Voice Symptoms Scale (VoiSS; Deary, Wilson, Carding & MacKenzie, 2003). A short form of the VHI, the VHI-10, has also been developed (Rosen, Lee, Osborne, Zullo & Murry, 2004). In addition, several instruments for specific populations are available. These include the Voice Outcome Survey (VOS; Gliklich, Glovsky & Montgomery, 1999), designed specifically for individuals with vocal fold paralysis and the Singing Voice Handicap Index (SVHI; Cohen et al., 2007). A description of each of these instruments is beyond the scope of this chapter, as is a review of the increasing number of translated and validated versions for people from non-English-speaking backgrounds, but readers are referred to recent reviews of these scales for further details (see, for example, Franic, Bramlett & Cordes Bothe, 2005; Zraick & Risner, 2008). In general, all of these instruments require the individual to rate, on Likert-type or visual analogue scales, the frequency or extent to which they experience particular voice impairments, activity and participation restrictions, and psychosocial problems associated with their voices. It is clear that these instruments have become standard tools for both diagnosis and assessment of treatment outcomes in clinical practice as well as research (Behrman, 2005; Zraick & Risner, 2008).

The self-report instruments listed above have been used in a large number of studies, most of which are focused on the psychometric characteristics of the tools, comparisons between instruments in terms of structure, content, validity and responsiveness, relationships between specific voice instruments and generic quality of life measures, and/or evaluation of the outcomes of interventions for voice disorders. In addition, there is a considerable body of research using these instruments with a primary purpose of delineating the impact of voice impairments or investigating relationships between the impact of voice impairments and factors such as the type of voice disorder, occupation, gender and age.

A smaller number of studies have used what are often labelled as generic health-related quality of life measures to investigate the impact of voice impairment. The most commonly used instrument is the Medical Outcomes Trust 36-Item Short Form Health Survey (SF-36) (Ware & Sherbourne, 1992). The SF-36 is a self-report questionnaire evaluating eight domains of physical and emotional health, social functioning and general health. Some items ask the individual to rate their health status, while others ask about the extent to which different health problems limit their work, social and physical activities.

Finally, a small number of studies have used psychometrically validated psychosocial measures such as the Centre for Epidemiological Studies-Depression Scale (CES-D; Radloff, 1977), the Hospital Anxiety Depression Scales (Zigmond & Snaith, 1983), the Perceived Stress Scale (Cohen & Williamson, 1988), the State-Trait Anxiety Inventory (STAI; Spielberger, Gorusch, Lushene, Vagg & Jacobs, 1983), the Self-rating of Depression Scale (SDS; Zung, 1967) and the Symptom Checklist (SCL-90; Derogatis, Lipman & Covi, 1973) to evaluate the specific psychosocial impacts of voice impairment.

Despite an explosion of research on the impact of voice disorders since the late 1990s, it remains difficult to reach clear conclusions about the impact of voice disorders at the individual level. The findings from this large body of research are little different from those of studies conducted prior to the advent of standardized voice specific self-report instruments. Again, the most consistent conclusion to date is that voice impairment is frequently associated with a range of moderate activity and participation restrictions across the domains of physical, vocational and social functioning as well as moderately compromised general health, mental health and psychosocial wellbeing (see, for example, Benninger, Ahuja, Gardner & Grywalski, 1998; Cohen, 2010; Rasch, Günther, Hoppe, Eysholdt & Rosanowski, 2005; Wilson, Deary, Millar & MacKenzie, 2002). Beyond this broad conclusion, inconsistent results are the norm and the available data on the specific impacts of voice impairment remain incomplete. It is therefore important to consider the reasons for this apparent lack of progress over the past decade or so. There are multiple reasons, only some of which can be addressed in any depth in this chapter.

The lack of clear evidence around the impact of voice impairment stems from a range of methodological limitations of past research, such as inadequate matching of participants with voice impairments with control participants, ad hoc or biased rather than systematic participant selection processes, failure to report basic participant characteristics such as duration, severity and type of voice impairment, and insufficient statistical power to detect differences between groups. Other limitations include the uneven attention to some types of voice disorders (e.g. muscle tension dysphonia, conversion dysphonia and aphonia, organic pathologies such as papilloma and vocal fold scar have received little research attention) and some categories of voice user (e.g. elderly people, call centre workers, singers and actors are rarely investigated) as well as investigation of heterogeneous groups of participants with widely varying types of voice disorders. More important, however, are the relative lack of sophistication in research approaches used to examine the impacts of voice impairment and the limitations in the self-report instruments used to measure activity and participation restrictions associated with voice impairment. Each of these two deficiencies of the current literature is outlined in further detail below.

Lack of sophistication in research approaches used to examine the impact of voice impairment

While it is clear that many individuals with voice disorders experience negative impacts as a result of their impairments, the current literature does not provide in-depth specification of those impacts. In addition to the limitations of the self-report instruments themselves as outlined below, a likely key reason for our limited understanding of potential impacts of voice impairment on activity and participation and psychosocial wellbeing is the dominance of one relatively unsophisticated research design and a dearth of in-depth qualitative research.

The dominant research design in this field is cross-sectional, descriptive and observational, mostly using only univariate approaches to data analysis. This research approach limits the extent to which the influence of a multitude of factors on the impact of voice disorders can be elucidated. Current research evidence suggests that many factors influence the way in which voice impairment impacts on the individual, but this evidence is full of contradictory findings and there has been almost no consideration of the interactions between these influencing factors or their relative importance in predicting the type and degree of negative impact. Some authors, for example, conclude that there are no differences in the negative impacts of voice disorders between men and women (see, for example, Bouwers & Dikkers, 2007; Hummel, Scharf,

Schuetzenberger, Graessel & Rosanowski, 2010). In contrast, other researchers have reported that women experience greater negative impacts as a result of voice disorders than do men (see, for example, Behlau, Hogikyan & Gasparini, 2007; Rasch et al., 2005). Potential factors requiring investigation through more sophisticated research approaches include type of voice disorder, self-perceived severity of voice impairment, expert-rated or instrumentally measured impairment, duration of voice impairment, occupational and social vocal demands, talkativeness, personality and other psychosocial factors, general health and co-existing chronic illness, and socio-demographic factors such as age, gender, socioeconomic status, cultural background and education level (Behlau et al., 2007; Benninger et al., 1998; Bouwers & Dikkers, 2007; Dietrich, Verdolini Abbott, Gartner-Schmidt & Rosen, 2006; Hummel et al., 2010; Spina, Maunsell, Sandalo, Gusmão & Crespo, 2009; Rasch et al., 2005; Yiu et al., 2011).

The dominance of cross-sectional descriptive research using univariate data analysis methods also limits the extent to which it is possible to tease out the consequences of voice impairment from pre-existing causal and contributing factors of the voice impairment or from coincidental activity and participation restrictions and compromised psychosocial wellbeing that may have nothing to do with voice impairment. This limitation is particularly important in the psychosocial domain, because there is reasonable evidence that poor psychosocial wellbeing and deficits in the processing of emotion are likely to contribute to the development of functional voice impairments (Baker, 2008, 2010; Baker & Lane, 2009). Cross-sectional descriptive research cannot determine whether compromised psychological wellbeing is the result of the voice impairment or its cause.

The dearth of qualitative research is another key limitation of the current literature on the impact of voice impairment. This may explain the very limited detail in the current literature on the specific impacts of voice impairment. Most studies in this area have used standardized self-report instruments such as the VHI (Jacobson et al., 1997) and the V-RQOL (Hogikyan & Sethuraman, 1998) to investigate activity and participation limitations. It is obvious that the impacts revealed through such studies will be limited to those listed on the instrument. As discussed below, the range of impacts included on these instruments is typically narrow and may not capture the possible types of impacts for every individual (Branski et al., 2010). Baylor, Yorkston and Eadie (2005) conducted one of the very few qualitative studies in this area. These researchers investigated the 'biopsychosocial consequences' of spasmodic dysphonia through in-depth interviews with six adults. Data collection and analysis was conducted within a phenomenological framework. These authors concluded that the impact of voice impairment is complex and highly individual, with multiple personal, social and impairment-related factors contributing to patterns of activity and participation restriction and psychosocial wellbeing. This conclusion, however, requires evaluation through further research; the credibility and dependability of the findings would be enhanced through purposive or theoretical sampling and by increasing the sample size so that saturation in the data is achieved. Another important outcome of this study was the development of a model of the consequences of living with spasmodic dysphonia. Although many previous studies have been conducted with the broad framework of the ICF (WHO, 2001), almost no other research on the impacts of voice impairment has been conducted within the framework of a specific model of the type developed by Baylor et al. (2005) and this constitutes yet another limitation of the current literature in this field.

Limitations of the self-report instruments used to measure the impact of voice impairment

Virtually all of the available self-report instruments designed to delineate the impact of voice impairment have been subject to psychometric evaluation and some of the findings of these evaluations have been positive (see, for example, Branski et al., 2010; Franic et al., 2005; Hogikyan & Sethuraman, 1998; Jacobson et al., 1997; Rosen, Murry, Zinn, Zullo & Sonbolian, 2000; Roy, Merrill, Gray & Smith, 2005; Steen et al., 2007; Zraick & Risner, 2008). This is the case for each of the generic tools specified above (i.e. V-RQOL, VHI, VHI-10, VAPP, VoiSS) and for one scale that is specific to vocal fold palsy (i.e. VOS). However, all current self-report instruments used to measure the impact of voice impairment in adults are associated with several shortcomings related to scale development processes, psychometric characteristics, and the adequacy with which they assess the breadth of domains of functioning that could be negatively affected by voice impairment (Behlau et al., 2007; Branski et al., 2010; Franic et al., 2005; Wilson et al., 2004). Branski et al. (2010) and Franic et al. (2005) have provided detailed evaluations of both scale development and psychometric properties, with the former constituting the only published systematic review of the development phase for self-report instruments that evaluate the impact of voice impairment. These reviews have demonstrated that shortcomings in relation to scale development include failure to draw on data from sufficient open-ended patient interviews to develop questionnaire items, inadequate coverage of the range of possible impacts of voice impairment, inadequate piloting of the questionnaires with patients and clinicians, failure to field-test revisions of the questionnaires based on statistical analyses of pilot data, failure to provide normative data with corresponding standardized scoring protocols, and failure to apply item reduction processes such as factor analysis and assessment for item redundancy. Shortcomings related to the psychometric properties of the scales include lack of statistical support for the purported factor structure of the instrument, failure to comprehensively evaluate validity (i.e. content and construct validity), and failure to demonstrate the responsiveness of the instrument to change, as well as the precision of the instrument for making clinical decisions.

Additional limitations of current self-report instruments from the perspective of this author include a lack of rigorous qualitative research to develop items on existing scales, inconsistent and incomplete application of the ICF model (WHO, 2001) in scale development, and some misleading use of terminology in the titles of the instruments. The lack of qualitative research in scale development is likely to have contributed to a narrow representation of possible impacts of voice impairment within existing scales. Although the ICF model has been used as the general framework for most of these instruments, it has not been applied consistently. For example, while the titles of some scales imply that they are designed to measure activity and participation or handicap, items concerned with voice impairment are also included and some scales barely touch on the participation domain. The use of the term 'quality of life', even when qualified as 'voice-related' is also potentially misleading. All of these instruments certainly measure factors that are likely to *contribute to* the individual's quality of life, but none directly assesses the perceived impact of voice impairments on the individual's general life satisfaction and wellbeing. The latter would be required to meet most of the currently accepted conceptualizations of quality of life (Bullinger, Anderson, Cella & Aaronson, 1993).

Impact of vocal impairment at the societal level

The impact of voice disorders at the societal level has received very little research attention, so it is not feasible to provide critical analysis of a body of research in this chapter. A small number of studies have documented the number of days lost to work associated with voice disorders in schoolteachers (e.g. Pemberton, Oates & Russell, 2010; Russell et al., 1998; Smith, Lemke, Taylor, Kirchner & Hoffman, 1998; Van Houtte, Claeys, Wuyts & Van Lierde, in press), as well as the proportion of adults with voice impairments who have consulted healthcare providers (e.g. Russell et al., 1998; Smith et al., 1998a). On the basis of these data, various estimates of the financial costs of voice disorders have been extrapolated. Verdolini and Ramig (2001), for example, estimated that the societal cost of voice disorders was approximately $US2.5 billion each year. Similarly, Pemberton et al. (in press) estimated that the cost of employing replacement teachers throughout Australia to cover absence for voice injury was over $AUS176 million annually. Morton and Watson (2001) also provide evidence of the potential societal impacts of voice disorders from the perspective of children's learning. Their study examined the effects of voice quality on the ability of upper primary school-aged children to process spoken language and on their learning in the classroom. Their qualitative and quantitative data indicated that dysphonia in teachers is likely to negatively affect children's language processing, their motivation and their attitudes towards teachers. These impacts of voice impairment may therefore negatively affect educational achievement in children.

Directions for future research

Although there is a substantial body of research addressing the impacts of voice impairment, much remains to be investigated through higher-quality systematic research. Research conducted over the past 10 to 15 years has provided evidence that individuals with voice impairments experience activity and participation restrictions and compromised psychosocial wellbeing, but beyond this general conclusion it is not yet possible to reach clear conclusions as to the specific types of negative impacts that may be experienced by people with voice disorders and the factors that influence the way in which voice impairment impacts on the individual and their family members, colleagues and employers. Even less is understood about the impacts of voice impairment at the societal level, mainly because virtually no systematic investigations at this level have been conducted.

Apart from the need for an increase in research activity concerned with the broader societal impacts of voice impairment, many shortcomings of previous research at the individual level warrant attention in future research. Only when those limitations are addressed will clinicians be able to accurately and comprehensively identify the potential impacts of voice impairment on their clients, to use that evidence to guide their intervention planning and to evaluate the effectiveness of their interventions.

Future researchers will ideally place their research more explicitly and consistently within modern conceptual frameworks of health and disability (Eadie et al., 2006; Worrall & Hickson, 2008). They will recognize that the impact of voice impairment is highly individual and more complex than previously thought, with many personal, environmental and impairment-related factors interacting to influence patterns of activity and participation in life roles and psychosocial wellbeing (Baylor et al., 2005; Baylor, Yorkston, Eadie, Miller & Amtmann, 2009). Rigorous qualitative research will be conducted, preferably taken to higher levels of theory development with approaches such as grounded theory. More sophisticated quantitative research will also be undertaken with prospective, longitudinal designs, intervention studies and multivariate approaches becoming more common. Future research will also investigate larger, more representative and properly matched groups of participants with and without voice impairments and focus on a wider range of voice disorders and categories of voice user. At an even more fundamental level, the development of self-report instruments to measure the impacts of voice impairments will be revisited by applying standard principles of scale development and psychometric evaluation (Branski et al., 2010; Franic et al., 2005). In-depth interviews with patients covering a wide range of life roles and communicative contexts will guide the development of item banks for new instruments. Those instruments will be developed using more contemporary psychometric models such as Item Response Theory (Baylor et al., 2009; Branski et al., 2010; Deary, Wilson, Carding, MacKenzie & Watson, 2010; Walshe, Peach & Miller, 2009). Finally, the content and construct validity of new instruments will be comprehensively evaluated.

Clinical implications

Because there is now a substantial body of evidence demonstrating that voice impairments are associated with negative impacts on activity and participation in life roles as well as on psychosocial wellbeing, it is clear that diagnostic processes, intervention planning and evaluations of the effectiveness of intervention must be guided by the clinician's and patient's understanding of those impacts. This imperative is in accord with contemporary conceptualizations of health and disability and with increasing acknowledgement that the patient's perspectives and insights into their own health condition and its consequences for their quality of life are critical to successful treatment (Hilari, Wiggins, Roy, Byng & Smith, 2003). As this review of the evidence has demonstrated, however, the available evidence on the impacts of voice impairment is incomplete and none of the currently available instruments designed to measure the consequences of vocal impairment is ideal for clinical application. Although previous reviews have reached some conclusions as to the relative merits of the available self-report instruments for measuring the impacts of voice impairment (see, for example, Branski et al., 2010; Eadie et al., 2006; Franic et al., 2005; Zraick & Risner, 2008), no particular instrument is consistently evaluated as superior and all have been shown to have limitations. Zraick and Risner (2008), in fact, conclude that 'the choice of which instrument to administer is largely based on clinician's preference' (p.188).

The lack of an ideal self-report tool does not mean that instruments such as the VHI, VHI-10, V-RQOL, VoiSS, VAPP, VOS and their cultural adaptations have no place in clinical practice. On the contrary, because these specific instruments have been shown to meet at least some of the standard criteria for scale development, because they all have some good psychometric properties and because they do not place an unreasonable burden on patients, they can play an important role, particularly in assisting clinicians to monitor overall change during intervention and to evaluate the outcomes of service delivery.

It remains clear, however, that the available self-report instruments are limited in the extent to which they can elucidate the impacts of voice impairment in sufficient depth or breadth for diagnosis and intervention planning for individual patients. While we await the development of improved self-report instruments, clinicians are also advised to undertake semi-structured in-depth interviews with each patient to explore the individual and complex impacts of their voice impairment. The interview could be structured around the ICF framework (WHO, 2001) and explore the patient's perceptions of the impact of their voice impairment on relevant dimensions of activities and participation listed within the ICF (e.g. general tasks and demands, communication, interpersonal interactions and relationships, etc.) as well as on their psychosocial wellbeing and overall life satisfaction. The interview could also explore the environmental factors listed within the ICF, such as the availability of social support from family, friends and work colleagues, attitudes of employers and colleagues, the physical characteristics of the voice use environment, and occupational health and safety policies of the workplace. Together with traditional measures of vocal impairment and data from one or more of the self-report instruments discussed earlier, data derived from the patient interview will provide the clinician with a rich data source on which to base intervention planning.

Conclusions

Since the late 1990s, there has been a strong research focus in the field of voice on the development of self-report instruments to evaluate the impacts of voice impairment on patients in terms of their activity and participation in all domains of life and on their psychosocial functioning. These instruments, including the VHI, VHI-10, V-RQOL, VoiSS, VAPP and the VOS, have rapidly become standard tools in clinical practice for both diagnosis and evaluation of treatment outcomes. These instruments have also been used extensively for research that aims to delineate the impacts of voice impairments on individuals, to evaluate the effectiveness of interventions for voice impairment, and to determine factors that influence the degree and type of impact that voice impairments have on individual patients.

While this large body of research has demonstrated that voice disorders are associated with moderately severe negative consequences for affected individuals' capacity to maintain their activity and participation in life roles and for their psychosocial wellbeing, progress over the past decade and a half has not been commensurate with the amount of research activity. There remains a great deal more to be learned about the precise nature of individual responses to voice impairment and the demographic, sociocultural, occupational, impairment-related and psychosocial factors that interact to produce the complex and highly individual patterns of activity and participation restriction and compromised emotional health that are often associated with voice disorders. In the meantime, clinicians should take heed of recent critical reviews of available self-report tools to select their preferred instrument(s) to guide both intervention planning and the evaluation of treatment outcomes. Clinicians should also consider using their knowledge of contemporary models of health and disability to explore, in depth, their patients' perceptions of the impacts of voice impairment on their lives. The insights derived from such interviews will provide clinicians with invaluable data on which to base their treatment planning.

References

Aronson, A.E. & Bless, D.M. (2009) *Clinical Voice Disorders*, 4th edition. New York: Thieme Medical Publishers, Inc.

Baker, J. (2008) The role of psychogenic and psychosocial factors in the development of functional voice disorders. *International Journal of Speech-Language Pathology, 10*, 210–230.

Baker, J. (2010) Women's voices: Lost or mislaid, stolen or strayed? *International Journal of Speech-Language Pathology, 12*, 94–106.

Baker, J., Ben-Tovim, D.I., Butcher, A., Esterman, A. & McLaughlin, K. (2007) Development of a modified classification system for voice disorders with inter-rater reliability study. *Logopedics Phoniatrics Vocology, 32*, 99–112.

Baker, J. & Lane, R.D. (2009) Emotion processing deficits in functional voice disorders. In K. Izdebski (Ed.) *Emotions in the Human Voice*, vol. 3, pp.105–136. San Diego, CA: Plural Publishing.

Baylor, C.R., Yorkston, K.M. & Eadie, T.L. (2005) The consequences of spasmodic dysphonia on communication-related quality of life: A qualitative study of the insiders' experiences. *Journal of Communication Disorders, 38*, 395–419.

Baylor, C.R., Yorkston, K.M., Eadie T.L., Miller, R.M. & Amtmann, D. (2009) Developing the communicative participation item bank: Rasch analysis results for a spasmodic dysphonia sample. *Journal of Speech, Language, and Hearing Research, 52*, 1302–1320.

Behlau, M., Hogikyan, N.D. & Gasparini, G. (2007) Quality of life and voice: Study of a Brazilian population using the voice-related quality of life measure. *Folia Phoniatrica et Logopaedica, 59*, 286–296.

Behrman, A. (2005) Common practices of voice therapists in the evaluation of patients. *Journal of Voice, 19*, 454–469.

Benninger, M.S., Ahuja, A.S., Gardner, G. & Grywalski, C. (1998) Assessing outcomes for dysphonic patients. *Journal of Voice, 12*, 540–550.

Bouwers, F. & Dikkers, F.G. (2007) A retrospective study concerning the psychosocial impact of voice disorders: Voice handicap index change in patients with benign voice disorders after treatment (measured with the Dutch version of the VHI). *Journal of Voice, 23*, 218–224.

Branski, R.C., Cukier-Blaj, S., Pusic, A., Cano, S.J., Klassen, A., Mener, D., Patel, S. & Kraus, D.H. (2010) Measuring quality of life in dysphonic patients: A systematic review of content development in patient-reported outcomes measures. *Journal of Voice, 24*, 193–198.

Bullinger, M., Anderson, R., Cella, D. & Aaronson, N.K. (1993). Developing and evaluating cross-cultural instruments: From minimum requirements to optimal models. *Quality of Life Research, 2*, 451–459.

Cohen, S.M. (2010) Self-reported impact of dysphonia in a primary care population: An epidemiological study. *Laryngoscope, 120,* 2022–2032.

Cohen, S.M., Jacobson, B.H., Garrett, C.G., Noordzij, J.P., Stewart, M.G., Attia, A., Ossof, R.H. & Cleveland, T.F. (2007) Creation and validation of the singing voice handicap index. *Annals of Otology, Rhinology and Laryngology, 116,* 402–406.

Cohen, S. & Williamson, G.M. (1988) Perceived stress in a probability sample of the United States. In S. Spacapan & S. Oskamp (Eds) *The Social Psychology of Health,* pp.31–67. Newbury Park, CA: Sage.

Colton, R.H., Casper, J.K. & Leonard, R. (2006) *Understanding Voice Problems: A Physiological Perspective for Diagnosis and Treatment,* 3rd edition. Baltimore, PA: Lippincott Williams & Wilkins.

Deary, I.J., Scott, S., Wilson, I.M., White, A., MacKenzie, K. & Wilson, J.A. (1997). Personality and psychological distress in dysphonia. *British Journal of Health Psychology, 2,* 333–341.

Deary, I.J., Wilson, J.A., Carding, P.N. & MacKenzie, K. (2003) VoiSS: A patient-derived Voice Symptom Scale. *Journal of Psychosomatic Research, 54,* 483–489.

Deary, I.J., Wilson, J.A., Carding, P.N., MacKenzie, K. & Watson, R. (2010) From dysphonia to dysphoria: Mokken scaling shows a strong, reliable hierarchy of voice symptoms in the Voice Symptom Scale questionnaire. *Journal of Psychosomatic Research, 68,* 67–71.

Derogatis, L.R., Lipman, R.S. & Covi, L. (1973) The SCL-90: An outpatient psychiatric rating scale: Preliminary report. *Psychopharmacology Bulletin, 9,* 13.

Dietrich, M., Verdolini Abbott, K., Gartner-Schmidt, J. & Rosen, C.A. (2006) The frequency of perceived stress, anxiety, and depression in patients with common pathologies affecting voice. *Journal of Voice, 22,* 472–488.

Eadie, T.L., Yorkston, K.M., Klasner, E.R., Dudgeon, B., Deitz, J.C., Baylor, C.R., Miller, R.M. & Amtmann, D. (2006) Measuring communicative participation: A review of self-report instruments in speech-language pathology. *American Journal of Speech- Language Pathology, 15,* 307–320.

Franic, D.M., Bramlett, R.E. & Cordes Bothe, A. (2005) Psychometric evaluation of disease specific quality of life instruments in voice disorders. *Journal of Voice, 19,* 300–315.

Gliklich, R., Glovsky, R.M. & Montgomery, W.M. (1999) Validation of a voice outcome survey for unilateral vocal cord paralysis. *Otolaryngology – Head and Neck Surgery, 120,* 153–158.

Goldman, S.L., Hargrave, J., Hillman, R.E., Holmberg, E. & Gress, C. (1996) Stress, anxiety, somatic complaints, and voice use in women with vocal nodules: Preliminary findings. *American Journal of Speech-Language Pathology, 5,* 44–54.

Hilari, K., Wiggins, R., Roy, P., Byng, S. & Smith, S. (2003) Predictors of health-related quality of life (HRQOL) in people with chronic aphasia. *Aphasiology, 17,* 365–381.

Hogikyan, N.D. & Sethuraman, G. (1998) Validation of an instrument to measure voice-related quality of life (V-RQOL). *Journal of Voice, 13,* 557–569.

Hummel, C., Scharf, M., Schuetzenberger, A., Graessel, E. & Rosanowski, F. (2010) Objective voice parameters and self-perceived handicap in dysphonia. *Folia Phoniatrica et Logopaedica, 62,* 303–307.

Jacobson, B.H., Johnson, A., Grywalski, C., Silbergleit, A., Jacobson, G., Benninger, M.S. & Newman, C.W. (1997) The Voice Handicap Index (VHI): Development and validation. *American Journal of Speech-Language Pathology, 6,* 66–70.

Liu, C.-Y., Yu, J-M., Wang, N.-M., Chen, R.-S., Chang, H.-C., Li, H.-Y., Tsai, C.-H., Yang, Y.-Y. & Lu, C.-S. (1998) Emotional symptoms are secondary to the voice disorder in patients with spasmodic dysphonia. *General Hospital Psychiatry, 20,* 255–259.

Ma, E.P.-M. & Yiu, E.M.-L. (2001) Voice activity and participation profile: Assessing the impact of voice disorders on daily activities. *Journal of Speech, Language, and Hearing Research, 44,* 511–524.

Mathieson, L. (2001) *The Voice and its Disorders,* 6th edition. London: Whurr Publishers Ltd.

Morton, V. & Watson, D.R. (2001) The impact of impaired vocal quality on children's ability to process spoken language. *Logopedics Phoniatrics Vocology, 26,* 17–25.

Murry, T., Cannito, M.P. & Woodson, G.E. (1994). Spasmodic dysphonia: Emotional status and botulinum toxin treatment. *Archives of Otolaryngology – Head and Neck Surgery, 120,* 310–316.

Oates, J. (2004) The evidence base for the management of individuals with voice disorders. In S. Reilly, J. Douglas & J. Oates (Eds) *Evidence Based Practice in Speech Pathology,* pp.110–139. London: Whurr Publishers Ltd.

Pemberton, C., Oates, J. & Russell, A. (2010) Voice care education: Preliminary evaluation of the Voice Care for Teachers package. *Journal of Health, Safety and Environment, 26(5),* 441–462.

Radloff, L.S. (1977) The CES-D scale: A self report depression scale for research in the general population. *Applied Psychological Measurement, 1,* 385–401.

Rasch, T., Günther, S., Hoppe, U., Eysholdt, U. & Rosanowski, F. (2005) Voice related quality of life in organic and functional voice disorders. *Logopedics Phoniatrics Vocology, 30,* 9–13.

Rosen, C.A., Lee, A.S., Osborne, J., Zullo, T. & Murry, T. (2004) Development and validation of the voice handicap index-10. *Laryngoscope, 114,* 1549–1556.

Rosen, C.A., Murry, T., Zinn, A., Zullo, T. & Sonbolian, M. (2000) Voice handicap index change following treatment of voice disorders. *Journal of Voice, 14,* 619–623.

Roy, N., Merrill, R.M, Gray, S.D. & Smith, E.M. (2005) Voice disorders in the general population: Prevalence, risk factors, and occupational impact. *Laryngoscope, 115,* 1988–1995.

Roy, N., Merrill, R.M., Thibeault, S., Parsa, R.A., Gray, S.D. & Smith, E.M. (2004). Prevalence of voice disorders in teachers and the general population. *Journal of Speech, Language, and Hearing Research, 47,* 281–293.

Russell, A., Oates, J. & Greenwood, K.M. (1998) Prevalence of voice problems in teachers. *Journal of Voice, 12,* 467–479.

Russell, A., Oates, J. & Greenwood, K.M. (2005) Prevalence of self-reported voice problems in the general population in South Australia. *Advances in Speech-Language Pathology, 7,* 24–30.

Sapir, S. (1993). Vocal attrition in voice students: Survey findings. *Journal of Voice, 7,* 69–74.

Sapir, S., Mathers-Schmidt, B. & Larson, G.W. (1996) Singers' and non-singers' vocal health, vocal behaviours, and attitudes towards voice and singing: Indirect findings from a questionnaire. *European Journal of Disorders of Communication, 31,* 193–209.

Scott, S., Robinson, K., Wilson, J.A. & MacKenzie, K. (1997) Patient-reported problems associated with dysphonia. *Clinical Otolaryngology, 22,* 37–40.

Smith, E., Gray, S.D., Dove, H., Kirchner, L. & Heras, H. (1997) Frequency and effects of teachers' voice problems. *Journal of Voice, 11,* 81–87.

Smith, E.M., Lemke, J., Taylor, M., Kirchner, H.L. & Hoffman, H. (1998a) Frequency of voice problems among teachers and other occupations. *Journal of Voice, 12,* 480–488.

Smith, E., Taylor, M., Mendoza, M., Barkmeier, J., Lemke, J. & Hoffman, H. (1998b) Spasmodic dysphonia and vocal fold paralysis: Outcomes of voice problems on work-related functioning. *Journal of Voice, 12,* 223–232.

Smith, E., Taylor, M., Mendoza, M., Lemke, J. & Hoffman, H. (1998c) Functional impact of nodules: A case-comparison study. *Journal of Voice, 12,* 551–558.

Smith, E., Verdolini, K., Gray, S., Nichols, S., Lemke, J., Barkmeier, J., Dove, H. & Hoffman, H. (1996) Effect of voice disorders on quality of life. *Journal of Medical Speech-Language Pathology, 4,* 223–244.

Spielberger, C.D., Gorusch, R.L., Lushene, R., Vagg, P. & Jacobs, G.A. (1983) *Manual for the State-Trait Anxiety Inventory (Form Y): Self-evaluation Questionnaire.* Palo Alto, CA: Consulting Psychologists Press.

Spina, A.L., Maunsell, R., Sandalo, K., Gusmão, R. & Crespo, A. (2009) Correlation between voice and life quality and occupation. *Brazilian Journal of Otorhinolaryngology, 75,* 275–279.

Steen, I.N., MacKenzie, K., Carding, P.N., Webb, A., Deary, I.J. & Wilson, J.A. (2007) Optimising outcome assessment of voice interventions, II: Sensitivity to change of self-reported and observer-rated measures. *Journal of Laryngology and Otology, 122,* 46–51.

Titze, I.R., Lemke, J. & Montequin, D. (1997) Populations in the U.S. workforce who rely on voice as a primary tool of trade: A preliminary report. *Journal of Voice, 3,* 254–259.

Van Houtte, E., Claeys, S., Wuyts, F. & Van Lierde, K. (in press) The impact of voice disorders among teachers: Vocal complaints, treatment-seeking behaviour, knowledge of vocal care, and voice-related absenteeism. *Journal of Voice*. DOI: 10:1016/j.jvoice.2010.04.008

Verdolini, K. & Ramig, L.O. (2001) Review; occupational risk for voice problems. *Logopedics Phoniatrics Vocology, 26*, 37–46.

Walshe, M., Peach, R.K. & Miller, N. (2009) Dysarthria Impact Profile: Development of a scale to measure psychosocial effects. *International Journal of Language and Communication Disorders, 44*, 693–715.

Ware, J.E. & Sherbourne, C.D. (1992) The MOS 36-Item Short Form Health Survey (SF-36) 1: Conceptual framework and item selection. *Medical Care, 30*, 473–483.

Wilson, J.A., Deary, I.J., Millar, A. & MacKenzie, K. (2002) The quality of life impact of dysphonia. *Clinical Otolaryngology, 27*, 179–182.

Wilson, J.A., Webb, A., Carding, P.N., Steen, I.N., MacKenzie, K. & Deary, I.J. (2004) The Voice Symptom Scale (VoiSS) and the Vocal Handicap Index (VHI): A comparison of structure and content. *Clinical Otolaryngology, 29*, 169–174.

World Health Organization (2001) *International Classification Functioning, Disability and Health (ICF)*. Geneva: World Health Organization.

Worrall, L.E. & Hickson, L. (2008) The use of the ICF in speech-language pathology research: Towards a research agenda. *International Journal of Speech-Language Pathology, 10*, 72–77.

Yiu, E.M.-L., Ho, E.M., Ma, E.P-M., Verdolini Abbott, K., Branski, R., Richardson, K. & Li, N.Y.-K. (2111) Possible cross-cultural differences in the perception of impact of voice disorders. *Journal of Voice, 25*, 348–353. DOI: 10:1016/j.jvoice.2009.10.005

Zigmond, A.S. & Snaith, R.P. (1983) The hospital anxiety and depression scale. *Acta Psychiatrica Scandinavica, 67*, 361–370.

Zraick, R.I. & Risner, B.Y. (2008) Assessment of quality of life in persons with voice disorders. *Current Opinion in Otolaryngology and Head and Neck Surgery, 16*, 188–193.

Zung, W.W. (1967) *The Measurement of Depression*. Milwaukee: Lakeside Laboratories.

15 Head and Neck Cancer

Mary T. Lee
City University London, UK

Introduction

Head and neck cancer is primarily a diagnosis affecting the over 50 age range. In order to understand issues related to quality of life, it is necessary to have some knowledge of the disease itself, as well as the treatment regimes used. Whether a person is treated curatively (i.e. disease eradication) or palliatively (i.e. disease control) will dictate type and timing of treatment and may impact how people rate quality of life. Quality of life is a rather all-encompassing concept that really only reflects the moment in time the person is completing the questionnaire or interview. This is particularly true in head and neck cancer, where there is heterogeneity of site of tumour, diversity, type and stage of treatment and/ or recovery that can have an effect on perceived health-related quality of life. As well, it makes it quite challenging to attribute precise outcomes to various available treatment options. However, with this in mind, the following is a whirlwind tour of current treatment options within head and neck cancer in order to facilitate understanding into the functional outcomes and the effect on aspects of patients' lives following treatment.

Head and neck cancer

Head and neck cancer refers to any malignancy in the upper aero-digestive tract, and includes tumours in the oral cavity, pharynx, larynx and oesophagus. Most recent cancer statistics indicate that there are over 5000 new cases a year in the UK, and over 400,000 worldwide (http://info.cancerresearchuk.org). More men than woman are diagnosed, although the ratio is decreasing. There has been a steady increase of 3% a year in the incidence of head and neck cancer in the UK since 1989 (http://info.cancerresearchuk.org). The highest risk is associated with the combination of smoking and drinking (Conway et al., 2009), although there is emerging evidence that there may be a genetic predisposition (Canova et al., 2010; Jeffries & Foulkes, 2001). The medical treatment for head and neck cancer comprises radiotherapy (conventional or IMRT – intensity modulated radiotherapy), chemotherapy, surgery as well as a combined modality approach, depending on a variety of medical, social, environmental and patient choice factors. Decisions regarding treatment are based on oncological principles encompassing survival likelihood, functional outcomes and quality of life.

In order to more clearly understand the effect of head and neck cancer, it is necessary to have some understanding of particular treatments, and their side effects. All treatment regimes have significant morbidities related to speech, swallow, taste and smell. The type and extent of the morbidity reflects the extent and site of cancer, as well as the specific treatment modality used. Combined treatment modalities usually result in a higher rate of morbidity. For speech, the effects range from mild dysarthria to non-verbal, requiring some alternative method of communication. For swallow, effects range from managing a full oral diet to completely non-oral requiring alternative feeding methods. Factors such as status of saliva production and management as well as oral motor competency contribute to both speech and swallow functioning, with morbidities in either or both areas affecting perceived quality of life.

Effect of treatment regimes

Surgery

Surgical management of head and neck cancer depends on the size and site of the tumour. Outcomes are related to whether or not there is primary closure or the use of a flap or graft to close the surgical defect, as well as to when and how much radiotherapy is received. Speech and swallow morbidities are increased with the use of flaps and grafts: all flaps and grafts are lacking in sensation, immobile and non-secretory. This has significant impact on the ability to manipulate the bolus during swallow, as well as manipulation of the articulators for speech. The literature reports worse outcomes for speech and swallow when flaps/grafts are used (Borggreven et al., 2005; Suarez-Cunqueiro et al., 2008), and patients report lower health-related quality of life related to cosmetic appearance, appetite loss, ability to eat in public and speech intelligibility (Allal, Nicoucar, Mach & Dulguerov, 2003; Zuydam, Lowe, Brown, Vaughan & Rogers, 2005).

Radiotherapy

Radiotherapy can occur on its own, pre- or post-surgically, and is comprised of either conventional three-dimensional conformal radiotherapy or intensity-modulated radiotherapy (IMRT). Acute morbidities associated with any radiotherapy to the head and neck include oro-pharyngeal mucositis, oedema, painful swallow, stenosis, loss of salivary function, inability to control secretions and changes in taste and appetite. Late morbidities include fibrosis, which reduces tissue pliability and elasticity, chronic sensitivity and dryness of mucous membranes (xerostomia) and reduced range of motion of oro-pharyngeal structures. Evidence suggests that IMRT reduces late effect morbidities; however, there is conflicting literature on whether or not this has an effect on quality of life (Scott-Brown, Miah, Harrington & Nutting, 2010). The literature focuses primarily on the functioning of the parotid glands post radiotherapy. The field of the radiotherapy beam invariably encompasses the parotid, which, once damaged, is unlikely to recover fully. The advantage of IMRT is that by varying the beam intensity across the radiation fields a high radiation dose can be delivered to the tumour while minimizing the dose delivered to nearby organs, thus reducing morbidity to healthy tissues within the vicinity of the disease.

Chemotherapy

Chemotherapy increases the morbidities of other treatment modalities. Although there is evidence that there are improved overall survival rates when chemotherapy is used in patients with oral and oro-pharyngeal cancers, functional outcomes are worse (Furness et al., 2010).

Organ preservation protocols

In an effort to preserve the organs, there is an increase in the use of radiation and/or chemo-radiation regimes in late-stage head and neck cancer. This assumes that sparing the organs associated with speech and swallow will also spare the function. A review by Rieger, Zalmanowitz and Wolfaardt (2006), in fact, suggests otherwise. They reviewed more than 50 articles looking at functional outcomes and quality of life specifically where organ preservation protocols had been used. They found higher swallow morbidity than speech, and that the swallow morbidities were long-standing, sometimes severe enough to warrant alternative non-oral feeding. This review suggests that preservation of the organ does not in fact translate to preservation of function.

Effect of head and neck cancer on life

Functional outcomes

There continues to be long-term objective and subjective deficits in speech and swallow affecting communication, eating and recreation following treatment for head and neck cancer (Meyer et al., 2004). Initially it is the cancer itself that contributes to deficits, particularly in swallow. Tumours in the oro-pharynx result in anatomical distortion of tissue, destruction, pain and neurological deficits. It is often the functional deficits in speech and/or swallow that are the motivator to seek medical advice. This implies that, before diagnosis and treatment even begins, there is an impaired physiological system.

Speech morbidities are related to intelligibility, both at word and sentence level, and are affected in comparison to an aged normed population, with the type of impairment related to the site of the cancer (McKinstry & Perry, 2003; Meyer et al., 2004). A large study with data from 1652 responders indicated that more than 60% of patients treated for head and neck cancer had resulting speech difficulties (Suarez-Cunqueiro et al., 2008). The main predictor of better speech outcomes following treatment was primary closure, involving no flaps or grafts (Zuydam et al., 2005).

Dysphagia remains prevalent in patients treated with surgery and any adjuvant or concomitant treatment (Garcia-Peris et al., 2007; Hammerlid & Taft, 2001), with up to 75% of people reporting ongoing problems (Suarez-Cunqueiro et al., 2008). The highest swallow morbidities are associated with surgery and adjuvant treatment, particularly for glossectomy. Severity of dysphagia correlates with lower health-related quality of life scores, anxiety and depression (Nguyen et al., 2005). The main predictors of good swallow outcomes were the absence of radiotherapy and primary closure (Zuydam et al., 2005).

Many patients continue to suffer from dry mouth (xerostomia) and this is included in factors relating to depression, as well as reduction in function of speech and swallow (Dirix, Nuyts, Vander Poorten, Delaere & Van den Bogaert, 2008). Xerostomia is a morbidity which does not recover and patients report dry mouth and/or sticky saliva as the single factor most affecting their enjoyment of life following treatment for head and neck cancer. Intervention strategies for xerostomia are rarely effective, which is one of the motivators for developing effective treatments that have less morbidity, such as IMRT (Dirix, Nuyts & Van den Bogaert, 2006).

Health-related quality of life (HRQL)

Most of the quality of life literature in head and neck cancer is health-related and likely reflects the ongoing medical implications of a diagnosis of cancer with the possibility of recurrence (Murphy, Ridner, Wells & Dietrich, 2007). This is reflected in the number of validated questionnaires in use, such as the European Organization for Research and Treatment of Cancer Quality of Life Questionnaire C30 (EORTC QLQ-C30) (Aaronson et al., 1993). Overall, it appears that HRQL in head and neck declines immediately after therapy, and returns towards baseline by one year, with the lowest scores occurring immediately following the conclusion of treatment (Hammerlid, Silander, Hornestam & Sullivan, 2001; Murphy et al., 2007). There is some evidence that patients treated with surgery alone, and those treated for early-stage tumours, report a better HRQL than those with late-stage tumours and adjuvant treatment (Chauker et al., 2009). The factors affecting this are not always obvious, and no doubt reflect an interaction between site and type of cancer and treatment, social support, coping strategies and psychological profile (Horney et al., 2011).

Consistent themes addressed in the literature include functional outcomes of speech and swallow and subjective questionnaire development highlighting the anatomical and physiological changes associated with head and neck cancer (Rogers, Ahad & Murphy, 2007). However, there is much conflicting evidence as to how or whether HRQL is related to functional outcomes (List & Stracks, 2000; Murphy et al., 2007). Therefore, the literature must be approached with careful consideration of methodology used, heterogeneity of the head and neck population and its treatment, which affects subject cohorts, as well as the measurement tools employed. Assumptions that impaired function necessarily relates to reduced quality of life should be avoided. A study by Hammerlid and Taft (2001) indicated that, even though patients still exhibited significant functional problems three years after completion of treatment, health-related quality of life as measured by a standardized questionnaire did not significantly differ from age-matched controls. They found that the significant factors negatively affecting health status were related to patient age, gender and site of original tumour. Tumour staging did not appear to affect long-term HRQL, nor did subsequent treatment. These rather surprising findings were supported in a separate study by Aarstad et al. (2006).

The biggest impact on health-related quality of life for head and neck cancer patients is most often seen in the first year following diagnosis, with slow recovery over the next several years (Hammerlid et al., 2001). The best predictor of 12-month global HRQL seems to be pre-treatment global HRQL (List & Stracks, 2000). In terms of late survival (10 years), a New Zealand study found that there was a significant decrease in overall HRQL compared with before treatment, or with years one and two post-treatment (Mehanna & Morton, 2006). This would suggest that HRQL decreases with survival; however, sample size was small and may have affected results. Along gender lines, females tend to rate emotional wellbeing as worse, whereas males rate social functioning as worse (Maciejewski et al., 2010). This is consistent with Lee, Gibson and Hilari (2010), who found that following total laryngectomy there were differences in male and female adjustment in both the social and emotional domains.

Employment and activities

Although the majority of people who are treated for cancer do return to work, this varies according to cancer and treatment type, as well as to factors associated with health status and education (Taskila & Lindbohm, 2007). For head and neck cancer there is a substantial proportion of patients (around 38%) who stop work prior to diagnosis (Buckwalter, Karnell, Smith, Christensen & Funk, 2007) as well as a concomitant reduction in physical activity (Rogers et al., 2008). Ongoing treatment and disease-related issues are most strongly associated with whether or not people return to work and re-establish some level of physical activity within the first year following completion of treatment (Rogers et al., 2006). Factors that contribute to patients' ability to sustain physical activity, as well as whether or not they stay at work, reflect an ongoing disability and are related primarily to fatigue, anxiety and oral dysfunction (Verdonck-de Leew, van Bleek, Leemans & de Bree, 2010; Rogers et al., 2008). Over 50% of survivors cite speech and eating as major issues in returning to work and reducing disability (Buckwalter et al., 2007; Verdonck-de Leew et al., 2010).

Treatment-related barriers, particularly those related to oral dysfunction and its effect on speech and swallow, as well as deterioration in social functioning, need to be specifically targeted within rehabilitation programmes in order to minimize disability, optimize enjoyment, and maximize potential for successful return to work.

Social and emotional wellbeing

It has been suggested in the literature that successful return to work and re-establishment of regular activities may be related to social wellbeing both in the workplace and in daily life (Taskila & Lindbohm, 2007).

As most practising clinicians have experienced, sometimes – despite all the positive prognostic signs – patients do not do well in rehab following the cancer treatments. It begs the question as to whether there are factors other than speech and swallow that influence rehabilitation outcomes. There is some emerging evidence that how a person copes and levels of distress may influence outcomes. Problems with depression have been highlighted by various support groups, including laryngectomy. Comments reflect a dawning realization that, although they have come through cancer treatment, the morbidities that remain are long term, resulting in a substantially different life as compared to pre-diagnosis. This is particularly true for total laryngectomy, where patients must learn to adjust to very different breathing, voice and swallow mechanisms (Graham, 2004). In investigations into why some patients do better than others in returning to pre-disease states, social support mechanisms and coping styles have been found to be major factors in predicting rehabilitation outcomes: 'Good' copers identified a wider social support network including health professionals and rated their communication/rehabilitation as positive. 'Poor' copers had a smaller network of family and fewer friends and tended to rate their communication negatively.

The size and type of support networks may therefore affect a laryngectomee's perception of their communication, which they then relate to the success of rehabilitation. Relic et al. (2001) found that, for laryngectomees, family support in particular was identified as the most important factor in overcoming the problems associated with the disease and treatment. Family support was also highly correlated with quality of life: the less the family support, the lower the participants rated their quality of life.

Coping styles and distress levels interact in complex ways and can affect HRQL (Aarstad, Beisland, Osthus & Aarstad, 2010). However, general health rating as well as HRQL is more affected by psychological factors: People who use avoidance and suppression strategies to manage anxiety tend to report lower ratings on quality of life questionnaires (Aarstad et al., 2010; Horney et al., 2010). Stages of treatment are also important: the use of avoidance/suppression strategies in patients who were receiving or recently completed treatment correlated with low health-related HRQL scores (Sherman, Simonton, Adams, Vural & Hanna, 2000). These studies highlight that psychological wellbeing is an important consideration when managing patients through and immediately following treatment, and clinicians should involve family and other support systems as much as possible. Morton (2003) adds further evidence to HRQL and its relationship to coping styles and distress in a longitudinal, cross-cultural study, where he found that measures of psychological distress were related to HRQL. In terms of coping styles, even when patients were still required to make significant adaptations for morbidities associated with swallow function, the perceived difficulties were rated as decreasing over time. This is further evidence that there may be a questionable relationship between functional outcome and HRQL (List & Stracks, 2000; Morton, 2003; Hammerlid & Taft, 2001; Murphy et al., 2007). The case study on oral cancer (see Case study 1 below) may be taken as an illustration of this. Of more significance in successful rehabilitation and improved health-related quality of life may be an individual's coping strategies combined with social and family support networks.

Clinical implications

It appears from the literature that psychological wellbeing and good support systems not only have a significant impact on quality of life, but result in a perceived improvement in functional outcomes. If this is indeed the case, then incorporating strategies for coping should be built into therapy programmes, as well as the management of the side effects. This could be incorporated into the immediate post-treatment period to include not only management of, for example, tracheostoma, mucus production and coughing, but also coping strategies. This is illustrated in the laryngectomy case study (see Case study 2, below), where anxiety regarding changes in respiration resulted in the patient using maladaptive strategies to cope. As well as addressing particular strategies to increase speech intelligibility, therapy should also contain aspects directed at developing communicative competence, confidence and strategies for managing anxiety to be included as goals and, indeed, outcomes. Rehabilitation should not only target safety during swallow, but include management strategies for social eating, which, again, are aimed at reducing the disability and potentially improving quality of life.

The multi-disciplinary team can be expanded to include mental health professionals, such as a clinical psychologist, or health counsellor, to screen and potentially treat patients for depression and/or anxiety. This may help to avert potential adjustment issues later and maximize the effect of rehabilitation programmes. Murphy (2009) concluded that, for quality of life and symptom management following treatment for head and neck cancer, 'Referral for appropriate supportive care and rehabilitative services is critical in order to minimize the acute and late effects of therapy and to maximize long-term function' (p.242).

Case study 1: Oral cancer

Miriam is a 70-year-old woman diagnosed with T4N2 squamous cell cancer (SCC) of the right floor of mouth. She was treated with chemotherapy, followed by surgery, which involved removal of part of the mandible, resection of floor of mouth with a free flap to close the defect, and a right modified neck dissection. Given the extent and nature of the disease, she underwent a full course of radiotherapy following surgery. Miriam has no family, a small circle of friends, and was living in a bedsit prior to diagnosis.

Swallow: Miriam was nil by mouth following her surgery, so was fed via a gastrostomy tube for two months, during which time she underwent radiotherapy. Acute effects of radiotherapy prevented any swallow rehabilitation. However, once these had subsided, Miriam commenced oral motor exercises aimed at increasing jaw opening, improving bolus control, improving pharyngeal constriction, and airway protection. She commenced to pureed diet with honey-thick fluids after another two months. She is now able to manage thin fluids but remains on a pureed diet. Due to lack of sensation in the right lower face, including the lip, Miriam continues to have a problem managing secretions and drooling. There have been no chest infections or any other contraindication for thin fluids.

Communication: Miriam's speech is severely impaired due to tethering of the tongue as a result of the free flap, impaired range of motion of jaw opening, and lip function. Intelligibility is moderately to severely reduced, depending on the familiarity of the listener and contextual clues. Articulation errors are consistent, so familiar listeners are able to decode Miriam's output with minimal effort; however, this is less effective in less than optimal communicative environments. Speech therapy focused on strategies for improving clarity of speech, such as overarticulation, slower rate, and use of consistent close sound substitutions.

Cont. overleaf

Daily life: Miriam was unable to return to her bedsit, as throughout her lengthy hospital stay her mobility decreased. There was concern regarding her ability to self-care; thus she now lives in a care facility. Miriam has significant facial disfigurements from the surgical reconstruction and, as a result, she rarely goes out in public. Efforts at linking her with support groups have been ineffective, and her only outlet remains regular checks in the cancer clinic, where she is seen by both the speech therapist and the counsellor. She continues to drink thin fluids and take a pureed diet, which she insists she prefers. She remains adamant that she is fine left by herself, as she doesn't then have to worry about people's reactions. Despite all her obvious problems, Miriam maintains she has a reasonable quality of life and has as much social contact now as she did prior to diagnosis and treatment.

Understanding the patient's support networks to ensure that there is opportunity for communication and to monitor/identify those patients who may become isolated is also important. This would necessarily involve not only multi-disciplinary teams within a tertiary acute hospital setting, but extend to the community in order to provide ongoing support both to the patient and to family/carers to ensure successful follow-up and carry-over of rehabilitation goals.

Case study 2: Laryngectomy

Stewart is a 55-year-old engineer diagnosed with T2N0 squamous cell cancer (SCC) of the glottis three years ago, treated with curative radiotherapy. At a routine ENT clinic follow-up appointment one year later, Stewart reported an ongoing hoarse voice. Biopsy confirmed recurrence of SCC of the glottis, fixed right vocal fold, and positive neck nodes on the right side. He underwent a total laryngectomy with myotomy and primary tracheo-oesophageal puncture (TEP) and a right modified neck dissection. Stewart has a supportive family and is planning on returning to work.

Respiration: Stewart has a permanent tracheo-stoma through which he breathes. He no longer has the warming, cleaning benefits of the nose and the upper respiratory tract. This has implications for mucus production and coughing, as external air is not filtered and enters the trachea directly. For a year following his laryngectomy, Stewart insisted on carrying a portable suctioning machine in order to clear his airway, as he was reluctant to cough in public.

Swallow: Following surgery, Stewart gradually increased food and fluid until he could manage a normal diet. It takes him longer to finish a meal, but his weight is stable. Initially he avoided public eating, because he was embarrassed at coughing through his stoma.

Voice: Stewart has been fitted with a voice prosthesis. His voice quality is loud, with varied intonation and normal phonation time. Intelligibility is more than 90% in all contexts, including the phone.

HRQL and distress: Stewart was initially very worried about his stoma becoming blocked with mucus and excessive public coughing. Working with members of the MDT, Stewart acknowledged his anxiety, understood that suctioning would create more mucus, and was able to replace the portable machine with the more appropriate Heat Moisture Exchange System, which reduces coughing and mucus production through the use of a filter system attached around the stoma. His coughing and mucus production reduced, as did his anxiety around a blocked airway. He now once again dines outside the home on a regular basis.

Daily life: Stewart's family has been by his side throughout his diagnosis, treatment and rehabilitation: his friends are frequent visitors. The speech therapist and Macmillan nurse have both helped Stewart adapt to the way his body works following treatment, as well as providing support for management of anxiety. At the completion of rehab, Stewart was 100% independent in care and maintenance of the physical aspects of post total laryngectomy, and could maximize his voice, swallow and respiration status. He returned to work, reports that he is satisfied with his voice, swallow and, although he still has some anxiety regarding his stoma, he does not view himself as 'disabled' or limited in his activities.

Directions for further research and impact for clinical practice

There is a paucity of prospective intervention studies within head and neck cancer. Most research focusing on the efficacy of intervention is retrospective, or commences once all medical treatment is completed. Partly this is due to the nature of the medical treatment, throughout which patients are ill, often hospitalized, which makes conforming to therapeutic regimes difficult if not impossible. However, further research addressing whether early pre-medical treatment intervention aimed at speech and swallow rehabilitation would have a long-term effect on the relevant function is required.

In terms of addressing the distress, anxiety and potential depression that this clinical population endures, it appears that reducing these parameters would have more of an impact on quality of life. However, there is a need for more evidence to understand how coping styles, personality and pre-treatment mental health status may potentially predict successful outcomes.

Defining 'successful' outcomes within head and neck cancer has mostly been related to functional outcomes, particularly in speech and swallow. Is this how patients define 'successful'? Some of the literature cited here would suggest that patients' perception of 'success' is related less to objective measurement of these aspects, and may rely more on social relationships, support systems and, again, psychological status. Our understanding of the interrelationship between these factors is relatively low. There has been an assumption that quality of life must be related to functional outcomes: This is equivocal at best and incorrect at worst. Clinical decisions based on this premise have to be revisited in light of what is emerging on the relationship between 'success' and other factors not necessarily related to function. As well, a more thorough understanding of how patients' wellbeing affects perception of function is necessary so that decisions regarding amount and type of services can be made with appropriate insight and knowledge into factors affecting successful outcomes within the head and neck population.

References

Aaronson, N.K., Ahmedzai, S., Bergman, B., Bulliger, M., Cull, A., Duez, N.J., Filiberti, A., Henning, F., Fleishman, S.B., Haes, J.C.J.M., Kaasa, S., Klee, M., Osoba, D., Razavi, D., Rofe, P.B., Schraub, S., Sneeuw, K., Sullivan, M. & Takeda, F. (1993) The European Organization for Research and Treatment of Cancer QLQ-C30: A quality of life instrument for use in international clinical trials in oncology. *Journal of National Cancer Institute*, *85(5)*, 365–367.

Aarstad, A.K., Beisland, E., Osthus, A.A. & Aarstad, H.J. (2010) Distress, quality of life neuroticism and psychological coping are related in head and neck cancer patients during follow-up. *Acta Oncology*, 15 September (Epub).

Aarstad, H.J., Aarstad, A.K., Lybak, S., Monge, O., Haugen, D.F. & Olofsson, J. (2006) The amount of treatment versus quality of life in patients formerly treated for head and neck squamous cell carcinoma. *European Archives of Otorhinolaryngology, 263(1)*, 9–15.

Allal, A., Nicoucar, K., Mach, N. & Dulguerov, P. (2003) Quality of life in patients with oropharynx carcinomas: Assessment after accelerated radiotherapy with or without chemotherapy versus radical surgery and postoperative radiotherapy. *Head Neck, 25*, 833–840.

Borggreven, P.A., Verdonck-de Leeuw, I., Langendijk, J.A., Doornaert, P., Koster, M.N., de Bree, R. & Leemans, R. (2005) Speech outcome after surgical treatment for oral and oropharyngeal cancer: A longitudinal assessment of patients reconstructed by a microvascular flap. *Head Neck, 27*, 785–793.

Buckwalter, A.E., Karnell, L.H., Smith, R.B., Christensen, A.J. & Funk, G.F. (2007) Patient reported factors associated with discontinuing employment following head and neck cancer treatment. *Archives of Otolaryngology Head Neck Surgury, 133(5)*, 464–470.

Canova, C., Richiardi, L., Merletti, F., Pentenero, M., Gervasio, C., Tanturri, G., Garzino-Demo, P., Pecorari, G., Talamini, R., Barzan, L., Sufaro, S., Franchini, G., Muzzolini, C., Bordin, S., Pugliese, G.N., Macri, E. & Simonato, L. (2010) Alcohol, tobacco and genetic susceptibility in relation to cancers of the upper aerodigestive tract in northern Italy. *Tumori, 96(1)*, 1–10.

Chauker, D.A., Walvekar, R.R., Das, A.K., Deshpande, M.S., Pai, P.S., Chaturvedi, P., Kakade, A. & D'Cruz, A.K. (2009) Quality of life in head and neck cancer survivors: A cross-sectional survey. *American Journal of Otolaryngology, 30(3)*, 176–180.

Conway, D.I., Hashibe, M., Boffetta, P., Wunsch-Filho, V., Muscat, J., La Vecchia, C. & Winn, D.M. (2009) Enhancing epidemiologic research on head and neck cancer: INHANCE – the International Head and Neck Cancer Epidemiology Consortium. *Oral Oncology, 45*, 743–746.

Dirix, P., Nuyts, S. & Van den Bogaert, W. (2006) Radiation induced xerostomia in patients with head and neck cancer: A literature review. *Cancer, 107(11)*, 2525–2534.

Dirix, P., Nuyts, S., Vander Poorten, V., Delaere, P. & Van den Bogaert, W. (2008) The influence of xerostomia after radiotherapy on quality of life: Results of a questionnaire in head and neck cancer. *Support Care Cancer, 16(2)*, 171–179.

Furness, S., Glenny, A.M., Worthington, H.V., Pavitt, S., Oliver, R., Clarkson, J.E., Maclusky, M., Chann, K.K. & Conway, D.I. (2010) The CSROC Expert Panel. Interventions for the treatment of oral cavity and oropharyngeal cancer: Chemotherapy. *Cochrane Database Systematic Review, 8–9*. CD006386.

Garcia-Peris, P., Paron, L., Velasco, C., de la Cuerda, C., Camblor, M., Breton, I., Herencia, H., Verdaguer, J., Navarro, C. & Clave, P. (2007) Long-term prevalence of oropharyngeal dysphagia in head and neck cancer patients: Impact on quality of life. *Clinical Nutrition, 26(6)*, 710–717.

Graham, M. (2004) Alaryngeal speech rehabilitation in a group setting. *Topics in Language Disorders, 24(2)*, 125–136.

Hammerlid, E., Silander, E., Hornestam, L. & Sullivan, M. (2001) Health-related quality of life three years after diagnosis of head and neck cancer – a longitudinal study. *Head Neck, 23(2)*,113–125.

Hammerlid, E. & Taft, C. (2001) Health-related quality of life in long-term head and neck cancer survivors: A comparison with general population norms. *British Journal of Cancer, 84(2)*, 149–156.

Horney, D.J., Smith, H.E., McGurk, M., Weinman, J., Herold, J., Altman, K. & Llewellyn, C.D. (2011) Associations between quality of life, coping styles, optimism, and anxiety and depression in pre-treatment patients with head and neck cancer. *Head and Neck, 33(1)*, 149–156.

Jeffries, S. & Foulkes, W.D. (2001) Genetic mechanisms in squamous cell carcinoma of the head and neck. *Oral Oncology, 37(2)*, 115–126.

Lee, M., Gibson, S. & Hilari, K. (2010) Gender differences in health-related quality of life following total laryngectomy. *International Journal of Language and Communication Disorders, 45(3)*, 287–294.

List, M.A. & Stracks, J. (2000) Evaluation of quality of life in patients definitively treated for squamous carcinoma of the head and neck. *Current Opinions in Oncology, 12(3)*, 215–220.

McKinstry, A. & Perry, A. (2003) Evaluation of speech in people with head and neck cancer: A pilot study. *International Journal of Language and Communication Disorders, 38(1)*, 31–46.

Maciejewski, O., Smeets, R., Gerhards, F., Kolk, A., Kloss, F., Stein, J.M., Kasaj, A., Koch, F., Grosjean, M., Riediger, D. & Yekta, S.S. (2010) Gender specific quality of life in patients with oral squamous cell carcinomas. *Head Face Medicine, 6*, 21. DOI: 10.1186/1746-160X-6-21.

Mehanna, H.M. & Morton, R.P. (2006) Deterioration in quality of life of late (10 years) survivors of head and neck cancer. *Clinical Otolaryngology, 13(3)*, 204–211.

Meyer, T.K., Kuhn, J.C., Campbell, B.H., Marbella, A.M., Myers, K.B. & Layde, P.M. (2004) Speech intelligibility and quality of life in head and neck cancer. *Laryngoscope, 114(11)*, 1977–1981.

Morton, R.P. (2003) Studies in quality of life of head and neck cancer patients: Results of a two-year longitudinal study and a comparative cross-sectional cross-cultural survey. *Laryngoscope, 113*, 1091–1103.

Murphy, B.A. (2009) Advances in quality of life and symptom management for head and neck cancer patients. *Current Opinion in Oncology, 21(3)*, 242–247.

Murphy, B.A., Ridner, S., Wells, N. & Dietrich, M. (2007) Quality of life in head and neck cancer: A review of the current state of the science. *Critical Review Oncology Hematology, 62(3),* 251–267.

Nguyen, N.P., Frank, C., Moltz, C.C., Vos, P., Smith, H.J., Karlsson, U., Dutta, S., Midyett, A., Barloon, J. & Sallah, S. (2005) Impact of dysphagia on quality of life after treatment of head and neck cancer. *International Journal of Radiation, Oncology, Biology and Physiology, 61(3),* 772–778.

Relic, A., Mazemda, P., Arens, C., Koller, M. & Glanz, H. (2001) Investigating quality of life and coping resources after laryngectomy. *European Archives of Oto-Rhino-Laryngology, 258(10),* 514–517.

Rieger, J., Zalmanowitz, J. & Wolfaardt, J. (2006) Functional outcomes after organ preservation treatment in head and neck cancer: A critical review of the literature. *International Journal of Oral Maxillofacial Surgery, 35,* 581–587.

Rogers, L.Q., Courneya, K.S., Robbins, K.T., Malone, J., Seiz, A., Koch, L. & Rao, K. (2008) Physical activity correlates and barriers in head and neck cancer patients. *Support Care Cancer, 16(1),*19–27.

Rogers, L.Q., Courneya, K.S., Robbins, K.T., Malone, J., Seiz, A., Koch, L., Rao, K. & Nagakear, M. (2006) Physical activity and quality of life in head and neck cancer survivors. *Support Care Cancer, 14(10),* 1012–1019.

Rogers, S.N., Ahad, S.A. & Murphy, A.P. (2007) A structured review and theme analysis of papers published on 'quality of life' in head and neck cancer: 2000–2005. *Oral Oncology, 43(9),* 843–868.

Scott-Brown, M., Miah, A., Harrington, K. & Nutting, C. (2010) Evidence-based review: Quality of life following head and neck intensity-modulated radiotherapy. *Radiotherapeutic Oncology, 2,* 249–255.

Sherman, C., Simonton, S., Adams, D.C., Vural, E. & Hanna, E. (2000) Coping with head and neck cancers at different stages of treatment. *Head and Neck, 22(8),* 787–793.

Suarez-Cunqueiro, M.M., Schramm, A., Schoen, R., Seoane-Lestón, J., Otero-Cepeda, X.L., Bormann, K.H., Kokemueller, H., Metzger, M., Diz-Dios, P. & Gellrich, N.C. (2008) Speech and swallowing impairment after treatment for oral and oropharyngeal cancer. *Archives of Otolaryngology and Head and Neck Surgery, 134(12),* 1299–1304.

Taskila, T. & Lindbohm, M.L. (2007) Factors affecting cancer survivors' employment and work ability. *Acta Oncology, 46(4),* 446–451.

Verdonck-de Leew, I.M., van Bleek, W.J., Leemans, C.R. & de Bree, R. (2010) Employment and return to work in head and neck cancer survivors. *Oral Oncology, 46(1),* 56–60.

Zuydam, A.C., Lowe, D., Brown, J.S., Vaughan, E.D. & Rogers, S.N. (2005) Predictors of speech and swallow function following primary surgery for oral and oropharyngeal cancer. *Clinical Otolaryngology, 30,* 428–437.

16 'You've got to realize when you have a stroke it's a stroke for life'[1]

Madeline Cruice and Naomi Cocks
City University London, UK
Tess Lancashire, Stuart Midgley
and the Morgan Family (Mary, David and Felicity)

Introduction

Healthcare providers' practice needs to be informed by the scientific evidence base and by an understanding of the lived experience of communication disability in order to provide meaningful and effective services that make a difference to their clients' and families' lives (Kovarsky, 2008). In recent years, there has been a substantial increase in the number of published qualitative or subjective experience reports of living with communication disability, in aphasia (e.g. Barrow, 2008; Hale, 2007; Parr, 2007), dysarthria (Walshe & Miller, 2011) and dysphonia (Baylor, Yorkston & Eadie, 2005). Although we could have reviewed this literature for this chapter, we chose a different route to illustrate the impact of communication disability through a collection of individuals' stories.

To this end, Madeline and Naomi spoke with five people who were interested in sharing their story with others. Tess's, Stuart's and the Morgans' stories do not represent the greater population with acquired communication disability – other sources such as those cited above provide this already. Instead, they are individual and family stories of living with a communication disability after stroke. Each person was guided to think broadly about his/her current life (what made it good/not so good), points in their journey since the stroke that represented insights or realisations, what s/he did to find peace or contentment, and anything in particular s/he wished to convey to the expected audience reading this book. Although the impact of communication disability

---

1   Tess Lancashire.

is the theme of this book, there was intentionally no interviewer-led emphasis on this during the interviews. Interviews lasted between 90 minutes and three hours, and were transcribed by speech and language therapy students Caroline, Eleanor, Emer, Alison, Jonathan, Keren, Kate and Rebecca (see Acknowledgements). Tess, Stuart and the Morgans then reviewed the typed transcripts with Madeline and Naomi, and in collaboration we selected and edited their stories. Each of their stories is unique, reflecting a style that represents them as a communicator and as a person.

Tess Lancashire

I am a 46-year-old woman who had her stroke 22 years ago, and the proud mother of a teenage son. For the past five years I have been the North London Aphasic Coordinator at Different Strokes.[2] In recent years, along with other members of the North London Different Strokes Group, I have been successful in obtaining funding to pay for a speech and language therapist (SLT) to provide group and individual therapy. I wanted to share my story, and my views and advice on stroke, aphasia, speech therapy and life in general.

My experience of aphasia and stroke

Aphasia is an invisible disability

Not everyone understands aphasia and as soon as they see you there's nothing there, it's a sort of invisible disability for me. So people just stare at you and you're trying to get the word out and you can't do it. But I've been finding ways of just taking the time, not panicking and just trying to get that word out. Sometimes even though it's still stuck, you find a way just to communicate it very subtly.

You communicate differently when you have aphasia

You can do communication in any form as far as I'm concerned, it literally can be anything. It can just be silence, you know, I mean, one thing again

---

2   Different Strokes is a UK charity that was set up in order to support younger stroke survivors.

I've noticed that you use your senses, when you're aphasic. You use your eyes, ears, smell, everything. It affects you straight away, it's almost like, I'm not deaf, but it's a bit like that. You kind of use your other senses. You pick up an awful lot. Sometimes you get it wrong I will admit, but it is this feeling you have. I think that's what a lot of aphasic people do and you can tell straight away what people are thinking. A lot of aphasic people have this kind of almost sixth sense.

The hidden side of communicating with aphasia

When I did the launch for the aphasia group, I had speakers coming, some very good ones, and I had to do the hosting and I was thinking 'Will I be able to do this?' and in my head I think I'd gone through the process God knows how many times about 'What am I going to say?' and 'I'll go from here to there and then I'll go from there to there', do you know what I mean and I had to keep doing this repetitive thing just to try and remind myself of how I was going to do this. But I suppose with the acting,[3] I was able to make it look ad hoc, very chilled out but really I'd been on this thing for weeks but I looked as if I'd only just started on this.

Silence and relaxation are important

I try and kick everyone out of the house, because suddenly being by yourself is really nice because you hear everything when you're aphasic. It does drive you up the wall, because it's like you are not just talking with one person, it's every single little thing around you and it's trying to focus on that one thing and trying to kick everyone away and all the voices and noises. So I do have a time when it's just me, me, me because that really is what you need. Or sometimes I have the radio on. I love radio, because just to hear the voices is quite nice and very relaxing. I find TV little bit sometimes too much, to get the real contentment. If I can just be… just be on a beach. I'm a naturist anyway, and there's just sea, blue sky. Because I don't read, I can't read. I'd like to be able to. So just having a gentle voice, or the gentle sea, and some warmth.

---

3   Tess was an actress in her younger days.

Having epilepsy affects everything

Well I have to be honest the epilepsy affects almost everything. And that affects your language again, sort of like being pushed back again. And also it takes again, about a week before you can get yourself back together properly and these things obviously for me they happen, I have like two every month, which I have to, again, try and find another way to kind of calm all that down. Rather than having a whole load of medication just to be sort of like a zombie, which I don't really fancy. It is things like that that will make you down because it does affect your speech. You can't go out because it is stressful having to get the language right or trying to get people to understand me. It's just too much so after having a seizure you just want to stay at home for a good few days.

My journey

Having aphasia can change the path you take in life

It pushes you into other areas and signposts you into things that you never probably thought you could do before. Because before you had your language and all of a sudden you don't have it.

Returning to education was important

I went to City Lit[4] and did a counselling skills course. They were excellent with working with people who had a language problem. I had an SLT[5] that helped me collate all the work I had to do.

When someone actually suggested about going to college and actually doing an actual course and I thought I can't do a course, there's no way. I remember feeling quite sick when I first went there, thinking I'm never going to do this. It really was a feeling of I can't do this. It was a two-year course but I carried on.

I managed to get my certificate and I was also awarded the London... I

---

4   An organization offering part-time evening, daytime and weekend courses for adults.

5   Speech and language therapist.

can't remember what it was called now, but it was to do with people that had been to college and done quite well.

That in one way, that was a big change for me, it really was. I noticed how more confident I was and I was really being able to have a proper connection with people.

But it did also make me look at things in my own life that weren't really working any more. It is sad when that happens because it was a time when my husband and I had to realize that we can't go any further and that's quite sad. But it also makes you a bit stronger because you're finding these things that are really not going to work and you become stronger and you just move onto that next bit. That was when I went travelling. It kind of spiralled off for me.

I think I was very lucky that I had this one particular guy who was encouraging me to go back into further education. I think that has made a big difference for me, it is not necessarily for everyone, but it certainly made a big difference for me.

Going travelling was and is important

I thought I'd never be able to travel. I did my travel around Australia. That was a big thing because that really made you have to become very independent. I took my son out of school so that was a big thing. I was going to have to do a lot of things I'd never done before, I was quite scared because of any medical problem I might have during that journey.

My reflections for service providers

It's a long road really, and that's something that I think people need to know. It's not an easy road either and you need all the proper support with it. And that's not just family, because they also have got their problems with it all, but professional experience as well. In the older days I think I got more support, I did get more support I have to be honest.

These days everything is just so fast, so quick. Sometimes just literally sitting down and just having a conversation or just making a connection about something that makes a big big difference. Whereas I think these days I think people are wanting to get all this service out but it doesn't always work, everything is so too fast. I think if everyone pulled back just for a bit it would make a big difference for stroke survivors because it is a slow process.

I certainly think that a lot of the speech and language therapy that's been given it just kind of stops. Then that's it. That's what we found when we set up the aphasic group. We also found out that a lot of people had a lot of psychological problems because things are just, everything has just gone and stopped.

In our group, we've got some people who've had a stroke a few years ago and some people who've had a stroke a long time ago and there is a big difference. Just because it's been a long time for stroke doesn't mean that they don't need that particular support, all it means is they've moved on to another part of their stroke.

There are people in the voluntary sector. There are groups, different groups but there is not much funding and people don't know where to go to get funding. People also do not always know where the groups are. It's just trying to network properly with people so that people who are just sitting at home and not really knowing where things are. It is important for people to easily be able to get information about the support that is available.

Starting our own aphasia group

It started certainly as something that was needed. Different Strokes is a group throughout the country there's about forty odd different groups anyway, some are aphasic and some are not. I think even within the group we knew that people very much wanted to have their own communication aphasic group. This group was important so that they could have connection with others. When we started we worked with students, SLT students, and that was okay for a while but they obviously then had to move on. We then had to think about getting grants. Local authority grants are just a no-no. So we had to find private grants, which luckily we managed to get. It was a small grant but we managed to get it and we were able to use that to pay for two SLTs but that itself was a very hard task to try and get them.

Finding the right speech and language therapist

It was really important that we got the right kind of SLT not just any old SLT. It's not just to do with the clinical thing, but it's someone who is involved in stroke who is very interested in clients doing the things themselves. Who empowers them I suppose. We wanted a SLT who wouldn't just work with speech problems but would find out whereabouts a client was going and see if they could help them achieve their goal. Now we have the group which is run by the SLT and we also offer one-to-one sessions. The actual group itself to me was extremely important, for other people they have other reasons for being involved in the aphasic group but it made a big big difference because people can then have their own communication and it makes a big big difference being able to do that. That was good.

The impact on families

My son is aware of life and death because of my stroke and epilepsy. As a result he is far more mature than other boys his age. He has saved my life on a number of occasions.

I know I talk about him quite a lot, but he means an awful lot to me. He always says how hilarious he thinks my aphasia is. He is now at that age where he's at school, he's 15 almost, he's an extremely intelligent boy and I think some of that has come simply because he's had to work with me to help me deal with things. In the shops sometimes I get mixed up with money. But he can gently and subtly do something to support me. But I think that that's been very good you know for all of us because he understands it all.

My son is also doing extremely well and that was a big achievement for me and he's doing some residential maths course in Cambridge University which is really good. I feel well that's alright because hopefully when it's the point where he wants to go to university they'll all go 'Oh hello it's [name of son]'.

Families also need support

I think that the fact that your language has gone, which means a lot to family, they see the person that they have known for all those years and all of sudden they're not there and it's really kind of difficult to understand where that person has gone.

I met this woman that came to the aphasic group who had her stroke at the same time as me and she had brought her sister deliberately because her sister had no understanding at all in the whole 20 years, she was aphasic this woman, and she wanted basically her sister to be in a group with other people that were aphasic so that she could see it and realize that it wasn't some wacko sort of thing. I spoke with this woman, and she said 'They have no understanding they don't understand they keep thinking it's just me but they can't understand where have I gone.' The fact that her sister coming in made a big big difference because she could really understand it and I think that when they see other people with different aphasia and stuff like that, they basically realize it is something that is maybe different to what it was before. It takes a lot of support through all of that happening, because it is a real shock.

My sisters won't talk to me any more, my own two sisters that are older, they won't talk to me. They've used other excuses and stuff like that, but they just see this where's Tess gone, and one minute you're that Tess and then all of a sudden you're something else, and then all of sudden, because I was getting a lot better I had kind of gone back to Tess. But I'm really a bit more, quite vibrant and they found that quite difficult. Again we need that proper support, because that goes along for a lifetime for a lot of people. It can get better if we have the proper support.

Final words

Just enjoy life, because I know that we're only here for so long, I do know that. That again, when you've had something that's like a life threatening thing you just think, I'm not going to spend all my time just moaning about it, I'm just going to basically just get on, because I know that I only have so much time in this world and I just want to have a really good day. Basically!

▬▬▬ Stuart Midgley

I'm 54, live in London, and have performed, written and directed fringe plays and storytelling since 1984. I've appeared at theatres throughout London, notably the Hen & Chickens Theatre Bar and Etcetera Theatre, and performed at Camden and Edinburgh Fringe Festivals. My work in the early 2000s included *Shame*, *Listen*, *Seepage*, *Winterval* and *Spinback*, and in earlier days I was involved in children's storytelling around schools. I had a stroke five years ago, which resulted in some significant changes in my life. Friends, most particularly Jennie McKeown, helped me to manage and live, especially in the early days after the stroke. Since the stroke, I've taken up ceramics at Westminster Adult Education, attend various conversation and support groups around London, and I want to write a play about my experience of stroke.

Because of significant dyspraxia after the stroke, it is effortful for Stuart to talk. He speaks in short sentences, meaning his story is essentially dialogue. Many of Madeline's turns (clarifications, confirmations) were not necessary for the reader and have been removed. Some, however, are needed, and are shown in italic to reflect her words. Furthermore, Stuart communicates a great deal through the use of his body (through gesture, facial expression, pantomime), and in order to represent this, these have shown in square brackets []. Despite the significant time and effort it takes Stuart to talk, he is a persistent communicator and a frequent storyteller. Whilst participating in the interviews for this book chapter, Stuart spoke to his good friend Querciolo Mazzonis. This prompted a spontaneous letter which is included here, although slightly edited to reduce length.

Life then and life today

Um, no because five years ago before I had... [points to right arm and leg]... I was very down. For two years... Yeah, um for instance five years ago when... [points to right arm and leg] I couldn't fall any lower [laughs]... *so this sounds like it was the lowest ever, yeah? We'll do a scale, this bit* [draws scale]. *It feels like it is down here* [points to bottom of scale]... I didn't do anything [mimes hanging himself, then shakes his head to indicate that this didn't happen]... It's um [points to mouth], it's with speaking [points to lowest point on scale]. Honestly, that's after I had that [points to right arm and leg] I couldn't speak. And I was in a chair... Yeah, see five years. At first I couldn't speak to my friends [laughs and shows frustrated face] and it's because five years, the first two of them [gestures difficulty eating with left hand] and then the last three I got over them.
   What about if you think about today?... so this is you when you were [points to low end of scale] *this is very unhappy. And this* [points to top end of scale] *is actually really happy, yeah? This is really kind of happy. Where would you put yourself today?...* [points to three-quarters of the way up the scale]... *And now this* [points to the more positive end of the scale] *is because you're speaking?* Yeah yeah yeah... *Are there other things that make you feel quite*

happy? I no longer get these thoughts inside my head [laughs]. Yeah yeah. Oh that was because John[6] who worked with... God! If you think we went to school together [raises arm to waist height, indicating they were young]... Yeah, and he said something very nasty um, he was 'above me'... He was always like that [laughs]... He didn't [mimes making a model] whereas I did the fine modelling,[7] he just sprayed it... And he ripped me off! [laughs]... *OK, so how does John fit in here then? Is he not around any more?*... Yeah... *OK, so him not being around any more.*

Yeah, yeah. No and I thought ten years is a mighty long time. Five years... just think of the other five years [laughs, extends timeline with five further pencil strokes and writes TOP at end]. *This is now* [pointing to halfway along timeline and writes 2010], *and this is what you're doing, always thinking forward?* Yeah.

Life now

Modelling... [rummages through papers to find examples of his work]... [finds college brochure]... [points to photo with ceramics] That's me... Yeah, I am doing it now. About three years I have been going there... Er, it's Maori [points to one sculpture], that one's [points to other sculpture suggesting to interviewer to guess]... *Um, Scandinavian?*... No... [both laugh]... *Well, it has no painting... is it just unpainted?*... Yeah... *What do you do with your work?* Yeah. If I could I would like to do something about this... [points to right arm and leg]... To tell other people with strokes they can do this [points to pictures of ceramics]... Yeah! I spose that's what I'd like to do with it.

Acting. Yeah. [shows paper] I was in that... Yeah. Comedy, not so much. Acting comedy. Acting, comedy [mimes a balance tipping each way]. *Bit of both?* Yeah... All my life... In Brixton. Started down there when I was 21... I want to write a play. Yeah. I got the right person... Unfortunately I can't write. That man can... I haven't told him about it yet [laughs]. *You said 'I want to write a play'. Why? What for?* To make the nurses and the doctors and of course anybody who wants to come there... it may be bit of a laugh, but not too much [laughs then makes very pensive expression and puts finger on bottom lip] *So maybe slightly... not black comedy, but maybe slightly... just a*

---

6   Business partner (pseudonym used).
7   Stuart made models for a living.

bit on edge... that will make you think. And I would like to be in it although I haven't done anything [pointing to right arm] since this [gesturing to arms and legs]... around five years.

Not so good... Oh it's going for a pint, with my mates. Although they still come round [mimes getting drunk]. It's not so often [points to right arm and leg]. Not speak so much... Not so good, that is because my... What am I? What am I? [points to right arm and leg and mouth, searching to express having had a stroke].

Communicating with others is frustrating but some people understand

Yeah. Um, nurses and doctors that's all I want to get through to... Yeah, because they don't know anything about... Some are nice, yeah. But... but some of them should not be working there [laughs]. Yeah, because instead of looking at me [mimes someone talking whilst looking away from the other person, then shows frustrated face with vocalization] Look at me! [laughs]. And talk slower. I have to go back maybe once a month. That's where they take blood out of my finger and then see... the doctor says how many... and take two more tablets. *So this happens quite frequently, then?* Yeah, yeah. And it will do for the rest of my life. *When the nurses don't communicate all that well with you, how does that make you feel?* Er... good when they understand something, bad when they don't understand anything.

What about people on the street? Or people in the supermarket? [laughs and makes wearied face] Yeah. Well, you can tell somebody that in their own family had something like this because then they will... ah [puts hand on heart]... Yeah.

Accessing information about services is difficult

Because... because half the time I was going to the main hospital, many many people and then I found, I found out that you should go to the Saint Christopher's... Yeah, yeah. For instance, there is lots of stroke units around. Their problem is how you go to get to them. Because, me and the other people about that go to... [opens his folio of personal information and points] yeah, YMCA, that is where we find... YMCA! [Looks at interviewer with baffled expression and laughs] it's the Different Strokes at YMCA... *They are the people where you find more information?* Yeah, yeah.

Querciolo Mazzonis's letter

Stuart for me is like a brother. I met Stu in the mid-1980s, through a common friend, in London and another time in Rome. Then, when I moved to London in 1990, I bumped into him again. Since that was the third time that we met occasionally, we decided to take fate into our hands and we exchanged telephone numbers.

In my 12 years as a Londoner, Stuart was the person I met socially more regularly – almost every week. I normally met him at his flat in Manchester Street, which was a gathering place for a group of Stu's friends. After any evening out (to the pub, to the theatre, for a walk in a London area, etc.), we would regularly return to Stu's place for an endless night of discussions (mostly political), jokes, drinks and joints. Stu has always been very generous: he was a point of reference for us, because he would listen and [give] advice to others' problems and because he would share everything (smoke, drink, food, and even money) he had (although, or perhaps precisely *because*, he was the person with less means among us). Stuart prizes friendship and love, and this is why he has always had people around him (together with the fact that he is arguably the funniest person I have ever met). Stu for me was (and still is) the mirror of my soul. Whenever I told him something about myself, or something that had happened to me, from his reaction I would learn about an aspect of my personality. Stuart is very capable to tell about the nature of people's intentions and he would respond to these very explicitly. Stuart obviously was (and is) not a saint and sometimes he would be very aggressive about behaviours (or even ideas) he disliked (areas he is sensitive about, for example, are money, selfishness and snobbery), attacking mercilessly the unfortunate friend who mistakenly stamped on his sensitivity. Although Stuart loves life, he had a tendency to depression and to perceive his life as rather negative. A metaphor he used to describe his situation was the guinea pig in the wheel: running all the time just to remain in the same place. Stuart was (and is! I've seen some sculptures he made after the stroke, which are just fantastic) an incredibly talented artist and some of us spent quite a few evenings trying to convince him to present a book with his work to some bloody companies. There was no way he would do it, partly for ideological reason (he is allergic to any form of what he would define as 'capitalism'), and mostly for psychological ones. Recently Stuart showed me some drawings he made when he was at school, at 14 or 15: they look like Van Gogh style, with the difference that Van Gogh wasn't that good at that age.

... One evening of Spring 2005 a friend called me. I did not expect his call and he had a serious voice: 'It's about Stuart'. For a fraction of a second I held my breath thinking 'He's dead'. After he told me about the stroke I cried, I was shocked, but at the same time I was very relieved that he was still alive and that I could still see him and talk to him. I went to visit him at the hospital. When he saw me he (the English, supposedly more reserved) cried, whereas I (the Italian, supposedly the opposite) tried to disguise my feelings by showing him some pictures of my daughter, whom he hadn't seen yet. As I discussed with others, paradoxically, Stuart looked much better than he used to because his face seemed more relaxed and even younger. The reason probably was that through the stroke Stuart got rid of a situation, which used to make him depressed: the abuse of drugs and alcohol, the feeling that he had to work like mad to survive (with no prospects and no pension), and (possibly) the fact that he had to leave his flat soon. Certainly, the situation in which he found himself was very hard to deal with. But at the same time, for the first time, Stuart had someone who took care of him and he had a positive prospect to fight for: the improvement of his health and his communication skills – and when Stuart finds a motivation, he is a very determined and positive person. That is what I (and some of his friends) sensed. Obviously I felt sad that the communication with Stuart became difficult, but Stuart was there, alive, we could still exchange opinions on everything, we could still make jokes, have nice walks (both in London and Rome) enjoy things like movies, food, drinks and joints. We only needed to learn how to do it, even if it required some patience and adaptation capacity. Stuart now has even learned new skills (such as swimming, something that he had never wanted to learn before), has regained his artistic ability (working with his left hand!) and he is writing theatre stuff (something that he used to postpone endlessly).

Of course there were difficulties. For me at the beginning it wasn't very easy to understand how to be materially helpful. This is partly a problem for anybody who suddenly finds his/her best friend with an illness, because things have to be adjusted, and we all have to face the obstacles created by our personalities. In addition, by that time I had returned to Rome, so I could not be around to help physically. And I wanted to do too much, I wanted to push people to do certain things that I thought were necessary. But my ideas were not necessarily shared by other friends of Stu, not because they were wrong, but because each one is different and was doing something different. It takes time to understand these issues when one is emotionally involved. Eventually, however, I feel that Stuart is still very much a presence in my life and I feel that he thinks the same about me.

▆▆▆▆▆▆ Mary, David and Felicity Morgan[8]

Mary (75 s) and David (78) live in South London in their own home, in the same street where they've been for the past 37 years. They have a daughter, Felicity, and a son, who also live in London, as well as grandchildren and great-grandchildren. At the age of 18, Mary was diagnosed with a degenerative condition of the spine, which cut short a promising career as a principal dancer with the Royal Ballet. She has never taken medication for the pain but manages it instead with will and determination. She found it difficult to walk as much as she liked to at the time of the interview, and believed this condition was catching up with her. She had a stroke three and a half years ago. David spent 10 years in the Fleet Air Arm of the Royal Navy, and then became a theatre technician coordinating specialist teams to ensure the hygiene of operating theatres across the UK. Felicity is in touch with them every day, and stays one night a week to assist with household cleaning and shopping. David and Felicity attend a regular stroke forum at the local hospital, where a volunteer visiting programme (befriending scheme) has now been implemented as a result of their suggestion. Mary and David have volunteered to share their experiences on several previous occasions (e.g. national news programmes, Stroke Association campaigns), and collectively shared a tremendous amount of their experience.

The impact of aphasia

The variability

Felicity: With Mum, the confusing thing is sometimes she will understand something perfectly and be able to express herself in one way, but then the next day, or even an hour later, or a bit later, it's completely different,

---

8   Their biographies are written in the third person because of the multiple people involved.

so you can't take it as read that just because she understands something at one point that she will the next time.

Mary: Yes you see so it all depends and what I am thinking is the other day, well every day when someone's talking to me, I answers and I think, I don't understand what they're talking about really but because I asked and them they think I know exactly what they saying, and I haven't got a clue.

The impact on conversation

David: We had an amusing time this morning going from here to Mitcham to the hairdresser's. She was trying to tell me what she experienced this morning at daybreak. And it took a 20-minute drive from here to the hairdresser's before I could understand what she was on about... [Mary laughs]... and she was trying to explain to me that she can see the moon. And you could see the moon and it was cloudy and suddenly the clouds opened and she could see the red sun rising and then the clouds closed again. But the problem with her trying to explain it to me is that she could not think of the right words for cloud, sun... She was saying no it was shining up there and I said, 'Stars?' No, there were no stars. 'Satellites?' No, not satellites.

Mary: It was beautiful, first thing in the morning and I sat there and I thought I bet you, you weren't ever seen any more today because there were that little one right up there [gesturing] and this is um not quite but that sort of colour [pointing to Felicity's jeans] and I thought I wish someone was here to have a look with me and so I just had to say[9] it on my own.

The exhaustion

David: It's mentally exhausting, um, trying to understand Mary at times, you know, to, and trying to, it, understand exactly what she's, um, trying to say at times, which you've heard for yourself... but sometimes you go all day long and you haven't understood a word hardly, you know, and that can be quite tiring.

Felicity: I think, as well, because it's so exhausting sometimes for you [talking to her mother] to listen and understand to explain things, so you might understand conversation but to say to you, 'Can you tell us what you had for dinner last night?', or what was something you like, and it's so

---

9   Mary means to use the word 'see'.

exhausting for you to... like with Dad... to explain for 20 minutes to try and get your point over and get us to understand that um it's just too much that you think, 'Oh never mind, forget it'.

Impact on relationships

David and Felicity: [Son] doesn't show up very often. The relationship's changed completely, him and Mum used to be really quite close before Mum's stroke, but for some reason or another he... I had a suspicion that he doesn't like to come over here because he gets upset when he sees her. I think that might be part of it. Mum was in hospital for six weeks and he only came to see her twice probably, but only for a very short time, and since then he just very rarely comes to see her, so I don't know, I think it's other things as well, but I think he does struggle with the changes with Mum since she's had the stroke.

David: A thing that has saddened Mary is, and Felicity knows too, is that Mary has created a, before the stroke over the years we've been here, she's created a little village atmosphere in the street here, whereas we all know each other um, I had five or six different sets of keys for neighbours that when they go away I can go in and pull the curtains, put the lights on... and we have at least two drinks parties a year, one just before Christmas and one during the summer... we haven't had one this year. All that seems to have gone and the fact is that Mary often had, would, er, be invited into the neighbours' for coffee or a chat and a cup of tea in the afternoons, but they'll acknowledge her in the street, 'Hello Mary, how are you?' and things like that. But she's never invited out now for these coffees because they're shy of her.

Mary: It's all changed completely as if they're ordinary, older ones and not mine now, yes, all those years, I'm not able to speak to them.

Felicity: They've been here for about 35, 37 years or something like that and so... there's only a couple of people that have been here that long, so as each new person's come Mum would make them a loaf of bread and take it along to them... And so it was a very neighbourly street, picnics on the common and nice things but, it, you found it really hurtful because although people will say, 'Oh, hi, Mary, you're doing fantastically well. Oh, I've got to go', and so they're not stopping to kind of have that quality time and that, you know... interaction with her any more.

Memories from early days after the stroke

Attitude and recovery

David: Just to show her determination, when she had the stroke she couldn't walk at all and she had physios coming in to give her beds, massage and moving her legs and things, and she had to have a bedpan and she said, 'To hell with this' and the next thing you know is, and even the nursing staff and the consultant said, 'How on earth is she doing it?' and she was up and going to the bathroom on her own... the consultant did say that the treatment[10] he had given her he didn't know how, why she was progressing so rapidly, the treatment he had given her, it takes patients anywhere from... two months to two years to have either be... by the state she had...

Spending time on the ward

Mary: Because when I wasn't allowed in the morning, you weren't to have anything important for you, you, you're there and the important people out and 'I'll see you now'... [therapy sessions in the morning meant no visitors were allowed]. Yes, yes, so what was I supposed to do, and I sit there, I used to sit there [uses body language and facial expression to show boredom] and and I couldn't see out [uses body language and facial expression to express trying to look out a window]. I thought I'm going to have a walk myself, so I did [laughs] and the man came along, and she said, 'Where have you been?', I said, 'Well I only walked'... 'I didn't know you were going, who told you you could go?' What am I supposed to do? I was saying this and of course I can't say it.

Realizing the consequences of stroke and aphasia

Mary: [Laughs] Oh yes, you see again I couldn't understand what I was saying [laughs]... because I didn't understand I wasn't able to speak [laughs] and the lady would come home and she said, 'How are you today?' and I said, 'I'm fine, how are you?' [laughs]... and then she'll say... [vocalizes and plays out a brief role play between two people]
Felicity: Yes, but I remember saying to you, because I didn't understand the extent of, of her stroke or anything and I remember asking you kinda

---

10   Mary had thrombolysis, more commonly known as 'clot busting drugs'.

simple questions and you were saying yes to me and I'd be saying... 'Do you want me to hold your hand?' 'Yes.' 'Do you want to go to the toilet?' 'Yes.' And so she was just repeating 'yes' and I, I took yes to mean yes, I didn't realize that that was all that she could say and that actually some of it was she didn't understand that I was asking her if she needed to go to the toilet... So it was confusing for us because we just didn't unders... realize at the time that you, you weren't understanding and you couldn't, you couldn't talk. You couldn't talk, you couldn't talk then.

Felicity: For me one of the turning points in my realization was because, as I say we didn't know anything about stroke or what to expect or anything, erm, and so because Mum's appeared to recover from being... you know, not being able to move at all and not being able to speak at all and swallow and everything to, within kind of a week, being up and about and physically being much better... and... I think it wasn't really until we started, there was a couple of things, when we used to take her down for occupational therapy or speech therapy or something, I used to think 'That's a bit odd, why is she...?' I know she can't talk very well yet but you know there was just this kind of... sort of character, sort of part of her character was accentuated because she'd been really quite rude to the speech therapists and abrupt.

Felicity, David and Mary: For instance, they'd ask you to do something and we'd spend maybe 15 or 20 minutes in the session, then [they'd] say, 'Okay, then, Mary, you know we're gonna take you back up to the ward now', and she'd say, 'Well, no, what, why, no I'm staying here' and she'd say, 'Well this is rubbish, this is rubbish', because she just wanted to do more and more. She wanted to continue. They used to say, 'Right, you can go home now', whatever for, I've only just begun!

Felicity and David: But when they were talking about whether Mum should go to the Wolfson[11] or whether she should come home or not, and those kind of things, and we started to talk about home and it was, she was confused because she didn't remember what home was. Felicity came here, and with a digital camera took photographs of the lounge and the bedrooms... and the stairs and the back garden, and the streets and the front door and everything and we were able to take them up and see if she remembered them. You did, you did, you started to, you started to remember. So for me, that, that, that point was hold on, this is much more than I understood about stroke, about just maybe being weaker on one

---

11   An inpatient rehabilitation centre.

side and obviously I'd learned that there was some speech difficulties that it, it was so much more than that and you know, for me it was like, alright, okay, this is gonna be very very different and you know, how do we, how do we do this, each step of the way, kinda learning.

Staff at hospital

David: Felicity and I found at each end of the ward there was a, a huge long connected corridor... glass-sided... with a glass roof, a long, long one and with windows you could open, and we used to take her out in the wheelchair and sit there and chat to her in, in the sunshine sort of thing, to get away from the ward, and there was one day we were sat there and matron said, 'You might as well have lunch out here then' and she got a little table for her and everything, yes [laughs].
Mary, Felicity and David: Except that lady, she got very angry because I, I could not understand how to read. Yeah, there was one, kind of quite early, distressing, Mum had just been put, she'd been moved from kinda the acute part of the hospital, the ward to the kind of longer stay and... she had difficulty adjusting to that move, really kind of being familiar with those surroundings and knowing where things were and it kind of set her back a little bit because the things that she knew weren't there any more, that she'd come to understand and there was a woman who, erm, came to ask, you know, what food they wanted, what she wanted for lunch... so she'd say to Mum. Yeah, that's right, we were there one day, I was there one lunchtime, can't remember now, and this woman came along and said, pushed in front of me, quite without manners, and said, 'Whadya want?/' [in rude tone] and I said, 'Can you hang on a minute, Mary's not able to read', and she said, 'Well, she won't get anything again' and I went spare. I said, 'Don't you realize she can't read and she can't speak'... and I made a formal complaint about it, Felicity and I, didn't we?

Concluding remarks

These stories illustrate the significant impact that stroke and acquired communication disability has had on these individuals, their families, their friends, and lives in general. For student and qualified healthcare providers reading these stories, the messages are strong. Individuals and their families need current, accessible and timely information on local services and support available after stroke. Therapy and therapeutic support are needed for longer than it is currently provided, or at different times when the person is ready, and families need to be involved. All professional staff need core requisite skills to communicate effectively and positively with individuals with communication disability. In addition, Tess's, Stuart's and the Morgans' stories highlight their determination, persistence and resourcefulness in how they manage the experiences that living with communication disability now requires. Their stories also serve as a reminder of the power of communication and one's voice, despite communication difficulties.

> *Acknowledgements*: Thanks are due to our team of eight speech and language therapy students – Caroline Bartrop, Eleanor Cornford, Emer Dowling, Alison Evans, Jonathan Fagan, Keren Lloyd, Kate Mackay and Rebecca Selley – for their tremendous commitment to transcribing several hours of video interviews, and for their thoughts and views on the process.

References

Barrow, R. (2008) Listening to the voice of living life with aphasia: Anne's story. *International Journal of Language and Communication Disorders, 43*(Suppl 1), 30–46.

Baylor, C., Yorkston, K. & Eadie, T. (2005) The consequences of spasmodic dysphonia on communication-related quality of life: A qualitative study of the insider's experiences. *Journal of Communication Disorders, 38*, 395–419.

Hale, S. (2007) *The Man who Lost His Language: A Case of Aphasia,* revised edition. London: Jessica Kingsley Publishers.

Kovarsky, D. (2008) Representing voices from the life-world in evidence-based practice. *International Journal of Language and Communication Disorders, 43*(Suppl 1), 47–57.

Parr, S. (2007) Living with severe aphasia: Tracking social exclusion. *Aphasiology, 21(1),* 98–123.

Walshe, M. & Miller, N. (2011) Living with acquired dysarthria: The speaker's perspective. *Disability and Rehabilitation, 33(3),* 195–203.